T0134673

Cancer Treatment and Research

Volume 172

Series editor

Steven T. Rosen, Duarte, CA, USA

More information about this series at http://www.springer.com/series/5808

Jeffrey Y.C. Wong · Timothy E. Schultheiss
Eric H. Radany

Editors

Advances in Radiation Oncology

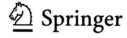

Editors
Jeffrey Y.C. Wong
Department of Radiation Oncology
City of Hope
Duarte, CA
USA

Eric H. Radany
Department of Radiation Oncology
City of Hope
Duarte, CA
USA

Timothy E. Schultheiss
Division of Radiation Physics, Department
  of Radiation Oncology
City of Hope
Duarte, CA
USA

ISSN 0927-3042   ISSN 2509-8497   (electronic)
Cancer Treatment and Research
ISBN 978-3-319-85098-6   ISBN 978-3-319-53235-6   (eBook)
DOI 10.1007/978-3-319-53235-6

Printed on acid-free paper

This Springer imprint is published by Springer Nature
The registered company is Springer International Publishing AG
The registered company address is: Gewerbestrasse 11, 6330 Cham, Switzerland

Preface

Radiation oncology is one of the first specialties to offer personalized approaches to cancer care using CT-based image guided therapy to sculpt dose to the unique anatomic characteristics of each patient's tumor and surrounding anatomy. Cancer medicine is now extending this personalized approach by tailoring treatment to the unique characteristics of each patient's cancer. The molecular signature of a tumor can now better predict prognosis and guide selection of appropriate therapy. Therapies are more targeted towards specific molecular targets for a given tumor type. The next decade will see a rapid expansion of this patient-specific approach through the incorporation of advances in our understanding of cancer biology, DNA damage and repair, cancer immunology, tumor microenvironment, tumor genomics and biomarkers, systems and mathematical biology, molecular imaging and molecular targeted therapeutics. In the future, radiotherapy will not only be image guided but also molecular and biologically guided, with therapy optimized not only to the anatomic features but also to the unique physiologic, biologic, phenotypic, and genotypic characteristics of a given cancer which predict prognosis and radiosensitivity. As the number of variables that predict for response increase, systems and mathematical oncologic modeling will be critical in analyzing and optimizing how these data are best used in the clinic.

Advances in newer imaging modalities such as multi-parametric MRI and PET using FDG and other novel agents allow for better visualization of these physiologic and phenotypic radio biomarkers to help better target therapy and assess response, and are now at the forefront of new image guided radiotherapy (IGRT) approaches. The next generation IGRT photon therapy devices will incorporate MRI guidance. CT image guidance and intensity modulation which transformed photon therapy delivery are now being integrated into proton and particle beam therapy.

These advances coupled with advances in the technologies to deliver radiation therapy have recently created new opportunities to treat patients with localized and metastatic disease. Tumors are no longer viewed simply as homogenous static collections of aberrant cells, but as a dynamic process with regions of changing viability and radiosensitivity that can vary over space and time. Intra-tumoral boost doses to these pockets of radioresistance are actively being explored. Radiotherapy is playing an increasingly important role in patients with metastatic disease in combination with systemic therapies. Patients with limited or oligometastatic disease may represent a subset of patients where a more aggressive use of IGRT to each metastatic site in combination with systemic therapies may prolong disease free intervals and possibly cure a subset of these patients. IGRT dose sculpting to large target regions is now possible and its use to deliver targeted total marrow irradiation has shown promise in patients with hematopoietic cancers undergoing hematopoietic stem cell transplantation. Molecular targeted or immunoguided systemically delivered radiopharmaceuticals also continue to show promise. Radiotherapy to tumor sites in combination with immunotherapy may have broader immune-stimulatory effects through localized changes in the tumor microenvironment and increased antigen presentation to antigen presenting cells.

In "Advances in Radiation Oncology", each chapter presents a concise review of these new and important areas, which will provide the practicing radiation oncologist with a fundamental understanding of each topic and an appreciation of its impact on the future of radiation oncology.

Duarte, USA   Jeffrey Y.C. Wong
                                                                   Timothy E. Schultheiss
                                                                        Eric H. Radany

Contents

Combining Radiotherapy and Immunotherapy

Onyinye Balogun and Silvia C. Formenti

Abstract

Traditionally, radiation therapy was viewed as a localized treatment to eliminate an "in field" tumor or metastasis or total body therapy, when used as a strategy to elicit immunosuppression in preparation for allogeneic transplant. Over the past decade, the purview of localized radiation therapy has been expanded to include a role as an adjuvant to immunotherapy. It is now recognized that radiation therapy to a tumor has the potential of converting it into an in situ vaccine, by releasing relevant epitopes and neo-antigens and inducing cell death signals that enable cross priming to activate tumor-specific T cells. Once successfully activated, the immune system contributes to the elimination of the irradiated tumor. If immunological memory is achieved, the patient's immune system can also reject systemic metastases, outside the radiation field (the "abscopal effect") and maintain durable tumor control. We summarize the current knowledge of radiation therapy's effects on the immune system, including results from preclinical and clinical trials, as well as future directions in combining radiotherapy and immunotherapy.

Keywords

Radiation therapy · Radiotherapy · Immunotherapy · Abscopal effect · Toll-like receptor · PD-1, PD-L1 · CTLA-4 · OX40 · CSF-1 · CSF-1R

O. Balogun (✉) · S.C. Formenti
Department of Radiation Oncology, 525 E 68th Street,
New York 10065, NY, USA
e-mail: onb9003@med.cornell.edu

S.C. Formenti
e-mail: formenti@med.cornell.edu

© Springer International Publishing AG 2017
J.Y.C. Wong et al. (eds.), *Advances in Radiation Oncology*,
Cancer Treatment and Research 172, DOI 10.1007/978-3-319-53235-6_1

1 Radiation Therapy Effects on the Immune System

Our group first introduced the concept of localized radiotherapy to convert the irradiated tumor into an in situ vaccine (Formenti and Demaria 2012; Demaria et al. 2004). In a series of experiments using immune competent BALB –C mice, two tumor nodules were induced by injection of 67NR mammary carcinoma cell lines. Local radiation therapy was then administered to only one of the two tumors. Mice were randomly assigned to: (1) no treatment; (2) local radiation to one tumor; (3) treatment with injection of Fms-like tyrosine kinase receptor 3 ligand (Flt3-L), a growth factor that stimulates production of dendritic cells (DCs) to enhance cross-priming or (4) irradiation of one tumor during treatment with Flt3-L. Flt3-L alone had no growth delay effects. Only when combined with radiation did Flt3-L cause growth delay of both the irradiated tumor as well as the non-irradiated contralateral tumor, i.e. radiation induced an abscopal effect. In addition, cytotoxic T-cells specific for 67NR were increased in the spleen of mice treated with both radiation therapy and Flt3-L compared to either agent alone. Without Flt3-L, there was no effect of radiation on the non-irradiated tumor. Moreover, radiation therapy elicited an antigen-specific response: irradiation of the primary 67NR mammary tumor with Flt3-L failed to affect an A20 lymphoma implanted as the second tumor

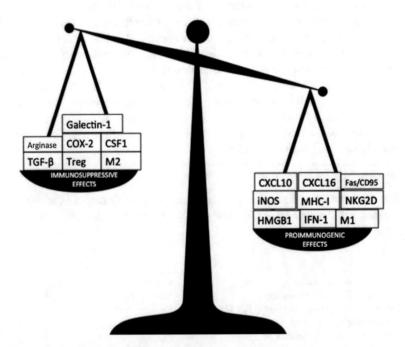

Fig. 1 Ideally, drug combinations should shift the balance between the pro-immunogenic and immunosuppressive effects of radiotherapy to favor its pro-immunogenic effects and or abrogate the immune-suppressive ones. Multiple strategies in each of these two directions are undergoing investigation pre-clinically and clinically

in the same mouse, demonstrating that the induced immune response was tumor-specific. In addition, the abscopal effect was abrogated in nude mice (who lack T cells) treated with the same experimental conditions. Subsequent studies have demonstrated that radiation therapy has both pro-immunogenic and immunosuppressive effects. Ongoing research aims at identifying strategies for tipping this balance in favor of the pro-immunogenic effects (Fig. 1).

1.1 Immunostimulatory Activity of Radiation Therapy

Radiation therapy has several effects on the immune system.

First, the cell-killing effect of radiation releases a series of signals that are relevant to immune rejection, resulting in cross-priming by DCs. The successful outcome of cross-priming after radiation therapy is limited by the number of intratumoral DCs (Pilones et al. 2014). Radiation is a powerful inducer of immunogenic cell death (ICD), a type of cellular demise that is sensed by the immune system, as it initiates immune rejection. The three hallmarks of ICD include: (1) translocation of calreticulin from the endoplasmic reticulum to the cell surface (Obeid et al. 2007); (2) release of the nuclear protein, high-mobility group box-1 (HMGB1) into the extracellular space and (3) release of adenosine triphosphate (ATP) which activates the inflammasome and causes interleukin (IL)-1β release (Apetoh et al. 2007; Galluzzi et al. 2007; Ghiringhelli et al. 2009; Ma et al. 2010).

Second, radiation therapy leads to DNA release from dying tumor cells. Delivery of tumor DNA to DCs activates the stimulator of interferon genes (STING) pathway and enhances interferon-1 (IFN-1) production by DCs (Deng et al. 2014; Woo et al. 2014). IFN-1 is necessary for the recruitment of DCs to tumors and their subsequent activation (Diamond et al. 2011; Fuertes et al. 2011). Activated DCs migrate to draining lymph nodes where they cross-present tumor-derived antigens to T-cells, resulting in anti-tumor T cell responses.

Moreover, radiation therapy promotes the release of chemokines that attract T-cells to tumors, enhancing trafficking. Studies revealed that radiation therapy induces expression and release of the chemokines CXCL10 and CXCL16 (Lugade et al. 2008; Matsumura et al. 2008). CXCL16 is a chemokine that binds to CXCR6 on Th1 and activated CD8+ effector T cells, and plays an important role in T-cell recruitment to sites of inflammation. Using 4T1, a poorly immunogenic mammary cancer murine cell line, Matsumura et al. (2008) demonstrated that irradiation of cells in vitro caused an over fourfold increase in CXCL16 mRNA. This effect peaked at 48 h after irradiation. In addition, when injected in a syngeneic immune-competent mouse, irradiation (12 Gy × 2) of 4T1 tumors induced CXCL16 in blood vessels and on the majority of tumor cells at immunohistochemistry, 48 h after tumor irradiation. In comparison, for un-irradiated tumors, immunohistochemistry for CXCL16 yielded only weak baseline CXCL16 immuno-reactivity in selected vessels and faint staining in tumor cells. These results provide evidence that irradiation can induce the secretion of key pro-inflammatory chemotactic factors that recruit antitumor effector T cells to the irradiated field.

Radiation therapy also increases the expression of major histocompatibility complex (MHC) class I proteins, necessary for antigen recognition by cytotoxic CD8+ T cells (CTLs) (Reits et al. 2006). MHC class I displays fragments of non-self antigens to cytotoxic T cells through the cytosolic/endogenous pathway. This effect of radiation is particularly important since tumors commonly escape recognition by the immune system via down-regulation or loss of the MHC-I molecules. In the GL261 preclinical mouse model of intracranial glioma, radiation therapy combined with granulocyte macrophage colony stimulating factor (GM-CSF) enhanced tumor infiltration by T cells and reversed MHC-I down-regulation of invasive glioma cells (Newcomb et al. 2006). In this model peripheral vaccination with GL261 tumor cells and GM-CSF (without radiation) resulted only in minimally improved survival of the treated mice compared to control animals. Conversely by recovering this basic mechanism of cross-presentation, radiation led to long-term survival in 80% of vaccinated mice, who also rejected challenge with the same tumors.

Similarly, radiation therapy increases the expression of Fas/CD95 (Chakraborty et al. 2003) and adhesion molecules which also participate in the mechanism of tumor cells recognition and elimination by CTLs. Radiation therapy also induces surface expression of NK group 2, member D (NKG2D) ligands such as UL-16 binding proteins, Rae-1 and MICA/B, which mediate tumor cell killing by both CTLs and natural killer cells (Kim et al. 2006). Tumor killing via NK cells is especially important when tumors have lost key components of the MHC-I complex rendering them unrecognizable by CTLs. Apart from direct cell killing, NK cells also enhance radiation sensitivity. Incubation with human NK cells prior to irradiation led to greater growth inhibition, radiation cytotoxicity and apoptosis among tumor cells from a variety of malignancies (Yang et al. 2013). Experiments using nasopharyngeal cancer cells revealed that incubation with NK cells led to an increase in the level of cytosolic Granzyme B, the molecule that initiates the proteolytic caspase cascade to cause cell death. Without radiation therapy, X-linked inhibitor of apoptosis protein (XIAP) inhibits apoptosis via the intrinsic mitochondrial apoptosis pathway by binding caspase-3. However, in the presence of radiation therapy, Smac is released from mitochondria and forms a complex with XIAP to enable Granzyme B-induced apoptosis.

Another radiation-induced mechanism that improves T-cell trafficking to the tumor involves reprogramming of the established immunosuppressive microenvironment by tumor-associated macrophages (TAMs). At baseline, most TAMs express the M2 phenotype (Stout et al. 2005), which promotes angiogenesis, tumor growth and metastasis while impairing T-cell function. In a mouse pancreatic cancer model, a single 2 Gy dose of radiation therapy caused significant expression of inducible nitric oxide synthetase (iNOS) in TAMs, eliciting what has been termed the M1 response (Klug et al. 2013). iNOS metabolizes L-arginine to produce L-citrulline and nitric oxide which promote immune and inflammatory reactions (Bansal and Ochoa 2003; Boucher et al. 1999). As a result, tumor macrophages normalized the tumor vasculature, recovering tumor perfusion and overcoming the barrier to T-cell infiltration of cancer-induced, abnormal vasculature.

Additional immunostimulatory effects of radiation therapy include upregulation of ICAM-1 (Ruocco et al. 2012), vascular cellular adhesion molecule 1 (VCAM-1) on tumor endothelium, which facilitates tumor infiltration by T, cells that produce interferon γ (IFN-γ) and tumor necrosis factor α (TNF-α).

1.2 Immunosuppressive Effects of Radiation Therapy

Although radiation therapy can function as an effective adjuvant for immunotherapy, it also has many identified immunosuppressive effects.

In contrast to the beneficial effects of low-dose radiation mentioned above, whereby a single low dose of radiation therapy induces tumor infiltration by TAMs that express iNOS, radiation also induces the expression of immunosuppressive enzymes such as arginase-1 and cycloxygenase-2 (COX-2) in TAMs (Tsai et al. 2007). Arginase converts L-arginine to polyamine precursors that can function as tumor growth factors (Chang et al. 2001). Moreover, depletion of L-arginine causes decreased expression of the T-cell receptor (TCR) signaling zeta chain (CD3zeta), impairs T cell proliferation and decreases cytokine output (Rodriguez et al. 2003). Similarly, COX-2 expression is associated with increased proliferation, invasion and angiogenesis (Fujita et al. 2002; Attiga et al. 2000; Wang et al. 2005). In murine prostate cancer cells, a single dose of 25 Gy led to a transient 1.4 and 2.3-fold increase in Arg-I and COX-2 mRNA, respectively, at 8 h. Beginning day 3, the Arg-I and COX-2 levels steadily rose to 1.5-fold and 5.6-fold, respectively, at 3 weeks. Increased iNOS expression began 3 days after irradiation and peaked at over 6-fold at 3 weeks. After fractionated radiation therapy (60 Gy in 15 fractions), COX-2 and Arg-I mRNA expression increased by the fifth fraction and was at least three-fold higher by the end of treatment. iNOS expression was not increased by the 10th fraction and only rose minimally by the final fraction (1.3 fold). Of note, low dose iNOS can promote angiogenesis in tumors while high doses have tumoricidal effects (Jenkins et al. 1995). These data suggest that the commonly used fractionated radiation therapy regimens may induce immune suppressive responses in tumors.

Importantly, single ablative doses of radiation (>10 Gy in one fraction) results in extensive endothelial cell death that may reduce vascular flow and impair effector T-cell trafficking to the tumor (Park et al. 2012). In addition, single high dose radiation therapy has been shown to promote a hypoxia-driven immunosuppressive environment in mouse melanoma models (Park et al. 2012; Hasmim et al. 2013).

Fractionated radiotherapy in classical therapeutic doses has been shown to increase additional mediators of immune suppression. First, it increases infiltration by myeloid-derived suppressor cells (MDSCs). This effect is mediated by colony stimulating factor 1 (CSF1), a chemokine that recruits MDSCs. In human and mouse prostate cancers, DNA damage caused by irradiation triggered ABL1 protein translocation to the nucleus and binding to the CSF1 promoter. These changes resulted in increased CSF1 gene transcription, which led to an increase in circulating MDSCs (Xu et al. 2013). Regulatory T cells are also increased after radiation therapy (Bos et al. 2013). These cells play a role in maintaining tolerance and suppressing antitumor immunity. Depletion of regulatory T-cells enhances the growth inhibitory effects of radiotherapy in murine carcinoma models (Bos et al. 2013).

Radiation is a powerful activator of transforming growth factor (TGF) β, that also contributes to immunosuppression. Reactive oxygen species, created by radiation therapy, cause TGFβ to dissociate from latency-associated peptide (LAP) (Barcellos-Hoff et al. 1994). In its active form, TGFβ inhibits stimulation of DCs and reduces priming of CD8+ T cells. In mouse breast carcinoma models, these inhibitory effects were overcome using antibodies that neutralized TGFβ (Vanpouille-Box et al. 2015). In mice bearing 4T1 breast cancers, intraperitoneal injection of 1D11, a TGF β neutralizing antibody, prior to irradiation led to a significant increase in the percentage of DCs, CD4+ and CD8+ T cells infiltrating the irradiated tumors. Moreover, in mice bearing two tumors, the combination of RT and 1D11, led to increased T cells infiltration of non-irradiated tumors suggesting that TGF β blockade may enable abscopal responses.

Finally, recent evidence implicates galectin-1, a carbohydrate-binding protein, as a barrier to the immune-mediated response to radiotherapy. In a syngeneic mouse model of non-small cell lung cancer, radiation induced galectin-1 secretion, leading to lymphopenia, due to a decrease in circulating CD3+ and CD8+ T cells through T-cell apoptosis (Kuo et al. 2014). These immune-suppressive effects were prevented with the use of thiodigalactosidase, a Gal-1 competitive inhibitor, or an anti-Gal-1 specific antibody.

Strategies to abrogate the immunosuppressive responses to radiation therapy may be necessary in order to best harness its potential for contributing to antitumor immunity.

2 Pre Clinical and Clinical Combinations of Radiotherapy and Immune Agents

2.1 Toll-like Receptor (TLR) Agonists

At the time tumors are discovered and the patient is diagnosed with cancer, multiple immunosuppressive mechanisms are in place that maintain their growth, making the tumor microenvironment immune-privileged (Joyce and Fearon 2015). For instance, macrophages, MDSCs and DCs, capable of suppressing T-cell activation, are often present in tumors.

Toll-like receptors (TLRs) activate innate immunity and initiate adaptive immune responses when stimulated by pathogen-derived and/or endogenous ligands (Adams 2009). Administration of synthetic TLR agonists has been shown to overcome some of the existing immunosuppressive barriers in established tumors by enhancing DC stimulation. Unmethylated C-G motifs (CpG) are single strand oligodeoxynucleotides that contain cytosines and guanines and they function as TLR9 agonists. They exert their effects on plasmacytoid DCs to induce IFN-α production, antigen presentation and upregulation of costimulatory molecules (Vollmer et al. 2004). They also stimulate cytokine production from Th1 cells (Wooldridge and Weiner 2003). In preclinical experiments, incubation of CpG with lymphoma cells led to the expression of costimulatory molecules, CD80 and CD86 as well as inhibition of proliferation (Li et al. 2007). The combination of intraperitoneal chemotherapy and intratumoral CpG injection in mice bearing B-cell lymphomas activated a CD8-dependent T cell immune response against local and systemic tumors, delayed tumor recurrence and prolonged survival of the mice. These results prompted a Phase I/II study of 15 patients with relapsed low-grade B-cell lymphoma (Brody et al. 2010). The study was designed to harness the anti-tumor vaccination properties of radiotherapy and intratumoral TLR9 in order to induce abscopal effects. A CpG-enriched TLR9 agonist was injected into the tumor site immediately before the first radiation therapy treatment, after the second treatment then weekly for 8 consecutive weeks. Radiation therapy consisted of 4 Gy administered consecutively daily in 2 Gy fractions. After a median follow-up of 33.7 months, there was one complete response, three partial responses and eight patients with stable disease for an overall response rate of 27%. Results were durable; the complete response lasted for 61 weeks while the 3 partial responses were maintained for 29, 64 and 111 weeks. Similarly, several patients had stable disease for up to 131 weeks. Like other immunotherapeutic treatments, clinical response peaked after ≥ 24 weeks. These remarkable results were obtained in a cohort of patients with a median of 3 prior failed therapies (range 1–6). Of note, the patient with a partial response lasting 64 weeks was re-treated with a higher dose of the TLR9 agonist, and then achieved a second PR within 12 weeks from re-treatment, which was faster than the initial PR that had occurred after 43 weeks. The development of flu-like symptoms during therapy and fewer prior therapies correlated with a greater magnitude of clinical response.

A series of immunological studies were conducted in this trial to elucidate the relationship with the clinical responses. These tests revealed a negative relationship between Treg induction and clinical response. Pre-treatment peripheral blood lymphocytes (PBLs) were cultured with autologous, irradiated, CpG-activated tumor B cells. At baseline, Treg levels among pre-treatment PBLs were low, with an average of 7.3%. After culture with autologous tumor cells, Treg proportion increased to an average 19.7% and was greater with CpG-activated tumor cells than with untreated tumor cells. The range of Treg increase varied, with 5 patients eliciting at least 4-fold increase and 9 patients eliciting ≤ 2-fold increase. Non-Treg inducers tended to have better clinical responses and significantly longer progression-free survival than Treg inducers. Interestingly, the baseline proportion of Tregs in patients' tumors and peripheral blood did not correlate with clinical outcomes, suggesting that it is the plasticity of Treg response after TLR agonists that matters. Additional experiments to modify Tregs include intratumoral injections of anti-CTLA-4 antibodies (Marabelle et al. 2013).

PBLs were also co-cultured with CpG-activated autologous tumor cells then assessed for activation markers such as CD-137, IL-2, interferon-γ and tumor necrosis factor. In some patients, disease regression correlated with improving immune response. However, these results were not statistically significant nor did all clinically responsive patients demonstrate tumor-reactive CD8+ T-cells.

The clinical availability of Imiquimod, a TLR agonist that specifically activates TLR7, which is expressed by both plasmacytoid DCs and CD11c+ myeloid-derived DCs, has made it an ideal candidate for clinical investigation (Stanley 2002). For instance, the combination of radiation therapy and TLR agonists is also being explored in breast cancer. In a preclinical syngeneic model using poorly immunogenic TSA mouse breast carcinoma cells, mammary adenocarcinoma were implanted subcutaneously, under the mouse skin, to mimic a chest wall recurrence of breast cancer (Dewan et al. 2012). Low-dose cyclophosphamide was delivered intra-peritoneally prior to the topical application of 5% imiquimod versus placebo cream to the skin overlying tumors, three times a week. A distinct subset of mice were also treated with cyclophosphamide which also reduces the proportion of circulating Tregs, to test the additional effect of this immune therapy. Radiation therapy was initiated 12 days after tumor injection and delivered in three consecutive daily fractions of 8 Gy. Either radiation therapy or imiquimod as single modalities resulted in some delay of tumor growth. However, radiation therapy in combination with imiquimod led to the regression of the majority of the tumors between days 25 and 30 as well as improved survival of the experimental animals, demonstrating synergy of the combination. Other experiments demonstrated that application of imiquimod and radiotherapy to the primary tumor led to tumor growth inhibition at a secondary un-irradiated site that had also been inoculated with TSA cells. Imiquimod/irradiated tumors demonstrated increased expression of two MHC class I alleles, intercellular adhesion molecule 1 (ICAM1) and infiltration by CD11c+ DCs, CD4+ and CD8+ T cells. Depletion of CD8+ T-cells suppressed these effects. Both CD8+ T-cells and CD8+ presenting DCs were key to the success of the combination that promoted both the priming and effector phases of anti-tumor T-cell responses. Importantly, when responding mice treated with low dose cyclophosphamide (a drug that reduces the number of regulatory T cells), radiation therapy and imiquimod were re-challenged with TSA cells after 90 days, they failed to develop tumors, showing long-term immunologic memory.

Based on these findings, an ongoing Phase I/II study of imiquimod, cyclophosphamide and radiation therapy for patients with breast cancer dermal or chest wall metastases is being conducted (ClinicalTrials.gov identifier: NCT01421017).

A previous Phase II trial in ten patients of single modality imiquimod for chest wall recurrences of breast cancer demonstrated a 20% ORR (Adams et al. 2012; Demaria et al. 2013). The current Phase I/II trial attempts to improve local and systemic anti-tumor immune response via the synergistic combination of imiquimod and radiation therapy. Radiation therapy is delivered to 1 area of skin metastases in 5 fractions of 6 Gy on Days 1, 3, 5, 8, and 10. As in the previous Phase II trial, imiquimod cream is applied topically 5 nights per week for 8 weeks, beginning on Day 1. During the Phase I portion, 6 patients completed treatment without any dose limiting toxicities. Phase II is currently underway with a target accrual of 25 additional patients. The primary endpoint is the response rate in untreated distant metastases, which will be assessed by immune-related response criteria. The local tumor responses, safety of the combination, immune-mediated rejection signatures and peripheral lymphocytes for antigen-specific T and B cell responses are also analyzed.

Imiquimod in combination with radiation therapy is also being used in a pilot study in diffuse intrinsic pontine glioma, a pediatric brain tumor with a poor prognosis (ClinicalTrials.gov identifier: NCT01400672). Patients will first receive 55.8 Gy over the course of 6–7 weeks directed to the intracranial tumor. Four weeks later, they will receive the first of 4 intradermal vaccines produced using the brain tumor initiating cell line GBM-6 as the antigen source. Vaccine will be injected at two separate sites every two weeks for 4 doses then every 4 weeks for up to 1 year. Imiquimod will be applied to the two vaccination sites 24 h after each injection. At the time of the 1st and 3rd vaccinations, 180 cGy fractions (for a total of 59.4 Gy) will be administered to the intracranial tumor with the intent to upregulate NKG2D ligands and enhance tumor killing by CTLs and NK cells.

2.2 Cancer Vaccines

In a Phase II clinical trial involving 30 prostate cancer patients with localized disease, the participants were randomized to receive standard definitive radiotherapy alone or in combination with a poxviral vaccine encoding prostate-specific antigen (PSA) (Gulley et al. 2005). Patients on the combination arm received recombinant vaccinia (rV) PSA plus rV containing the T-cell costimulatory molecule B7.1 (rV-B7.1) followed by monthly booster vaccines with recombinant fowlpox PSA. The vaccines were given with local GM-CSF and low-dose systemic interleukin-2. Standard external beam radiation therapy was given between the fourth and the sixth vaccinations. Overall, treatment with the combination was well tolerated. Of nineteen patients enrolled on the combination arm, seventeen patients completed all eight vaccinations. An increase in PSA-specific T cells of at least 3-fold was noted in 13 of 17 patients. No T-cell increases were detected in patients on the radiotherapy-only arm. There was also evidence of de novo generation of T cells to well-described prostate-associated antigens that were not part of the vaccine. This observation suggests that radiation therapy enabled the mechanism of antigenic spread, enabling vaccine-elicited T-cells to better access the tumor, and induce T-cell mediated killing, with release of additional antigens and priming of new T-cell reactivity. These cascading effects support the role of combining radiotherapy with tumor- directed vaccines.

2.3 GM-CSF

Similar to the experiments already described with Flt3-L used to stimulate DC production during radiation (Demaria et al. 2004), GM-CSF can also potentiate cross-presentation of antigens released from the irradiated tumor. T cells, macrophages, endothelial cells and fibroblasts secrete GM-CSF in response to immune stimuli. At low concentrations, GM-CSF stimulates macrophage proliferation while moderate concentrations elicit dendritic cell proliferation and maturation (Burgess and Metcalf 1980).

To translate our preclinical experience with Flt3-L (2) to the clinic, we designed a proof-of-principle trial that substituted Flt3-L with GM-CSF, which was available for clinical use. Abscopal responses were detected in 26.8% of patients with metastatic cancer who received radiotherapy (35 Gy in 10 fractions) and concurrent GM-CSF injected subcutaneously daily for two weeks, beginning with the second week of radiotherapy (Golden et al. 2015). Median overall survival was significantly better in abscopal responders than in patients without abscopal responses (20.98 months vs. 8.33 months). Of note, abscopal responders presented with lower baseline median neutrophil to lymphocyte ratio than non-responders (2.29 vs. 4.24). This finding is consistent with previous reports that a neutrophil to lymphocyte ratio greater than 4 is a poor prognostic marker (2014). Overall, treatment was well tolerated. The most common side effects were Grade 1 fatigue (35 patients), Grade 1 dermatitis (13 patients) and Grade 1 nausea/vomiting (19 patients). Importantly, this trial demonstrates that despite advanced metastatic disease and extensive pre-treatment, patients can derive benefit from localized radiation and immunotherapy.

2.4 TGF-β Antagonist

As previously described, reactive oxygen species created by radiation therapy cause TGFβ to dissociate from its latency-associated peptide (LAP) (Barcellos-Hoff et al. 1994). TGFβ induction has multiple concurrent effects: it promotes DNA damage response and modulates radiosensitivity (Bouquet et al. 2011), and inhibits the antigen-presenting function of DCs (Wrzesinski et al. 2007). In preclinical models of metastatic breast cancer, radiation therapy combined with TGFβ neutralizing antibodies induced T-cell mediated rejection of the irradiated tumor as well as the un-irradiated metastases (Vanpouille-Box et al. 2015). Of note, neither TGFβ blockade nor radiation therapy alone had an effect on lung metastases. Conversely, radiation combined with TGFβ blockade led to complete regression of 81% of the primary irradiated tumors as well as significant growth inhibition of contralateral non-irradiated tumors and lung metastases. Microarray analysis of primary tumors treated with radiation therapy and TGFβ blockade revealed that the top 20 upregulated pathways were immune-related and the top 3 gene networks were involved in recruitment of CTLs and the activation of immune effector function genes and IFNγ pathways. Finally, use of PD-1 blocking antibody in addition to radiation therapy and TGFβ blockade improved the rate of complete regression

(75%) and enhanced survival rates, compared to radiation therapy with TGFβ blockade (44%) or with anti-PD-1 (25%), respectively.

These findings suggest that TGFβ blockade enables CD8+ T cell priming, which improves both local and distant tumor control but, optimal preclinical results could only be achieved by overcoming adaptive immune resistance mediated by PD-L1 expression, supporting a therapeutic strategy that targets multiple immune pathways in combination with radiation therapy. We recently completed a Phase 2 trial investigating the combination of radiation therapy and fresolimumab, a human monoclonal TGFβ antibody, is underway in metastatic breast cancer patients. The primary endpoint is the abscopal response rate at 15 weeks (ClinicalTrials.gov identifier: NCT01401062). After completion of this trial, we plan to test the addition of anti-PD1 to the combination.

2.5   CTLA-4 Blockade

Cytotoxic T-lymphocyte-associated protein 4 (CTLA-4) or CD152 is a costimu-latory molecule that is expressed on T-cells. It functions as an immune checkpoint, to down-regulate an immune response. Anti-CTLA4 predominantly inhibits T-regulatory cells (Treg cells), thereby increasing the CD8 T-cell to Treg (CD8/Treg) ratio. Preclinical models of breast and colon carcinoma have demon-strated synergy between anti-CTLA-4 antibody and radiation therapy (Demaria et al. 2005; Dewan et al. 2009). In 4T1 breast carcinoma murine models, anti-CTLA-4 antibody alone did not affect primary tumor growth or mouse sur-vival; radiation therapy only delayed tumor growth without influencing survival (Demaria et al. 2005). However, the combination of radiation therapy and anti-CTLA-4 antibody led to local tumor growth inhibition as well as inhibition of lug metastases and improved survival. Experiments by Ruocco et al. (2012) revealed one of the mechanisms underlying these observations. Anti-CTLA-4 antibody alone enhanced T cell motility and reduced contact time with tumor cells. However, combining anti-CTLA-4 antibody with radiation therapy promoted MHC-I and NKG2D dependent CD8+ T cell arrest in contact with tumor cells and inhibited cell growth (Ruocco et al. 2012). Expression of the NKG2D ligand retinoic acid early inducible-1 (RAE-1) was increased in irradiated 4T1 cells, enabling a more effective immunological synapse.

Clinical translation of the synergy of radiation and anti-CTLA-4 blockade has been reported with cases of abscopal responses in patients with melanoma and non-small cell cancer who received both radiation and ipilimumab, a monoclonal antibody against CTLA-4 (Golden et al. 2013; Grimaldi et al. 2014; Hiniker et al. 2012; Postow et al. 2012). Ipilimumab and irradiation of a liver metastasis elicited a dramatic response within the radiotherapy field and at distant metastases in a 64-year-old man with metastatic lung adenocarcinoma (Golden et al. 2013). Despite multiple lines of chemotherapy and radiation to the chest, the patient was rapidly progressing with multiple metastases in the lung, liver and bones. Radiation therapy to a metabolically active hepatic metastasis was treated with 30 Gy in 5 fractions, with Ipilimumab administered the day after the first radiation fraction then every three weeks for a total of 4 infusions. Four months after treatment, the irradiated lesion and all other metastases had dramatically decreased, and eventually resolved. The patient has remained disease free 3 years later, without any other treatment.

Recently, a phase I dose escalation trial in patients with metastatic melanoma demonstrated partial responses in 18% of study participants and stable disease in another 18% (Twyman-Saint Victor et al. 2015). Patients with lung or bone metastases received 8 Gy × 2 or 8 Gy × 3 to an index lesion while those with liver or subcutaneous metastases received 6 Gy × 2 or 6 Gy × 3. Three to five days after radiation therapy, all patients received ipilimumab every three weeks for four doses. Preclinical models revealed that resistance to this treatment combination was due to T-cell exhaustion and upregulation of PD-L1 on melanoma cells. Among patients on this trial, high PD-L1 expression in the melanoma cells prohibited response to the treatment regimen and was associated with rapid disease progression and persistent T-cell exhaustion. While the findings could also demonstrate PD-L1 expression as a sign of T cell activation, it is possible that anti-CTLA4 and anti-PD-L1/PD-1 therapies may need to be combined with radiation in order to improve systemic response.

At present, there are multiple trials underway that explore the combination of radiation therapy and ipilimumab. One example is a Phase 2 trial in metastatic non-small cell lung cancer patients. Patients receive ipilimumab within 24 h of starting radiation therapy (6 Gy × 5 or 9.5 Gy × 3) to an index lesion. Ipilimumab is given every three weeks for a total of four doses. The primary endpoint is the abscopal response rate (ClinicalTrials.gov identifier: NCT02221739).

2.6 PD-1/PD-L1

Programmed cell death protein 1 is an immunoglobulin receptor that is expressed on the surface of T- and pro-B cells. It binds two ligands, PD-L1 and PD-L2, to mediate T cell inhibition. PD-L1 is upregulated as a part of radiation-induced antitumor immune response within cancer cells and infiltrating myeloid cells of irradiated mouse tumors (Deng et al. 2014). This up-regulation requires IFNγ (Chen et al. 2012). In multiple preclinical models, blockade of PD-1 or PD-L1 in conjunction with radiation therapy improved antitumor responses. In a mouse model of glioblastoma multiforme (Zeng et al. 2013), mice treated with combination anti-PD-1 therapy plus radiation therapy (10 Gy × 1) demonstrated improved survival compared with either modality alone: median survival of 53 days in the radiation therapy plus anti-PD-1 arm, 25 days in the control arm, 27 days in the anti-PD-1 antibody arm, and 28 days in the radiation arm. Also, long-term survivors were only seen in the combined treatment arm with 15–40% of animals alive at day 180+ after treatment. On a molecular level, combined treatment led to a decrease in Tregs and an increase in tumor infiltration by cytotoxic CD8+ T cells compared with the single modality arms.

Table 1 Active clinical trials evaluating the combination of radiation therapy and anti-PD-1/PD-L1

Clinicaltrials.gov identifier	Disease	Phase	Design	Primary endpoint	Radiation dose/timing	Institution(s)
NCT02407171	Stage IV melanoma or NSCLC	I/II	Phase I: anti-PD-1 Q2 wks with RT initiated at time of progression on anti-PD-1 agent	ORR	30 Gy in 5 fractions, dose-escalation to 30 Gy in 3 fractions	Yale University
NCT02400814	Stage IV NSCLC	I	Arm 1: concurrent RT and anti-PD-L1 Arm 2: induction anti-PD-L1 Q3 weeks with RT added at beginning of course 3	AEs, ORR, PFS	5 fractions over 1.5–2 weeks; dose unspecified	UC Davis
NCT02599779	Stage IV RCC	II	Arm A: RT at progression Arm B: RT prior to second course of pembrolizumab	PFS	1–3 most clinically significant lesions to receive RT, dose unspecified	Sunnybrook Health Sciences Centre
NCT02383212	Advanced malignancies	I	Monotherapy, dual, triple and quadruple combination cohorts	AEs, DLTs	9 Gy × 3	Multiple Centers in the United States
NCT02642809	Metastatic esophageal cancers	0	Pembrolizumab within 1 week after brachytherapy completion, given Q3 weeks	AEs	16 Gy in 2 fractions separated by 7-10 days between fractions	Washington University

PFS Progression free survival
ORR Overall response rate
AE Adverse event
DLT Dose limiting toxicity

Several clinical trials exploring the combination of anti-PD-1/PD-L1 and radiation therapy are underway (Table 1).

3 Optimizing Radiation Dose and Fractionation

The optimal radiation therapy regimens to induce its pro-immunogenic effects while minimizing its immunosuppressive consequences remain to be defined. However, experiments in mouse carcinoma models suggest that hypo-fractionated radiotherapy may be superior to single ablative doses, in strategies aimed at generating immune mediated anti-tumor effects both in the irradiated field and systemically.

For instance, a comparison of three radiotherapy regimens (20 Gy × 1, 8 Gy 3 or 6 Gy × 5) in syngeneic mice injected with TSA mouse breast carcinoma cells at two separate sites, revealed that 8 Gy × 3 best induced complete regression of the "primary" irradiated tumor as well as significant growth inhibition ("abscopal effect") of the second tumor site outside the radiotherapy field (Dewan et al. 2009). In this experiment, mice with palpable tumors were randomly assigned to three different radiotherapy regimens: no radiotherapy, 20 Gy × 1, 8 Gy × 3, or 6 Gy × 5 fractions in consecutive days with or without a murine monoclonal antibody against CTLA-4. Although all three of the radiotherapy regimens similarly inhibited growth of the irradiated primary tumor, all radiotherapy regimens failed to inhibit growth of the secondary tumors outside the radiation field when used alone.

In contrast, the combination of CTLA-4 and radiation of 8 Gy × 3 or 6 Gy × 5 fractions achieved an abscopal effect. Conversely, the abscopal effect was minimal if a single dose of 20 Gy to the primary tumor was used. The frequency of CD8+ T cells showing tumor-specific IFN-gamma production was proportional to the inhibition of the secondary tumor. Similar experiments were conducted in the MCA38 mouse colon carcinoma model with comparable results.

While evidence suggests that single high dose radiation therapy may be more effective than fractionated radiation therapy for the in-field control of some tumor types, none of these experiments tested abscopal effects. In experiments using the B16 mouse melanoma cell line, a single dose of 15 Gy was more effective at priming antitumor T cells than 3 Gy given for 5 consecutive days (Lugade et al. 2005). Similarly, a single 20 Gy dose was more effective at eliciting an antitumor T cell response than 5 Gy given four times over the course of 2 weeks (Lee et al. 2009). These findings suggest that pathways eliciting memory and abscopal effects may differ from those recruiting the immune response to contribute to local control of cancer, within the irradiated field.

4 Future Directions

4.1 CSF-1/CSF-1R

Macrophage-colony stimulating factor 1 (CSF-1) signals through its receptor (CSF-1R) to promote the differentiation of macrophages and dendritic cells. Analysis of human pancreatic cancers has revealed elevated expression of CSF-1 compared to normal tissues and expression of CSF-1R within the tumor stroma (Pyonteck et al. 2012; Zhu et al. 2014). In preclinical pancreatic cancer studies, CSF1 neutralizing antibodies led to a 60% decrease in tumor-associated macrophages (TAMs), especially within the CD206^{Hi} TAMs subset, that have been associated with poor outcomes in human pancreatic cancer (Zhu et al. 2014; Ino et al. 2013). CD206^{Hi} TAMs were decreased by >90% after 8 days of treatment whereas there were 45% fewer CD206^{Low} TAMs. CD206^{Hi} TAMs also express higher levels of CSF-1R so they may be especially sensitive to this treatment strategy. In addition, blockade of CSF1R curbed tumor infiltration by MDSCs (myeloid derived suppressor cells), a cell population that can exert immunosuppressive effects. Of note, CSF1R blockade led to increased CTLA-4 expression. Therefore, dual targeting of CTLA-4 and CSF1R may be needed to optimize response. In murine pancreatic cancer models, combining CTLA-4 and CSF1R antagonists led to a >90% reduction in tumor progression (Zhu et al. 2014).

CSF-1R blockade may also enhance the anti-tumor effects of radiation therapy. In human glioblastoma xenograft models, treatment with radiation therapy and PLX3397, a small molecule inhibitor of CSF-1R, increased median survival compared to radiation therapy alone (Stafford et al. 2016). Moreover, CSF-1R inhibition precluded CD11b+ myeloid-derived cells from differentiating into immunosuppressive, pro-angiogenic TAMs.

Blockade of CSF1R may also improve the efficacy of radiotherapy in prostate cancer. In a preclinical prostate cancer model, irradiation of the primary tumor led to a systemic increase in MDSCs and intratumoral increases in MDSCs, TAMs and CSF-1 (Xu et al. 2013). Similarly, in prostate cancer patients, serum levels of CSF increased after radiation therapy. When combined with a CSF1R inhibitor, radiation therapy suppressed tumor growth more effectively than either therapy alone. These results indicate that CSF-1R targeting can dampen the immunosuppressive modulation of the tumor milieu generated by irradiation. This strategy may also be of future application in breast cancer where CSF-1/CSF-1R signaling was shown to recruit TAMs, while blockade of this pathway inhibited TAMs and improved treatment outcomes in transgenic mice (DeNardo et al. 2011).

4.2 OX40

OX40 (CD134) is a co-stimulatory molecule and member of the tumor necrosis factor receptor superfamily. It is expressed on the surface of T cells and binds

OX40L (CD252) that is expressed on activated antigen presenting cells (Aspeslagh et al. 2016). OX40 activation exerts effects on diverse components of the immune system. OX40 agonistic antibodies increase effector T-cell survival (Lei et al. 2013; Ruby et al. 2008) and OX40 activation prevents the production of new Tregs and impairs their suppressive functions (Kroemer et al. 2007; Vu et al. 2007). However, in the absence of IFN-γ and IL-4, OX40 activation can stimulate the proliferation of Tregs (Ruby et al. 2009). In preclinical models of lung cancer, radiation therapy combined with OX40 agonists led to improved survival (Yokouchi et al. 2008) and immune rejection when mice were re-challenged with same tumor inoculation (Gough et al. 2010). In these experiments, combination therapy stimulated the recruitment of tumor antigen-specific OX40+ T cells to draining lymph nodes. Similar results were obtained in preclinical combinations of anti-OX40 with radiotherapy for glioma in C57Bl/6 mice. Moreover, the 50-80% of mice treated with the combination therapy in an intracranial experimental glioma model had durable responses and significant survival benefit (Kjaergaard et al. 2005). At present, there are ongoing clinical trials examining radiotherapy and OX40 agonist antibody combinations in metastatic breast cancer (NCT01862900) and metastatic prostate cancer (NCT01303705).

5 Conclusion

Over the past decade, many discoveries have elucidated radiation therapy's inter-action with the immune system. Traditionally, the 4Rs (reassortment, reoxygena-tion, repair and repopulation) have been used to describe the principles underlying radiation therapy's ability to elicit tumor cell kill. Preclinical studies and clinical trials suggest that a 5th R, immune mediated rejection, should be added, in recognition of the contribution of the immune system to the effects of ionizing radiation (Golden and Formenti 2014). However, radiation alone is often insuffi-cient to overcome the existing immunosuppressive tumor microenvironment. Moreover, it also elicits immunosuppressive effects by itself, such as infiltration of MDSCs and Tregs that may at least in part abrogate its immunostimulatory func-tions. Research aiming at shifting the balance in favor of a proimmunogenic global effect of radiation is ongoing.

The renaissance of cancer immunotherapy and the availability of multiple tar-geting strategies offer an unprecedented opportunity for therapeutic investigations that include radiotherapy. Combination of radiotherapy and these agents can shift the balance in favor of immune stimulation and overcome obstacles surrounding promotion of cross-priming and stimulation of CTLs. These combinatorial strate-gies have significant potential to improve the therapeutic efficacy of both radiation and immunotherapy, and establish long-term immunological memory with impli-cations on metastatic dormancy and equilibrium.

References

Adams S (2009) Toll-like receptor agonists in cancer therapy. Immunotherapy 1(6):949–964

Adams S et al (2012) Topical TLR7 agonist imiquimod can induce immune-mediated rejection of skin metastases in patients with breast cancer. Clin Cancer Res 18(24):6748–6757

Apetoh L et al (2007) Toll-like receptor 4-dependent contribution of the immune system to anticancer chemotherapy and radiotherapy. Nat Med 13(9):1050–1059

Aspeslagh S et al (2016) Rationale for anti-OX40 cancer immunotherapy. Eur J Cancer 52:50–66

Attiga FA et al (2000) Inhibitors of prostaglandin synthesis inhibit human prostate tumor cell invasiveness and reduce the release of matrix metalloproteinases. Cancer Res 60(16): 4629–4637

Bansal V, Ochoa JB (2003) Arginine availability, arginase, and the immune response. Curr Opin Clin Nutr Metab Care 6(2):223–228

Barcellos-Hoff MH et al (1994) Transforming growth factor-beta activation in irradiated murine mammary gland. J Clin Invest 93(2):892–899

Bos PD et al (2013) Transient regulatory T cell ablation deters oncogene-driven breast cancer and enhances radiotherapy. J Exp Med 210(11):2435–2466

Boucher JL, Moali C, Tenu JP (1999) Nitric oxide biosynthesis, nitric oxide synthase inhibitors and arginase competition for L-arginine utilization. Cell Mol Life Sci 55(8–9):1015–1028

Bouquet F et al (2011) TGFbeta1 inhibition increases the radiosensitivity of breast cancer cells in vitro and promotes tumor control by radiation in vivo. Clin Cancer Res 17(21):6754–6765

Brody JD et al (2010) In situ vaccination with a TLR9 agonist induces systemic lymphoma regression: a phase I/II study. J Clin Oncol 28(28):4324–4332

Burgess AW, Metcalf D (1980) The nature and action of granulocyte-macrophage colony stimulating factors. Blood 56(6):947–958

Chakraborty M et al (2003) Irradiation of tumor cells up-regulates Fas and enhances CTL lytic activity and CTL adoptive immunotherapy. J Immunol 170(12):6338–6347

Chang CI, Liao JC, Kuo L (2001) Macrophage arginase promotes tumor cell growth and suppresses nitric oxide-mediated tumor cytotoxicity. Cancer Res 61(3):1100–1106

Chen J et al (2012) Interferon-gamma-induced PD-L1 surface expression on human oral squamous carcinoma via PKD2 signal pathway. Immunobiology 217(4):385–393

Demaria S et al (2004) Ionizing radiation inhibition of distant untreated tumors (abscopal effect) is immune mediated. Int J Radiat Oncol Biol Phys 58(3):862–870

Demaria S et al (2005) Immune-mediated inhibition of metastases after treatment with local radiation and CTLA-4 blockade in a mouse model of breast cancer. Clin Cancer Res 11(2 Pt 1): 728–734

Demaria S et al (2013) The TLR7 agonist imiquimod as an adjuvant for radiotherapy-elicited in situ vaccination against breast cancer. Oncoimmunology 2(10):e25997

DeNardo DG et al (2011) Leukocyte complexity predicts breast cancer survival and functionally regulates response to chemotherapy. Cancer Discov 1(1):54–67

Deng L et al (2014) STING-dependent cytosolic DNA sensing promotes radiation-induced type i interferon-dependent antitumor immunity in immunogenic tumors. Immunity 41(5):843–852

Dewan MZ et al (2009) Fractionated but not single-dose radiotherapy induces an immune-mediated abscopal effect when combined with anti-CTLA-4 antibody. Clin Cancer Res 15(17):5379–5388

Dewan MZ et al (2012) Synergy of topical toll-like receptor 7 agonist with radiation and low-dose cyclophosphamide in a mouse model of cutaneous breast cancer. Clin Cancer Res 18(24): 6668–6678

Diamond MS et al (2011) Type I interferon is selectively required by dendritic cells for immune rejection of tumors. J Exp Med 208(10):1989–2003

Formenti SC, Demaria S (2012) Radiation therapy to convert the tumor into an in situ vaccine. Int J Radiat Oncol Biol Phys 84(4):879–880

Fuertes MB et al (2011) Host type I IFN signals are required for antitumor CD8+ T cell responses through CD8{alpha} + dendritic cells. J Exp Med 208(10):2005–2016

Fujita H et al (2002) Cyclooxygenase-2 promotes prostate cancer progression. Prostate 53(3): 232–240

Galluzzi L et al (2007) Cell death modalities: classification and pathophysiological implications. Cell Death Differ 14(7):1237–1243

Ghiringhelli F et al (2009) Activation of the NLRP3 inflammasome in dendritic cells induces IL-1beta-dependent adaptive immunity against tumors. Nat Med 15(10):1170–1178

Golden EB, Formenti SC (2014) Is tumor (R)ejection by the immune system the "5th R" of radiobiology? Oncoimmunology 3(1):e28133

Golden EB et al (2013) An abscopal response to radiation and ipilimumab in a patient with metastatic non-small cell lung cancer. Cancer Immunol Res 1(6):365–372

Golden EB et al (2015) Local radiotherapy and granulocyte-macrophage colony-stimulating factor to generate abscopal responses in patients with metastatic solid tumours: a proof-of-principle trial. Lancet Oncol 16(7):795–803

Gough MJ et al (2010) Adjuvant therapy with agonistic antibodies to CD134 (OX40) increases local control after surgical or radiation therapy of cancer in mice. J Immunother 33(8):798–809

Grimaldi AM et al (2014) Abscopal effects of radiotherapy on advanced melanoma patients who progressed after ipilimumab immunotherapy. Oncoimmunology 3:e28780

Gulley JL et al (2005) Combining a recombinant cancer vaccine with standard definitive radiotherapy in patients with localized prostate cancer. Clin Cancer Res 11(9):3353–3362

Hasmim M et al (2013) Cutting edge: Hypoxia-induced Nanog favors the intratumoral infiltration of regulatory T cells and macrophages via direct regulation of TGF-beta1. J Immunol 191(12): 5802–5806

Hiniker SM et al (2012) A systemic complete response of metastatic melanoma to local radiation and immunotherapy. Transl Oncol 5(6):404–407

Ino Y et al (2013) Immune cell infiltration as an indicator of the immune microenvironment of pancreatic cancer. Br J Cancer 108(4):914–923

Jenkins DC et al (1995) Roles of nitric oxide in tumor growth. Proc Natl Acad Sci U S A 92(10): 4392–4396

Joyce JA, Fearon DT (2015) T cell exclusion, immune privilege, and the tumor microenvironment. Science 348(6230):74–80

Kim JY et al (2006) Increase of NKG2D ligands and sensitivity to NK cell-mediated cytotoxicity of tumor cells by heat shock and ionizing radiation. Exp Mol Med 38(5):474–484

Kjaergaard J et al (2005) Active immunotherapy for advanced intracranial murine tumors by using dendritic cell-tumor cell fusion vaccines. J Neurosurg 103(1):156–164

Klug F et al (2013) Low-dose irradiation programs macrophage differentiation to an iNOS(+)/M1 phenotype that orchestrates effective T cell immunotherapy. Cancer Cell 24(5):589–602

Kroemer A et al (2007) OX40 controls functionally different T cell subsets and their resistance to depletion therapy. J Immunol 179(8):5584–5591

Kuo P et al (2014) Galectin-1 mediates radiation-related lymphopenia and attenuates NSCLC radiation response. Clin Cancer Res 20(21):5558–5569

Lee Y et al (2009) Therapeutic effects of ablative radiation on local tumor require CD8+ T cells: changing strategies for cancer treatment. Blood 114(3):589–595

Lei F et al (2013) Regulation of A1 by OX40 contributes to CD8(+) T cell survival and anti-tumor activity. PLoS ONE 8(8):e70635

Li J et al (2007) Lymphoma immunotherapy with CpG oligodeoxynucleotides requires TLR9 either in the host or in the tumor itself. J Immunol 179(4):2493–2500

Lugade AA et al (2005) Local radiation therapy of B16 melanoma tumors increases the generation of tumor antigen-specific effector cells that traffic to the tumor. J Immunol 174(12):7516–7523

Lugade AA et al (2008) Radiation-induced IFN-gamma production within the tumor microenvironment influences antitumor immunity. J Immunol 180(5):3132–3139

Ma Y et al (2010) Chemotherapy and radiotherapy: cryptic anticancer vaccines. Semin Immunol 22(3):113–124

Marabelle A et al (2013) Depleting tumor-specific Tregs at a single site eradicates disseminated tumors. J Clin Invest 123(6):2447–2463

Matsumura S et al (2008) Radiation-induced CXCL16 release by breast cancer cells attracts effector T cells. J Immunol 181(5):3099–3107

Newcomb EW et al (2006) The combination of ionizing radiation and peripheral vaccination produces long-term survival of mice bearing established invasive GL261 gliomas. Clin Cancer Res 12(15):4730–4737

Obeid M et al (2007) Calreticulin exposure dictates the immunogenicity of cancer cell death. Nat Med 13(1):54–61

Park HJ et al (2012) Radiation-induced vascular damage in tumors: implications of vascular damage in ablative hypofractionated radiotherapy (SBRT and SRS). Radiat Res 177(3): 311–327

Pilones KA et al (2014) Invariant natural killer T cells regulate anti-tumor immunity by controlling the population of dendritic cells in tumor and draining lymph nodes. J Immunother Cancer 2 (1):37

Postow MA et al (2012) Immunologic correlates of the abscopal effect in a patient with melanoma. N Engl J Med 366(10):925–931

Pyonteck SM et al (2012) Deficiency of the macrophage growth factor CSF-1 disrupts pancreatic neuroendocrine tumor development. Oncogene 31(11):1459–1467

Reits EA et al (2006) Radiation modulates the peptide repertoire, enhances MHC class I expression, and induces successful antitumor immunotherapy. J Exp Med 203(5):1259–1271

Rodriguez PC et al (2003) L-arginine consumption by macrophages modulates the expression of CD3 zeta chain in T lymphocytes. J Immunol 171(3):1232–1239

Ruby CE et al (2008) IL-12 is required for anti-OX40-mediated CD4 T cell survival. J Immunol 180(4):2140–2148

Ruby CE et al (2009) Cutting edge: OX40 agonists can drive regulatory T cell expansion if the cytokine milieu is right. J Immunol 183(8):4853–4857

Ruocco MG et al (2012) Suppressing T cell motility induced by anti-CTLA-4 monotherapy improves antitumor effects. J Clin Invest 122(10):3718–3730

Stafford JH et al (2016) Colony stimulating factor 1 receptor inhibition delays recurrence of glioblastoma after radiation by altering myeloid cell recruitment and polarization. Neuro Oncol 18(6):797–806

Stanley MA (2002) Imiquimod and the imidazoquinolones: mechanism of action and therapeutic potential. Clin Exp Dermatol 27(7):571–577

Stout RD et al (2005) Macrophages sequentially change their functional phenotype in response to changes in microenvironmental influences. J Immunol 175(1):342–349

Templeton AJ et al (2014) Prognostic role of neutrophil-to-lymphocyte ratio in solid tumors: a systematic review and meta-analysis. J Natl Cancer Inst 106(6): p. dju124

Tsai CS et al (2007) Macrophages from irradiated tumors express higher levels of iNOS, arginase-I and COX-2, and promote tumor growth. Int J Radiat Oncol Biol Phys 68(2):499–507

Twyman-Saint Victor C et al (2015) Radiation and dual checkpoint blockade activate non-redundant immune mechanisms in cancer. Nature 520(7547):373–377

Vanpouille-Box C et al (2015) TGFbeta is a master regulator of radiation therapy-induced antitumor immunity. Cancer Res 75(11):2232–2242

Vollmer J et al (2004) Characterization of three CpG oligodeoxynucleotide classes with distinct immunostimulatory activities. Eur J Immunol 34(1):251–262

Vu MD et al (2007) OX40 costimulation turns off Foxp3 + Tregs. Blood 110(7):2501–2510

Wang W, Bergh A, Damber JE (2005) Cyclooxygenase-2 expression correlates with local chronic inflammation and tumor neovascularization in human prostate cancer. Clin Cancer Res 11(9): 3250–3256

Woo SR et al (2014) STING-dependent cytosolic DNA sensing mediates innate immune recognition of immunogenic tumors. Immunity 41(5):830–842

Wooldridge JE, Weiner GJ (2003) CpG DNA and cancer immunotherapy: orchestrating the antitumor immune response. Curr Opin Oncol 15(6):440–445

Wrzesinski SH, Wan YY, Flavell RA (2007) Transforming growth factor-beta and the immune response: implications for anticancer therapy. Clin Cancer Res 13(18 Pt 1):5262–5270

Xu J et al (2013) CSF1R signaling blockade stanches tumor-infiltrating myeloid cells and improves the efficacy of radiotherapy in prostate cancer. Cancer Res 73(9):2782–2794

Yang KL et al (2013) Reciprocal complementation of the tumoricidal effects of radiation and natural killer cells. PLoS ONE 8(4):e61797

Yokouchi H et al (2008) Anti-OX40 monoclonal antibody therapy in combination with radiotherapy results in therapeutic antitumor immunity to murine lung cancer. Cancer Sci 99(2):361–367

Zeng J et al (2013) Anti-PD-1 blockade and stereotactic radiation produce long-term survival in mice with intracranial gliomas. Int J Radiat Oncol Biol Phys 86(2):343–349

Zhu Y et al (2014) CSF1/CSF1R blockade reprograms tumor-infiltrating macrophages and improves response to T-cell checkpoint immunotherapy in pancreatic cancer models. Cancer Res 74(18):5057–5069

SBRT and the Treatment of Oligometastatic Disease

Jeffrey M. Lemons, Michael W. Drazer, Jason J. Luke
and Steven J. Chmura

Abstract

For patients with metastatic cancer, there is significant variation in the amount of time from diagnosis to disease progression or death. For physicians, predicting the duration of this interval can be difficult. The clinical course for these patients is dependent on myriad factors including the primary histology, size, and location of metastatic lesions. Attempts have been made to model prognosis based on other factors such as response to neoadjuvant chemotherapy and volume of disease. A distinct clinical state of metastases with low volume disease and few organs affected was coined "oligometastases." It is hypothesized this state may be amenable to local therapy to improve outcomes. After long term follow up, patients with this limited metastatic progression appear to have relatively good outcomes, with some long-term survivors, after aggressive treatment with local therapy combined with systemic therapy. In the past 20 years since the conception of the oligometastatic hypothesis, there have been advances in surgical and radiation therapy techniques resulting in reduced toxicities. Additionally, developments in systemic therapy have prolonged survival for

J.M. Lemons (✉) · S.J. Chmura
The University of Chicago Department of Radiation and Cellular Oncology,
5841 S. Maryland Avenue, MC 9006, Chicago, IL 60637, USA
e-mail: jlemons1@radonc.uchicago.edu

S.J. Chmura
e-mail: schmura@radonc.uchicago.edu

M.W. Drazer · J.J. Luke
The University of Chicago Department of Medicine Section of Hematology/Oncology,
5841 S. Maryland Avenue, MC 2115, Chicago, IL 60637, USA
e-mail: mdrazer@medicine.bsd.uchicago.edu

J.J. Luke
e-mail: jluke@medicine.bsd.uchicago.edu

© Springer International Publishing AG 2017
J.Y.C. Wong et al. (eds.), *Advances in Radiation Oncology*,
Cancer Treatment and Research 172, DOI 10.1007/978-3-319-53235-6_2

patients with metastatic disease. Herein we discuss the history and rationale for local treatment of oligometastases and delve into the implementation of stereotactic body radiotherapy (SBRT) to this evolving treatment paradigm.

Keywords

Radiation · SBRT · SABR · Oligometastases · Metastatic cancer · Radiation treatment planning

Abbreviations

AAPM	American Association of Physicists in Medicine
BED	Biologically effective dose
CTV	Clinical target volume
DFS	Disease free survival
GTV	Gross tumor volume
ITV	Internal target volume
MOSART	Multi-organ site ablative radiation therapy
MRI	Magnetic resonance imaging
OAR	Organ at risk
OS	Overall survival
PD1	Programmed Death 1
PDL1	Programmed Death Ligand 1
PET CT	Positron emission tomography computed tomography
PTV	Planning target volume
RTOG	Radiation therapy oncology group
RT	Radiation therapy
SABR	Stereotactic ablative radiotherapy
SBRT	Stereotactic body radiotherapy
SRS	Stereotactic radiosurgery
WBRT	Whole brain radiation therapy

1 The Oligometastatic Hypothesis

Once a solid cancer is found to have metastasized to a distant organ, discussions between doctors and their patients change (Aitini and Aleotti 2006). These difficult conversations focus on palliative treatments, as opposed to curative measures. This common approach in oncology implies tumor cells are present in both macro- and micrometastases as soon as the malignancy has spread distantly and therefore cannot be completely eradicated. As such, systemic therapy is the mainstay of treatment for patients with metastatic disease.

Breast cancer was the original model for the metastatic sequence of solid tumors. In the early 1900s, William Stewart Halsted pioneered the paradigm of radical treatment for localized breast cancer (Halsted 1907). He contended cancer spreads sequentially, from a single location to regional lymph nodes, before eventually spreading to distant organs. Expanding on the work of Keynes (1954), Bernard Fisher presented an "alternative hypothesis." suggesting breast cancer is a systemic disease at the time of diagnosis and local therapy is unlikely to impact the chance of overall survival (Fisher 1980). Fisher postulated cancer disseminated at the onset, not in a contiguous progression as Halsted had suggested. Samuel Hellman offered a third model for breast cancer spread, the "spectrum theory" (Hellman 1994) implying cancer presents on a spectrum of localized disease to wide spread distant metastases. In his theory, Hellman indicated metastatic sites, either nodal or distant, could be a source of further disease spread. Shortly after proposing the spectrum theory, Hellman and Weichselbaum described an intermediate state between local and widespread disease which they coined "oligometastases" (Hellman and Weichselbaum 1995).

2 Biology of Oligometastases

In their original publication, Hellman and Weichselbaum stated "… in the light of the emerging information on the multistep nature of cancer progression, we propose the existence of a clinical significant state of *oligometastases*. For certain tumors, the anatomy and physiology may limit or concentrate these metastases to a single or a limited number of organs." Since the original "seed and soil" hypothesis by Stephan Paget in 1889 (Paget 1889), the biological progression of localized malignancy to distant spread has been further elucidated (Fidler 2003). This process includes local proliferation and angiogenesis with subsequent loss of cellular adhesion and increased motility. This leads to the interaction of malignant cells with platelets and other intravascular cells, which are transported throughout the circulatory system. This cell cluster will arrest in organs with adherence to the vessel wall followed by extravasation into tissue. Tumor cells will evade the host defense to establish a microenvironment, proliferate, and undergo angiogenesis in order to develop a marcometastasis.

It has been suggested patients with oligometastatic disease consist of deposits grown from sloughed cancer cells from the primary site, but have limited further metastatic and proliferation potential (Reyes and Pienta 2015). A plethora of preclinical in vitro and in vivo studies have shown a wide variation in the phenotypes of cells isolated from different primary and distant malignant tumor sites. Biologic basis for the clinical discrepancy between widespread and oligometastatic disease may include different primary tumor microenvironments, fitness of the migrant cancer cells, and the hospitality of host sites (Pienta et al. 2013).

Patients with a limited number of indolent metastatic deposits in different anatomic locations may represent the only trace of malignancy that remains. The natural history of cancer in this limited state may behave differently than the clinical course of a patient with diffuse metastatic disease. This crucial point of the oligometastatic theory suggests metastases-directed therapy through surgery and/or radiation combined with systemic therapy offers hope for patients previously deemed "incurable." The theoretical curative potential of treating oligometastases makes aggressive treatment for these patients enticing.

3 Defining "Oligo" Metastases

There is not a consensus definition of what constitutes "oligo" with respect to counting the number of metastases (Treasure 2012). Most studies have defined the oligometastatic state to be a limited distant hematogenous spread of disease, generally involving 1–5 metastatic lesions. Furthering the oligometastic hypothesis, Niibe et al. described oligorecurrence to distinguish patients with controlled primary tumors who experienced improved outcomes compared to patients with uncontrolled primary disease (Niibe and Hayakawa 2010). The process of counting metastases to define oligometastatic disease is predicated upon the reliability of imaging studies used for staging. Novel imaging modalities have become readily available, including PET-CT and MRI, which allow for increased ability to evaluate patients for the presence of metastatic disease. For example, pretreatment work up with PET-CT for lung cancer leads to increased detection of occult metastases in 19% of patients (MacManus et al. 2001). Beyond medical imaging, there is a developing body of literature demonstrating the utility of circulating tumor cells to evaluate metastatic disease (Krebs et al. 2011). This creates a clinical predicament, how you look for metastases may ultimately determine the presence or absence of the oligometastatic state. Mathematical modeling to predict presence of additional occult metastases has been proposed (Kendal 2014), but has not been widely adopted. Additionally, biological prognostic tools are currently being studied and are discussed in more detail later on in this chapter.

With the aforementioned caveats, cancers presenting with presenting with fewer metastases have a distinct clinical behavior relative to patients with increased burden of disease. In prostate cancer, patients with five or fewer metastatic deposits have similar survival to patients with no evidence of metastatic disease at 5 years (73% vs. 75%) and 10 years (36% vs. 45%) (Singh et al. 2004). Furthermore, patients with more than five lesions exhibited a 5-year survival of 45% with only 18% of patients alive at 10 years. Early stage breast cancer patients who experience oligorecurrent disease, with less than five sites of disease, have improved median survival (108 vs. 22 months) compared to patients with greater than five sites of disease (Dorn et al. 2011).

A limited number of reports inform the incidence of oligometastatic presentation or recurrence. A retrospective series determined breast cancer relapses were isolated to the liver and/or one other organ in 59% of patients (Pentheroudakis et al. 2006). Data from prospective trials performed for the first line treatment of metastatic breast cancer indicate up to 91% of patients enrolled had ≤ 4 metastases at time of enrollment (Albain et al. 2008). Memorial Sloan Kettering Cancer Center published a series of patients with sarcoma and found 19% of patients presented with isolated pulmonary metastases as their first site of failure (Gadd et al. 1993).

4 Surgical Resection of Limited Metastases

In the mid 20th century, anecdotal evidence demonstrated metastatic renal adeno-carcinoma to lung could be controlled long term with surgical resection of meta-static deposits (Barney 1945). There is a strong body of evidence supporting local treatment for limited metastatic disease in the setting of intracranial metastases. Randomized trials have demonstrated improvements in disease control and overall survival for patients treated with surgical resection or stereotactic radiosurgery (SRS) in addition to whole brain radiation therapy (WBRT) (Patchell et al. 1990; Andrews et al. 2004). Outside of the brain, there is surgical data demonstrating long-term disease control and survival in patients treated with metastectomy from sarcoma (van Geel et al. 1996) and breast cancer (Hanrahan et al. 2005) amongst other primary tumors. Patients presenting with spinal cord compression from solid tumors who undergo surgical decompression in addition to radiation have improved ambulatory function, continence, and survival compared to radiation monotherapy (Patchell et al. 2005).

Fong et al. published their experience with metastectomy of hepatic oliog-metastases for 456 patients with colorectal cancer treated between 1985 and 1991 (Fong et al. 1997). The treatment was well tolerated with low mortality and a post resection median survival of 46 months and 38% 5-year survival. A later publi-cation showed 22% of these patients achieved 10-year survival and were effectively cured of their disease (Fong et al. 1999). Subsequent studies (Simmonds et al. 2006) lead to hepatic resection for oligometastases from colorectal cancer becoming the standard of care in the absence of a prospective clinical trial in an era prior to oxaliplatin and ironotecan chemotherapy backbones. Long-term survival post lung metastectomy has also been published. The International Registry of Lung Metastases reported outcomes of surgical resection of lung metastases on 5206 patients with metastases from a variety of primary tumor histologies. The series demonstrated 15-year survival rates of 22% (Pastorino et al. 1997). Intriguingly, patients with fewer metastases and a longer disease-free interval fared even better. There is preliminary evidence to suggest a subset of patients with limited metastatic disease may be curable with localized treatment beyond chemotherapy.

5 Using SBRT for Extracranial Oligometastases

In general, SBRT is less invasive than surgical resection and can be used to treat anatomic locations that may not be surgically accessible. SBRT is an attractive treatment modality for oliogmetastases since it is rapidly deployable, allowing limited interruptions in systemic therapy. Advancements in radiation treatment planning and delivery platforms have improved the quality and reliability of delivering ablative doses of radiation. However, there is a scarcity of high quality prospective randomized trials evaluating the use of SBRT in this setting. Multiple groups have analyzed retrospective case series or performed single arm dose escalation studies in an effort to better understand the clinical history of oligometastases which have been treated with ablative radiation therapy.

Investigators at the University of Chicago recently updated their series of 61 patients with five or less extracranial metastases who were treated on a dose escalation trial in which all known sites of metastasis were treated with ablative RT (Wong et al. 2016). At a median follow up of 2.3 years (6.8 years for survivors), Kaplan-Meier estimates of treated metastases control were 51% at 2 years and 44% at 5 years. 13 patients (21.3%) were alive at last follow up and 11.5% of patients never progressed after protocol therapy. Treatment was well tolerated with only 2 patients experiencing acute grade 3 toxicity and 6 patients with late grade 3 toxicity. There were no grade 4 or higher toxicities. The University of Rochester prospectively analyzed the role of SBRT in the treatment of one to five oligometastases, present in one to three organs. Patients with breast cancer showed a 2-year overall survival of 74% with 52% of patients free from widespread distant metastasis, and local control rate at 2 years of 87%. Long term (6 year) overall survival was 47% in this subset of patients 87% local control achieved. These values were all significantly higher than rates of disease control achieved for patients with metastases from non-breast primary tumors. On multivariate analysis, patients with bone metastases or single metastatic lesion experienced significantly improved survival. This study offers insight into selecting patients who may experience therapeutic benefit from the utilization of SBRT for oligometastases. It appears the patients most likely to garner benefit from SBRT include individuals with breast cancer primary tumors, single bony metastases, and stable to responsive disease prior to SBRT.

The largest published series evaluating outcomes after SBRT for oligometastases comes from Vrije University in Brussels, Belgium (de Vin et al. 2014). Their study included 309 patients with ≤5 metastases, 209 of whom were treated with SBRT to 430 extracranial lesions. 82.6% of extracranial lesions were treated with 10 fractions of 4 or 5 Gy. The majority (74%) of patients had a single anatomic site of disease with 46.3% of patients having only one metastatic lesion and 29.8% of patients having two lesions. The most common sites of disease were brain (34.6%), lymph node (28.5%), liver (24.9%), or lung (18.1%). Patients with a solitary extracranial metastasis had a median survival time of 40 months, whereas patients with two to five sites of disease achieved a median survival of 26 months. In an

Table 1 Select studies of SBRT for multisite oligometastases

Publication	Year	Number of patients	Median follow-up (months)	RT dose	Metastases control	Overall survival
University of Chicago (Wong et al. 2016)	2016	61	82	24–48 Gy in 3 fractions	44% at 5y	32% at 5y
University of Rochester (Milano et al. 2012)	2012	121	85	50 Gy in 10 fractions	67% at 2y	28% at 4y
Vrije University (de Vin et al. 2014)	2014	309	12	40–50 Gy in 10 fractions	33% at 2y	32% at 3y

attempt to build a prognostic model for patient selection, de Vin et al. determined male sex, nonadenocarcinoma histology, presence of intracranial metastases, and synchronous presentation of metastases were associated with inferior outcomes. Stratifying patients by number of risk factors showed patients with two or fewer risk factors had a median overall survival of 23 months compared to 9 months for patients with three risk factors and 4 months if all four risk factors were present. Table 1 outlines the studies with the longest follow-up and highest patient numbers.

6 First, Do No Harm?

The safety of SBRT to a distinct anatomic site of oligometastatic disease has been explored. A multi-institutional phase I/II study investigated the use of SBRT for oligometastatic cancer to lung (Rusthoven et al. 2009). Thirty-eight patients with an assortment of primary cancers were treated with SBRT on a dose escalation trial of 48–60 Gy in 3 fractions. The majority of patients (82%) were treated to 1 or 2 lesions with no extrathoracic metastases in 87% of patients. Local progression was only observed in 1 patient conferring a local control rate of 96% at 2 years. Two year overall survival was 39 and 63% of patients had distant progression. Treatment was well tolerated with no grade 4–5 toxicity. Only three of the 38 patients experienced grade 3 toxicity.

Berber et al. published the largest series exploring the use of SBRT for liver metastases (Berber et al. 2013). 153 patients with 363 metastases were treated to a dose between 31.3 and 46.5 Gy in 3 or 5 fractions. With a mean follow-up of 25.2 months, the overall local control rate was 62% and 1 year overall survival was 62%. Treatment was well tolerated with no grade 4–5 toxicity and only 3.2% of patients experiencing grade 3 toxicity. Other series exploring treatment of liver metastases with SBRT have shown grade 3–5 toxicity rates up to 18% (Carey Sampson et al. 2006). In one published experienced, three of 31 patients experienced grade 5 toxicity (Blomgren et al. 1995).

The use of SBRT for spinal metastases was studied in a multi-institutional phase II/III trial, RTOG 0631. Phase II results included 44 patients with 4 cervical, 21 thoracic and 19 lumbar sites treated with a single fraction of 16 Gy (Ryu et al. 2014). There was high quality treatment delivery with on 26% of patients with minor deviations in target coverage and spinal cord dose constraint met in 100% of patients. Treatment was well tolerated with only one patient experiencing grade 3 neck pain and no grade 4–5 events. The phase III component is randomizing patients to receive single fraction high dose SBRT (16 or 18 Gy) compared to standard palliation with a single fraction of 8 Gy with a primary end point of pain control at 3 months post treatment. A recent multi-institutional series of 541 patients (594 tumors) treated with spine SBRT showed a total of 34 patients (5.7%) had a new or progressive vertebral compression fracture following SBRT, with a median time to fracture of 3 months (Jawad et al. 2016). Preexisting fracture, solitary metastasis, and higher prescription dose (≥ 38.4 Gy) were associated with increased risk of fracture.

In summary, these limited data suggest for some patients with limited metastatic disease, local treatment of macroscopic tumor sites is generally well tolerated and may improve disease free intervals, and potentially, overall survival for select patients.

7 SBRT Treatment Planning

There is no absolute definition for high dose ablative radiation for extracranial disease. Stereotactic body radiotherapy (SBRT) and stereotactic ablative radiation (SABR) are used interchangeably. AAPM TG 101 suggested SBRT is typically comprised of 1–5 fractions of 6–30 Gy doses per fraction (Benedict et al. 2010). As summarized above, early studies evaluating the use of radiation therapy consisted of a more prolonged treatment course of hypofractionated radiation. The optimal radiation dose is influenced by several factors including the number and location of target lesions. Desired local disease control must be balanced with respecting surrounding normal tissue tolerance. In early stage lung cancer, there are data showing improved local control when the biologically effective dose (BED) is greater or equal to 105 Gy (Grills et al. 2012; Kestin et al. 2014). Excellent rates of local disease control with use of high BED SBRT has been shown in the oligometastatic setting (Salama et al. 2012). NRG-BR001 outlines a location-adapted approach for multi-organ site ablative radiation therapy (MOSART) SBRT (Table 2).

In order to provide high precision SBRT, accurate patient positioning and immobilization is required. Respiratory motion analysis and management is imperative, particularly for lesions in the lung or liver, which exhibit significant movement with respiration (Benedict et al. 2010). GTV, CTV, ITV, and PTV volumes should be delineated depending on the anatomic location of the tumor and clinical scenario. There are many commercially available treatment delivery systems to enable reliable, high fidelity SBRT. The prescription isodose surface is chosen such that 95% of the target volume (PTV) is conformally covered by the

Table 2 MOSART prescription doses used in NRG-BR001

Metastatic location	Initial starting dose	Dose limiting toxicity dose
Lung—peripheral	45 Gy in 3 fractions	42 Gy in 3 fractions
Lung—central	50 Gy in 5 fractions	47.5 Gy in 5 fractions
Mediastinal/cervical lymph node	50 Gy in 5 fractions	47.5 Gy in 5 fractions
Liver	45 Gy in 3 fractions	42 Gy in 3 fractions
Spinal/paraspinal	30 Gy in 3 fractions	27 Gy in 3 fractions
Osseous	30 Gy in 3 fractions	27 Gy in 3 fractions
Abdominal-pelvic (lymph node/adrenal gland)	45 Gy in 3 fractions	42 Gy in 3 fractions

A phase 1 study of stereotactic body radiotherapy (SBRT) for the treatment of multiple metastases

Table 3 Recommended treatment plan evaluation parameters

PTV volume (cc)	Ratio of 50% prescription isodose volume to PTV volume (R50%)	Maximum dose at 2 cm from PTV as % of prescription dose (D2 cm) (%)
1.8	<7.5	<57.0
3.8	<6.5	<57.0
7.4	<6.0	<58.0
13.2	<5.8	<58.0
22.0	<5.5	<63.0
34.0	<5.3	<68.0
50.0	<5.0	<77.0
70.0	<4.8	<86.0
95.0	<4.4	<89.0
126.0	<4.0	<91.0
163.0	<3.7	<94.0

prescription isodose surface. When evaluating target coverage, doses less than 95% of the prescription dose are restricted to the outside edges of the PTV. The prescription isodose surface selected used should typically be $\geq 60\%$ and $\leq 90\%$ of the dose maximum within the PTV. Treatment plans must be optimized to limit the high dose spillage to surrounding tissue. To assess the dose fall off, the ratio of prescription isodose volume to the PTV volume should be kept below 1.5 with a goal of 1.2. Moreover, the ratio of the 50% prescription isodose volume to the PTV (R50%) and the maximum dose a 2 cm (D2 cm) should be minimized. Suggested guidelines are outlined in Table 3. Priority should be placed on limiting radiation exposure to surrounding organs at risk, particularly for organs with grave potential toxicities (e.g. spinal cord). One, three, and five fraction SBRT OAR dose limits proposed in NRG BR002 (Table 4) are tabulated below. Circumferential irradiation of gastrointestinal tract structures (esophagus, duodenum, bowel, and rectum) should be avoided.

Table 4 Organ-at-risk (OAR) dose limits used in NRG-BR002

Organ	1 fraction		3 fractions		5 fractions		Avoidance endpoint (Reference)
	Volume	Total dose (Gy)	Volume	Total dose (Gy)	Volume	Total dose (Gy)	
Spinal cord	<0.35 cc	10	<0.03 cc	22.5	<0.03 cc	28	Myelitis (RTOG 0631, 0915, Timmerman)
	<10% partial cord	10			<0.35 cc	22	
	<1.2 cc	8	<1.2 cc	13	<1.2 cc	15.6	
	<0.03 cc	14					
Brachial plexus	<0.03 cc	17.5	<0.03 cc	26	<0.03 cc	32	Neuropathy (RTOG 0813, 0915, Timmerman)
	<3 cc	14	<3 cc	22	<3 cc	30	
Cauda equina	<0.03 cc	16	<0.03 cc	24	<0.03 cc	32	Neuropathy (RTOG 0631, AAPM TG-101, Timmerman)
	<5 cc	14	<5 cc	21.9	<5 cc	30	
Sacral plexus	<0.03 cc	18	<0.03 cc	24	<0.03 cc	32	Neuropathy (RTOG 0631, AAPM TG-101, Timmerman)
	<5 cc	14.4	<5 cc	22.5	<5 cc	30	
Trachea and bronchus	<0.03 cc	20.2	<0.03 cc	30	<0.03 cc	40	Stenosis/fistula (RTOG 0813, 0915, Z4099, Timmerman)
	<4 cc	17.4	<5 cc	25.8	<5 cc	32	
Esophagus	<0.03 cc	15.4	<0.03 cc	27	<0.03 cc	35	Stenosis/fistula (RTOG 0631, 0813, 0915, Z4099, Timmerman)
	<5 cc	11.9	<5 cc	17.7	<5 cc	27.5	
Heart/pericardium	<0.03 cc	22	<0.03 cc	30	<0.03 cc	38	Pericarditis (RTOG 0631, 0813, Z4099, Timmerman)
	<15 cc	16	<15 cc	24	<15 cc	32	
Great vessels	<0.03 cc	37	<0.03 cc	45	<0.03 cc	53	Aneurysm (RTOG 0631, 0813, 0915, Z4099, Timmerman)
	<10 cc	31	<10 cc	39	<10 cc	47	
Skin	<0.03 cc	27.5	<0.03 cc	33	<0.03 cc	38.5	Ulceration (Z4099, Timmerman)
	<10 cc	25.5	<10 cc	31	<10 cc	36.5	
Stomach	<0.03 cc	22	<0.03 cc	30	<0.5 cc	35	Ulceration/fistula (Timmerman)
	<5 cc	17.4	<10 cc	22.5	<5 cc	26.5	
Duodenum	<0.03 cc	17	<0.03 cc	24	<0.5 cc	30	Ulceration (RTOG 0631, Timmerman)
	<5 cc	11.2	<10 cc	15	<5 cc	18.3	
	<10 cc	9					

(continued)

Table 4 (continued)

Organ	1 fraction		3 fractions		5 fractions		Avoidance endpoint (Reference)
	Volume	Total dose (Gy)	Volume	Total dose (Gy)	Volume	Total dose (Gy)	
Bowel	<0.03 cc	29.2	<0.03 cc	34.5	<0.03 cc	40	Colitis/fistula (Z4099, Timmerman)
	<20 cc	18	<20 cc	24	<20 cc	28.5	
Rectum	<0.03 cc	44.2	<0.03 cc	49.5	<0.03 cc	55	Proctitis/fistula (Timmerman)
	<3.5 cc	39	<3.5 cc	45	<3.5 cc	50	
	<20 cc	22	<20 cc	27.5	<20 cc	32.5	
Bladder	<0.03 cc	25	<0.03 cc	33	<0.03 cc	38	Cystitis/fistula (AAPM TG-101, Timmerman)
	<15 cc	12	<15 cc	16.8	<15 cc	20	
Ureter	<0.03 cc	35	<0.03	40	<0.03 cc	45	Stenosis (Timmerman)
Penile bulb	<3 cc	16	<3 cc	25	<3 cc	30	Impotence (Timmerman)
Femoral heads	<10 cc	15	<10 cc	24	<10 cc	30	Necrosis (Timmerman)
Bile duct	<0.03 cc	30	<0.03 cc	36	<0.03 cc	41	Stenosis (Timmerman)
Renal hilum/vascular trunk	<15 cc	14	<15 cc	19.5	<15 cc	23	Malignant hypertension (Timmerman)
Rib	<0.03 cc	33	<0.03 cc	50	<0.03 cc	57	Pain/fracture (Timmerman)
	<5 cc	28	<5 cc	40	<5 cc	45	
Lung	<37% lung volume	8	<15% lung volume	20	<37% lung volume	13.5	Pneumonitis/lung function (RTOG 0618, 0813, Z4099, Timmerman)
			<37% lung volume	11			
	<1500 cc	7	<1500 cc	10.5	<1500 cc	12.5	
	<1000 cc	7.6	<1000 cc	11.4	<1000 cc	13.5	
Total kidney	<200 cc	9.5	<200 cc	15	<200 cc	18	Renal function (Timmerman)
Liver	<700 cc	11	<700 cc	17.1	<700 cc	21	Liver function (Z4099, Timmerman)

8   Future Directions

8.1   Combining SBRT with PD-1 Blockade

An intact immune system is important for controlling the neoplastic process. To enhance their proliferative transformation, tumors garner the ability to evade this immune regulation (Vinay et al. 2015). After decades of interest, but limited clinical relevance in solid tumors, the use of cancer immunotherapy has entered the mainstream over the past decade. With the identification of regulatory immune receptor to ligand interactions which influence immunity, "checkpoint" blocking monoclonal antibodies have become standard of care in multiple tumors (Pardoll 2012). The first of these approaches to enter clinical usage was the inhibition of cytotoxic T lymphocyte antigen 4 (CTLA4) being approved for the treatment of metastatic melanoma (Hodi et al. 2010). Since then, CTLA4 blockade has been studied in several other primary tumors including non-small cell lung cancer (Lynch et al. 2012).

Subsequent to the development of CTLA4 blocking antibodies, cancer immunotherapy has gained a broader usage with the production of monoclonal antibodies against the Programmed Death 1 (PD1): Programmed Death Ligand (PDL1) axis. The PD1:PDL1 interaction appears to be a major immune-evasion pathway up-regulated by some tumors to suppress anti-tumor immunity. Preliminary data suggests a potential synergistic effect on tumor response using PD-1 blockade in combination with radiotherapy (Drake 2012; Deng et al. 2014). This effect was observed in both tumors within the radiation field as well as distant tumors, suggesting the beneficial effects of radiation on the immune response have systemic impact. Clinical case reports have shown this abscopal response in sites distant from radiation while patients are receiving CTLA4 blocking immunotherapy (Postow et al. 2012).

Tumor cell death after high dose per fraction SBRT appears to be mediated through pathways beyond DNA damage and may enhance immune surveillance of tumors (Liang et al. 2013). The mechanism for this enhanced effect seems to include, at least in part, increased tumor antigen exposure, improved antigen presentation, and T cell function as well as modulation of immunosuppressive cell populations such as T regulatory cells and myeloid derived suppressor cells (Gaipl et al. 2014).

Beyond synergistic mechanisms of modulating the immune response, direct tumor debulking by radiation may also be particularly well suited as an adjunct to immunotherapy. Radiation to sites of bulk tumor would be presumed to improve the overall response rate of combination therapy. Additionally, reports of SBRT combinations with systemic therapies have suggested time to progression is delayed (Milano et al. 2012; Iyengar et al. 2014). Anti-PD1 antibody treatment may particularly be boosted by this approach. Clinical reports of the drug pembrolizumab suggest lower disease burden at the time of treatment initiation has been associated with higher response rate and one year survival in advanced melanoma (Joseph et al. 2014). Several phase I studies are ongoing to evaluate treatment with SBRT to various metastatic sites in patients with advanced solid tumors in conjunction with immune modulators (NCT02608385) (Bernstein et al. 2016).

8.2 Biological Prognostic and Predictive Tools

There have been recent advancements in the use of biologic markers to forecast disease behavior in oligometastatic patients. One such technology, microRNA classifiers, may help assess tumor biology and predict clinical outcomes. Significant differences in expression of microRNA200c occur between polymetastatic and oligometastatic phenotypes, with polymetastatic phenotypes expressing significantly higher levels of microRNA200c (Lussier et al. 2011). Using an oligometastatic-polymetastatic xenograft model, the group demonstrated oligometastatic cell lines could be induced to progress in a polymetastatic manner via the enhancement of microRNA200c. In the clinical setting, microRNA expression analysis in patients treated with pulmonary metastastectomy identified patterns that predicted higher rates of progression and lower rates of survival (Lussier et al. 2012). Wong et al. performed a microRNA expression analysis on 17 patients treated on their institutional protocol showing differential survival for patients exhibiting high and low classifier scores. Overexpression of a subset of microRNAs, miR-517a, miR-519c, and miR-521 directly correlated with poor long-term outcomes and increased cell proliferation. These data suggest certain tumors may exhibit an indolent nature, supporting Hellman and Weichselbaum's original hypothesis. A priori selection of patients with indolent tumors may justify local therapy to interrupt further metastatic potentiation. These developments emphasize the importance of prospectively collecting biological and clinical outcomes in the treatment of oligometastases on a randomized controlled clinical trial.

9 Ongoing Clinical Trials

Several ongoing studies are accruing patients to assess the use of SBRT for oligometastases (Reyes and Pienta 2015). SABR-COMET is an international randomized phase II trial enrolling patients with up to 5 metastases (NCT01446744). All patients will be treated with standard of care chemotherapy and randomized to SBRT directed to all known oligometastases or no SBRT with the primary endpoint designed to detect a difference in in overall survival (Palma et al. 2012). The UK and Australia are conducting CORE trial (conventional care or radioablation in the treatment of extracranial metastases) (Aitken et al. 2014). This is a phase II trial enrolling patients with three or less extracranial metastases with metastatic non-small cell lung cancer, breast cancer, or prostate cancer with a primary endpoint of progression free survival. Patients are randomized to either standard of care with systemic therapy or standard of care systemic therapy combined with SBRT.

Also in the UK, the Stereotactic Ablative Radiotherapy for Oligometastatic Non-small Cell Lung Cancer (SARON) trial is evaluating the use of systemic chemotherapy with or without radial RT to primary disease and up to 3 metastatic sites (NCT02417662). In prostate cancer, the Surveillance or metastasis-directed Therapy for OligoMetastatic Prostate cancer recurrence (STOMP) trial is currently ongoing. With a primary endpoint of androgen deprivation therapy free survival, the investigators are randomizing patients with metastatic disease to local therapy (surgery or radiation) or active clinical surveillance (NCT01558427). NRG Oncology has sponsored NRG-BR001 "A Phase 1 Study of Stereotactic Body Radiotherapy (SBRT) for the Treatment of Multiple Metastases" (NCT02206334). To parlay off the results of the phase I study, NRG-BR002 is a phase II/III trial comparing standard of care treatment to standard of care in addition to SBRT for women with 1–2 breast cancer metastases (NCT02364557). The trial is powered to address progression-free survival in the phase II study, and the study will automatically expand to a phase III design in the event a benefit in progression-free survival is observed in the phase II component.

10   A Cautionary Tale

With no randomized data to show the therapeutic benefit of SBRT for the treatment of extracranial oligometastases, the field may be in danger of putting the "cart before the horse." Despite the lack of high quality evidence, local treatment for oligometastases has become the de facto standard of care (Bartlett et al. 2015; Lewis et al. 2015). This sets the stage for a phenomenon known as a "medical reversal," when a widely adopted and accepted intervention is later found to have no clinically significant benefit (Prasad and Cifu 2013; Prasad et al. 2013). In oncology we are keenly aware of widespread implementation of an unproven therapy. Based on promising observational studies in the late 1980s and 1990s, it became commonplace to treat locally advanced and metastatic breast cancer with high dose chemotherapy followed by autologous hematopoietic stem-cell transplantation (Belanger et al. 1991). The proliferation of transplant clinics was sparked by a 1995 randomized study showing improvements in DFS and OS, which was later retracted (Bezwoda et al. 1995; Vickers and Christos 2000, 2001). Clinical trials published in the 2000s showed contrary findings, which prompted a steep decline in the use of transplant in breast cancer (Antman et al. 1997; Tallman et al. 2003; Berry et al. 2011). There has been an exponential rise in publications referencing oligometastases (Fig. 1) since the original publication by Hellman and Weichselbaum in 1995. To prevent another medical reversal, we encourage the prospective collection of data, preferably on a clinical trial. These data will allow us to conduct high quality analyses to answer clinical questions in order to best serve our patients now, and for years to come.

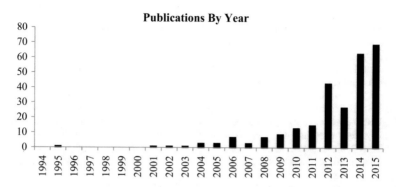

Fig. 1 Number of publications, by year, with "oligometastasis", "oligometases", or "oligometastatic" in title

References

Aitini E, Aleotti P (2006) Breaking bad news in oncology: like a walk in the twilight? Ann Oncol 17(3):359–360

Aitken K, Ahmed M, Hawkins M, Nutting C, Khoo V (2014) 214 A trial in design: CORE—conventional care or radioablation in the treatment of extracranial metastases. Lung Cancer 83 (Supplement 1):S79

Albain KS, Nag SM, Calderillo-Ruiz G, Jordaan JP, Llombart AC, Pluzanska A, Rolski J, Melemed AS, Reyes-Vidal JM, Sekhon JS, Simms L, O'Shaughnessy J (2008) Gemcitabine plus Paclitaxel versus Paclitaxel monotherapy in patients with metastatic breast cancer and prior anthracycline treatment. J Clin Oncol 26(24):3950–3957

Andrews DW, Scott CB, Sperduto PW, Flanders AE, Gaspar LE, Schell MC, Werner-Wasik M, Demas W, Ryu J, Bahary JP, Souhami L, Rotman M, Mehta MP, Curran WJ Jr (2004) Whole brain radiation therapy with or without stereotactic radiosurgery boost for patients with one to three brain metastases: phase III results of the RTOG 9508 randomised trial. Lancet 363 (9422):1665–1672

Antman KH, Rowlings PA, Vaughan WP, Pelz CJ, Fay JW, Fields KK, Freytes CO, Gale RP, Hillner BE, Holland HK, Kennedy MJ, Klein JP, Lazarus HM, McCarthy PL, Saez R, Spitzer G, Stadtmauer EA, Williams SF, Wolff S, Sobocinski KA, Armitage JO, Horowitz MM (1997) High-dose chemotherapy with autologous hematopoietic stem-cell support for breast cancer in North America. J Clin Oncol 15(5):1870–1879

Barney JJ (1945) A twelve-year cure following nephrectomy for adenocarcinoma and lobectomy for solitary metastasis. Trans Am Assoc Genitourin Surg 37:189–191

Bartlett EK, Simmons KD, Wachtel H, Roses RE, Fraker DL, Kelz RR, Karakousis GC (2015) The rise in metastasectomy across cancer types over the past decade. Cancer 121(5):747–757

Belanger D, Moore M, Tannock I (1991) How American oncologists treat breast cancer: an assessment of the influence of clinical trials. J Clin Oncol 9(1):7–16

Benedict SH, Yenice KM, Followill D, Galvin JM, Hinson W, Kavanagh B, Keall P, Lovelock M, Meeks S, Papiez L, Purdie T, Sadagopan R, Schell MC, Salter B, Schlesinger DJ, Shiu AS, Solberg T, Song DY, Stieber V, Timmerman R, Tomé Wa, Verellen D, Wang L, Yin F-F (2010) Stereotactic body radiation therapy: the report of AAPM Task Group 101. Med Phys 37:4078–4101

Berber B, Ibarra R, Snyder L, Yao M, Fabien J, Milano MT, Katz AW, Goodman K, Stephans K, El-Gazzaz G, Aucejo F, Miller C, Fung J, Lo S, Machtay M, Sanabria J (2013) Multicentre results of stereotactic body radiotherapy for secondary liver tumours. HPB (Oxford) 15 (11):851–857

Bernstein MB, Krishnan S, Hodge JW, Chang JY (2016) Immunotherapy and stereotactic ablative radiotherapy (ISABR): a curative approach? Nat Rev Clin Oncol

Berry DA, Ueno NT, Johnson MM, Lei X, Caputo J, Smith DA, Yancey LJ, Crump M, Stadtmauer EA, Biron P, Crown JP, Schmid P, Lotz JP, Rosti G, Bregni M, Demirer T (2011) High-dose chemotherapy with autologous hematopoietic stem-cell transplantation in metastatic breast cancer: overview of six randomized trials. J Clin Oncol 29(24):3224–3231

Bezwoda WR, Seymour L, Dansey RD (1995) High-dose chemotherapy with hematopoietic rescue as primary treatment for metastatic breast cancer: a randomized trial. J Clin Oncol 13 (10):2483–2489

Bezwoda et al. (2001) Retraction. J Clin Oncol 19(11):2973

Blomgren H, Lax I, Naslund I, Svanstrom R (1995) Stereotactic high dose fraction radiation therapy of extracranial tumors using an accelerator. Clinical experience of the first thirty-one patients. Acta Oncol 34(6):861–870

Carey Sampson M, Katz A, Constine LS (2006) Stereotactic body radiation therapy for extracranial oligometastases: does the sword have a double edge? Semin Radiat Oncol 16 (2):67–76

de Vin T, Engels B, Gevaert T, Storme G, De Ridder M (2014) Stereotactic radiotherapy for oligometastatic cancer: a prognostic model for survival. Ann Oncol 25(2):467–471

Deng L, Liang H, Burnette B, Beckett M, Darga T, Weichselbaum RR, Fu YX (2014) Irradiation and anti-PD-L1 treatment synergistically promote antitumor immunity in mice. J Clin Invest 124(2):687–695

Dorn PL, Meriwether A, LeMieux M, Weichselbaum RR, Chmura SJ, Hasan Y (2011) Patterns of distant failure and progression in breast cancer: implications for the treatment of oligometastatic disease. Int J Radiat Oncol Biol Phys 81(2, Supplement 1):S643

Drake CG (2012). Combination immunotherapy approaches. Ann Oncol 23(Suppl 8): viii41–46

Fidler IJ (2003) The pathogenesis of cancer metastasis: the 'seed and soil' hypothesis revisited. Nat Rev Cancer 3(6):453–458

Fisher B (1980) Laboratory and clinical research in breast cancer–a personal adventure: the David A. Karnofsky memorial lecture. Cancer Res 40(11):3863–3874

Fong Y, Cohen AM, Fortner JG, Enker WE, Turnbull AD, Coit DG, Marrero AM, Prasad M, Blumgart LH, Brennan MF (1997) Liver resection for colorectal metastases. J Clin Oncol 15 (3):938–946

Fong Y, Fortner J, Sun RL, Brennan MF, Blumgart LH (1999) Clinical score for predicting recurrence after hepatic resection for metastatic colorectal cancer: analysis of 1001 consecutive cases. Ann Surg 230(3):309–318; discussion 318–321

Gadd MA, Casper ES, Woodruff JM, McCormack PM, Brennan MF (1993) Development and treatment of pulmonary metastases in adult patients with extremity soft tissue sarcoma. Ann Surg 218(6):705–712

Gaipl US, Multhoff G, Scheithauer H, Lauber K, Hehlgans S, Frey B, Rodel F (2014) Kill and spread the word: stimulation of antitumor immune responses in the context of radiotherapy. Immunotherapy 6(5):597–610

Grills IS, Hope AJ, Guckenberger M, Kestin LL, Werner-Wasik M, Yan D, Sonke J-J, Bissonnette J-P, Wilbert J, Xiao Y, Belderbos J (2012) A collaborative analysis of stereotactic lung radiotherapy outcomes for early-stage non-small-cell lung cancer using daily online cone-beam computed tomography image-guided radiotherapy. J Thoracic Oncol 7:1382–1393

Halsted WS (1907) I. The results of radical operations for the cure of carcinoma of the breast. Ann Surg 46(1):1–19

Hanrahan EO, Broglio KR, Buzdar AU, Theriault RL, Valero V, Cristofanilli M, Yin G, Kau S-WC, Hortobagyi GN, Rivera E (2005) Combined-modality treatment for isolated recurrences of breast carcinoma: update on 30 years of experience at the University of Texas M.D. Anderson Cancer Center and assessment of prognostic factors. Cancer 104:1158–1171

Hellman S (1994) Karnofsky memorial lecture. Natural history of small breast cancers. J Clin Oncol 12(10):2229–2234

Hellman S, Weichselbaum RR (1995) Oligometastases. J Clin Oncol 13(1):8–10

Hodi FS, O'Day SJ, McDermott DF, Weber RW, Sosman JA, Haanen JB, Gonzalez R, Robert C, Schadendorf D, Hassel JC, Akerley W, van den Eertwegh AJ, Lutzky J, Lorigan P, Vaubel JM, Linette GP, Hogg D, Ottensmeier CH, Lebbe C, Peschel C, Quirt I, Clark JI, Wolchok JD, Weber JS, Tian J, Yellin MJ, Nichol GM, Hoos A, Urba WJ (2010) Improved survival with ipilimumab in patients with metastatic melanoma. N Engl J Med 363(8):711–723

Iyengar P, Kavanagh BD, Wardak Z, Smith I, Ahn C, Gerber DE, Dowell J, Hughes R, Abdulrahman R, Camidge DR, Gaspar LE, Doebele RC, Bunn PA, Choy H, Timmerman R (2014) Phase II trial of stereotactic body radiation therapy combined with erlotinib for patients with limited but progressive metastatic non-small-cell lung cancer. J Clin Oncol 32(34):3824–3830

Jawad MS, Fahim DK, Gerszten PC, Flickinger JC, Sahgal A, Grills IS, Sheehan J, Kersh R, Shin J, Oh K, Mantel F, Guckenberger M (2016) Vertebral compression fractures after stereotactic body radiation therapy: a large, multi-institutional, multinational evaluation. J Neurosurg Spine 24(6):928–936

Joseph RW, Elassaiss-Schaap J, Wolchok JD, Joshua AM, Ribas A, Hodi FS, Hamid O, Robert C, Daud A, Hwu W-J, Kefford R, Hersey P, Weber JS, Patnaik A, Alwis DPD, Perrone AM, Kang SP, Ebbinghaus S, Anderson KM, Gangadhar TC (2014) Baseline tumor size as an independent prognostic factor for overall survival in patients with metastatic melanoma treated with the anti-PD-1 monoclonal antibody MK-3475. J Clin Oncol 32(5s):abstr 3015

Kendal WS (2014) Oligometastasis as a predictor for occult disease. Math Biosci 251:1–10

Kestin L, Grills I, Guckenberger M, Belderbos J, Hope AJ, Werner-Wasik M, Sonke JJ, Bissonnette JP, Xiao Y, Yan D (2014) Dose-response relationship with clinical outcome for lung stereotactic body radiotherapy (SBRT) delivered via online image guidance. Radiother Oncol 110:499–504

Keynes G (1954) Carcinoma of the breast, the unorthodox view. Proc Cardiff M So. 40

Krebs MG, Sloane R, Priest L, Lancashire L, Hou JM, Greystoke A, Ward TH, Ferraldeschi R, Hughes A, Clack G, Ranson M, Dive C, Blackhall FH (2011) Evaluation and prognostic significance of circulating tumor cells in patients with non-small-cell lung cancer. J Clin Oncol 29(12):1556–1563

Lewis SL, Porceddu S, Nakamura N, Palma DA, Lo SS, Hoskin P, Moghanaki D, Chmura SJ, Salama JK (2015) Definitive stereotactic body radiotherapy (SBRT) for extracranial oligometastases: an International Survey of >1000 radiation oncologists. Am J Clin Oncol

Liang H, Deng L, Chmura S, Burnette B, Liadis N, Darga T, Beckett MA, Lingen MW, Witt M, Weichselbaum RR, Fu YX (2013) Radiation-induced equilibrium is a balance between tumor cell proliferation and T cell-mediated killing. J Immunol 190(11):5874–5881

Lussier YA, Khodarev NN, Regan K, Corbin K, Li H, Ganai S, Khan SA, Gnerlich JL, Gnerlich J, Darga TE, Fan H, Karpenko O, Paty PB, Posner MC, Chmura SJ, Hellman S, Ferguson MK, Weichselbaum RR (2012) Oligo- and polymetastatic progression in lung metastasis(es) patients is associated with specific microRNAs. PLoS ONE 7(12):e50141

Lussier YA, Xing HR, Salama JK, Khodarev NN, Huang Y, Zhang Q, Khan SA, Yang X, Hasselle MD, Darga TE, Malik R, Fan H, Perakis S, Filippo M, Corbin K, Lee Y, Posner MC, Chmura SJ, Hellman S, Weichselbaum RR (2011) MicroRNA expression characterizes oligometastasis(es). PLoS ONE 6(12):e28650

Lynch TJ, Bondarenko I, Luft A, Serwatowski P, Barlesi F, Chacko R, Sebastian M, Neal J, Lu H, Cuillerot JM, Reck M (2012) Ipilimumab in combination with paclitaxel and carboplatin as first-line treatment in stage IIIB/IV non-small-cell lung cancer: results from a randomized, double-blind, multicenter phase II study. J Clin Oncol 30(17):2046–2054

MacManus MP, Hicks RJ, Matthews JP, Hogg A, McKenzie AF, Wirth A, Ware RE, Ball DL (2001) High rate of detection of unsuspected distant metastases by pet in apparent stage III non-small-cell lung cancer: implications for radical radiation therapy. Int J Radiat Oncol Biol Phys 50(2):287–293

Milano MT, Katz AW, Zhang H, Okunieff P (2012) Oligometastases treated with stereotactic body radiotherapy: long-term follow-up of prospective study. Int J Radiat Oncol Biol Phys 83 (3):878–886

Niibe Y, Hayakawa K (2010) Oligometastases and oligo-recurrence: the new era of cancer therapy. Jpn J Clin Oncol 40(2):107–111

Paget S (1889) The distribution of secondary growths in cancer of the breast. 1889. Cancer Metastasis Rev 8(2):98–101

Palma DA, Haasbeek CJ, Rodrigues GB, Dahele M, Lock M, Yaremko B, Olson R, Liu M, Panarotto J, Griffioen GH, Gaede S, Slotman B, Senan S (2012) Stereotactic ablative radiotherapy for comprehensive treatment of oligometastatic tumors (SABR-COMET): study protocol for a randomized phase II trial. BMC Cancer 12:305

Pardoll DM (2012) The blockade of immune checkpoints in cancer immunotherapy. Nat Rev Cancer 12(4):252–264

Pastorino U, Buyse M, Friedel G, Ginsberg RJ, Girard P, Goldstraw P, Johnston M, McCormack P, Pass H, Putnam JB Jr, International Registry of Lung M (1997) Long-term results of lung metastasectomy: prognostic analyses based on 5206 cases. J Thorac Cardiovasc Surg 113 (1):37–49

Patchell RA, Tibbs PA, Regine WF, Payne R, Saris S, Kryscio RJ, Mohiuddin M, Young B (2005) Direct decompressive surgical resection in the treatment of spinal cord compression caused by metastatic cancer: a randomised trial. Lancet 366(9486):643–648

Patchell RA, Tibbs PA, Walsh JW, Dempsey RJ, Maruyama Y, Kryscio RJ, Markesbery WR, Macdonald JS, Young B (1990) A randomized trial of surgery in the treatment of single metastases to the brain. N Engl J Med 322(8):494–500

Pentheroudakis G, Fountzilas G, Bafaloukos D, Koutsoukou V, Pectasides D, Skarlos D, Samantas E, Kalofonos HP, Gogas H, Pavlidis N (2006) Metastatic breast cancer with liver metastases: a registry analysis of clinicopathologic, management and outcome characteristics of 500 women. Breast Cancer Res Treat 97(3):237–244

Pienta KJ, Robertson BA, Coffey DS, Taichman RS (2013) The cancer diaspora: metastasis beyond the seed and soil hypothesis. Clin Cancer Res 19(21):5849–5855

Postow MA, Callahan MK, Barker CA, Yamada Y, Yuan J, Kitano S, Mu Z, Rasalan T, Adamow M, Ritter E, Sedrak C, Jungbluth AA, Chua R, Yang AS, Roman RA, Rosner S, Benson B, Allison JP, Lesokhin AM, Gnjatic S, Wolchok JD (2012) Immunologic correlates of the abscopal effect in a patient with melanoma. N Engl J Med 366(10):925–931

Prasad V, Cifu A (2013) In reply I-reversal of medical practices. Mayo Clin Proc 88(10):1183–1184

Prasad V, Vandross A, Toomey C, Cheung M, Rho J, Quinn S, Chacko SJ, Borkar D, Gall V, Selvaraj S, Ho N, Cifu A (2013) A decade of reversal: an analysis of 146 contradicted medical practices. Mayo Clin Proc 88(8):790–798

Reyes DK, Pienta KJ (2015) The biology and treatment of oligometastatic cancer. Oncotarget 6 (11):8491–8524

Rusthoven KE, Kavanagh BD, Burri SH, Chen C, Cardenes H, Chidel MA, Pugh TJ, Kane M, Gaspar LE, Schefter TE (2009) Multi-institutional phase I/II trial of stereotactic body radiation therapy for lung metastases. J Clin Oncol 27(10):1579–1584

Ryu S, Pugh SL, Gerszten PC, Yin FF, Timmerman RD, Hitchcock YJ, Movsas B, Kanner AA, Berk LB, Followill DS, Kachnic LA (2014) RTOG 0631 phase 2/3 study of image guided stereotactic radiosurgery for localized (1–3) spine metastases: phase 2 results. Pract Radiat Oncol 4(2):76–81

Salama JK, Hasselle MD, Chmura SJ, Malik R, Mehta N, Yenice KM, Villaflor VM, Stadler WM, Hoffman PC, Cohen EEW, Connell PP, Haraf DJ, Vokes EE, Hellman S, Weichselbaum RR (2012) Stereotactic body radiotherapy for multisite extracranial oligometastases: final report of a dose escalation trial in patients with 1 to 5 sites of metastatic disease. Cancer 118:2962–2970

Simmonds PC, Primrose JN, Colquitt JL, Garden OJ, Poston GJ, Rees M (2006) Surgical resection of hepatic metastases from colorectal cancer: a systematic review of published studies. Br J Cancer 94(7):982–999

Singh D, Yi WS, Brasacchio RA, Muhs AG, Smudzin T, Williams JP, Messing E, Okunieff P (2004) Is there a favorable subset of patients with prostate cancer who develop oligometastases? Int J Radiat Oncol Biol Phys 58(1):3–10

Tallman MS, Gray R, Robert NJ, LeMaistre CF, Osborne CK, Vaughan WP, Gradishar WJ, Pisansky TM, Fetting J, Paietta E, Lazarus HM (2003) Conventional adjuvant chemotherapy with or without high-dose chemotherapy and autologous stem-cell transplantation in high-risk breast cancer. N Engl J Med 349(1):17–26

Treasure T (2012) Oligometastatic cancer: an entity, a useful concept, or a therapeutic opportunity? J R Soc Med 105(6):242–246

van Geel AN, Pastorino U, Jauch KW, Judson IR, van Coevorden F, Buesa JM, Nielsen OS, Boudinet A, Tursz T, Schmitz PI (1996) Surgical treatment of lung metastases: The European Organization for Research and Treatment of Cancer-Soft Tissue and Bone Sarcoma Group study of 255 patients. Cancer 77:675–682

Vickers A, Christos P (2000) Bezwoda: evidence of fabrication in original article. J Clin Oncol 18 (15):2933

Vinay DS, Ryan EP, Pawelec G, Talib WH, Stagg J, Elkord E, Lichtor T, Decker WK, Whelan RL, Kumara HM, Signori E, Honoki K, Georgakilas AG, Amin A, Helferich WG, Boosani CS, Guha G, Ciriolo MR, Chen S, Mohammed SI, Azmi AS, Keith WN, Bilsland A, Bhakta D, Halicka D, Fujii H, Aquilano K, Ashraf SS, Nowsheen S, Yang X, Choi BK, Kwon BS (2015) Immune evasion in cancer: mechanistic basis and therapeutic strategies. Semin Cancer Biol 35(Suppl):S185–198

Wong AC, Watson SP, Pitroda SP, Son CH, Das LC, Stack ME, Uppal A, Oshima G, Khodarev NN, Salama JK, Weichselbaum RR, Chmura SJ (2016) Clinical and molecular markers of long-term survival after oligometastasis-directed stereotactic body radiotherapy (SBRT). Cancer

MRI Guided Radiotherapy

Daniel A. Low

Abstract

Magnetic Resonance Imaging (MRI) has been a part of radiation therapy for many years, but its role is expanding. MR provides soft tissue contrast that is superior to what can be obtained with computed tomography (CT), the modality used most often to support radiation therapy treatment simulation. There are a number of critical challenges to employing MR for simulation imaging, namely the reduced spatial fidelity, and the lack of a direct relationship between MR image values and electron density, a quantity needed for dose calculations, as well as a difference between MR image values and the attenuation of kV X-rays, used to aid in patient positioning. These challenges are being met by clinics and companies, to the extent that the exclusive use of MR for simulation is now possible in a number of treatment sites. While MR has been used for simulation, it has only recently been introduced into the treatment room. Integrating MR with patient positioning and monitoring before and during treatment, respectively, would potentially improve radiation therapy treatment accuracy, enabling tighter uncertainty margins and ultimately improving outcomes. The challenges of integrating a MRI system with radiation treatment delivery have been recently met by radiation therapy equipment manufacturers, providing the radiation oncology community with an opportunity to deliver radiation doses with unparalleled accuracy.

Keywords

Magnetic Resonance Imaging · Radiation Therapy · Magnetic Resonance Image-Guided Radiation Therapy

D.A. Low (✉)
200 Medical Plaza Way, Suite B265, Los Angeles, CA 90095, USA
e-mail: Dlow@mednet.ucla.edu

1 Radiation Therapy Workflow and Where MR Can and Does Help

At its most basic, radiation therapy workflows include simulation, treatment planning, and treatment. Simulation is mainly conducted using computed tomography (CT) imaging. CT imaging provides distinct advantages that make it most suitable for radiation therapy workflows. CT has outstanding spatial integrity. Modern CT scanners are fast and provide nearly artifact-free images. The CT values themselves, termed Hounsfield Units, are rescaled linear attenuation coefficients of the X-ray energies employed during the CT scans, typically 120 or 140 kV. Radiation therapy employs megavoltage X-rays for imaging, which interact primarily via the Compton effect. The Compton effect is sensitive to a material's electron density, and it is fortuitous that for human tissues, the relationship between HU and relative electron density is nearly monotonic. Therefore, the CT image can be directly used to estimate human tissue electron densities for purposes of dose distribution calculations.

The treatment itself often involves the use of X-rays for imaging tissue positions and comparing against the intended positions. Because the X-ray images are acquired with similar X-ray energies as the CT simulation scan, they can be directly compared to digitally reconstructed radiographic images. Similarly, on-board cone-beam CT images provide similar, although not exactly the same, image features as the CT simulations, the differences being mainly due to the impact of scattered radiation on the cone-beam CT images. The only image-based process that does not utilize the similarity between the images acquired at simulation and at the machine are those using fiducial markers. When fiducial markers are used, the only requirements are spatial integrity and marker conspicuity.

Given that CT simulators are relatively inexpensive and provide such valuable information for radiation therapy treatment planning, the question arises, what is missing that could be provided by other imaging technology? We need only to look at stereotactic treatments of the brain to find the main limitation of CT simulation. Treatment planning of the brain requires that the brain tumor boundaries be visible on the images to allow for segmentation (contouring) and subsequent dose planning. Because CT is sensitive only to the linear attenuation coefficient, soft tumors that exist within soft tissues typically have poor conspicuity. This is true for cancers in the brain. Figure 1 shows a CT simulation and two MR images of a patient with metastatic cancer in the brain. The tumors are not visible in the CT and are quite clear in the MRI.

When MRI was first developed, it was clear that it could be employed for radiation therapy treatment planning of the brain. Treatments were universally conducted employing invasive immobilization, where a metal ring was attached to the patient skull using pins (Fig. 2a). The tumor localization was conducted by attaching a fiducial frame to the ring. The frame (Fig. 2b) typically had rods that were visible on MR and CT. The rod geometry was known to the treatment planning system and the rod images were localized in the CT and MRI scans.

(a)   (b)

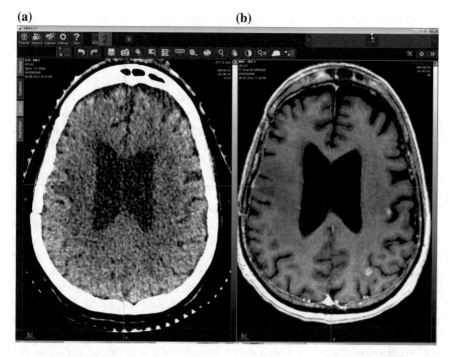

Fig. 1 **a** CT scan of the brain. **b** MR scan of the brain. There are two small metastatic lesions clearly visible in the MR scan that are invisible in the CT scan

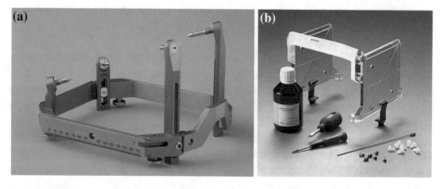

Fig. 2 **a** Invasive immobilization system frame (Leksell). **b** Jig used for MR alignment of immobilization frame coordinate system. Location of tubes, filled with contrast agent, are known to the treatment planning system. Contrast agent is localized in the images to align them to the frame coordinate system. This is used to accurately target the tumor at the radiation producing machine (GammaKnife). Images from the Elekta Leksell sales website

The treatment planning software used the imaged rod positions to determine the stereotactic coordinate system with in the patient's skull. In the early MRI days, the spatial fidelity of the imagers was relatively poor, so the digitized frame positions also served as quality assurance that the MRI image spatial fidelity was adequate for treatment planning.

As 3D conformal therapy was developed in the 1990s, use of MRI to segment tumors became more practical. Tools such as fusion were developed to overlay the CT and MRI images to enable the use of CT for electron density and DRR generation while taking advantage of MRI's soft tissue contrast. If invasive immobilization was not employed, a rigid coordinate system could not be straightforwardly generated. The fusion process in the brain typically aligned the bony anatomy, visible as high HU values and low image values (due to the very rapid T1 times in the bone) in the CT and MR images, respectively. Often, structures other than the bones, such as the ventricles, were used to align, guide, or verify registration. The potential for image distortion in the MR images was managed by comparing the locations of structures visible in both image datasets.

Fusion in other parts of the body was more challenging. The MR and CT images were taken at different sessions, and often with different patient setups. Often, the MR image was a diagnostic image that was acquired for diagnostic purposes, so the patient position differed from that used for treatment. In these cases, fusion was made more difficult by the internal tissue distortions caused by patient posture differences. These differences were exacerbated because diagnostic MR couches tended to be more rounded than therapy couches, which were and are flat. Many clinics elected to develop their own flat couch inserts, and vendors began to provide professionally produced flat couch inserts for their MR scanners, to make the MR patient positioning more consistent with the CT simulation positioning.

2 MR Simulation

More recently, the concept of MR simulation has been developed. MR simulation, as defined here, is the use of MR images as the primary image dataset for treatment planning. This does not preclude other images, such as PET, but it would exclude processes that also acquire CT simulation images, processes that can be more accurately described as MR + CT simulation.

Why would one employ MR simulation (also called MR-only simulation)? The benefits include the improved soft tissue contrast and the ability to acquire multiple image datasets that highlight the tissue boundaries, and differentiate different tissue types, even within a specific tumor (Fig. 3). The benefit of MR simulation is that only one simulation process is needed. In the MR + CT simulation workflow, two simulations are scheduled and conducted, requiring that the patient appear for two sessions. The images themselves must be fused, involving further clinical effort and providing additional opportunities for error.

Because of these potential benefits, a number of clinics are expanding their use of MR simulation. Figures 4 and 5 show examples of different sites employing MR simulation from Devic (2012).

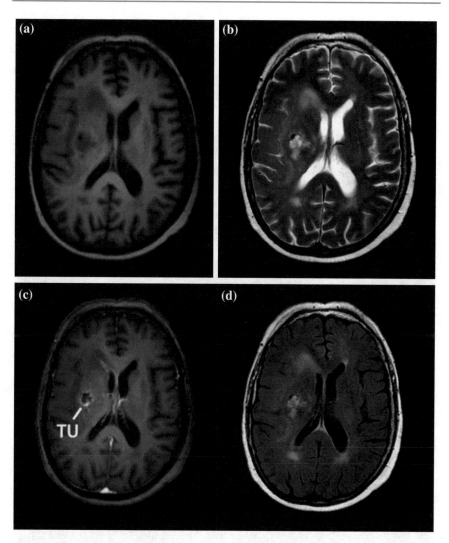

Fig. 3 Patient with Glioblastoma scanned using 4 different MR protocols. **a** T1 weighted. **b** T2 weighted. This shows fluids as very bright. The tumor is readily visualized in this image. **c** Contrast-enhanced T1. The tumor contrast has improved. **d** T2 weighted with fluid-attenuated inversion recovery (FLAIR). Images are from Schmidt and Payne (2015)

There are a number of challenges inherent in employing MR simulation. The MRI scanner bore is generally smaller than a CT simulator. CT simulators started out as slightly modified diagnostic CT scanners, but the CT manufacturers realized early that increasing the bore size was critical for radiation oncology. Unlike most diagnostic CT applications, the patient position was specified by the ideal position during treatment, which often employed extended arm postures. The first wide bore CT scanner had an 85 cm diameter bore and some current units have

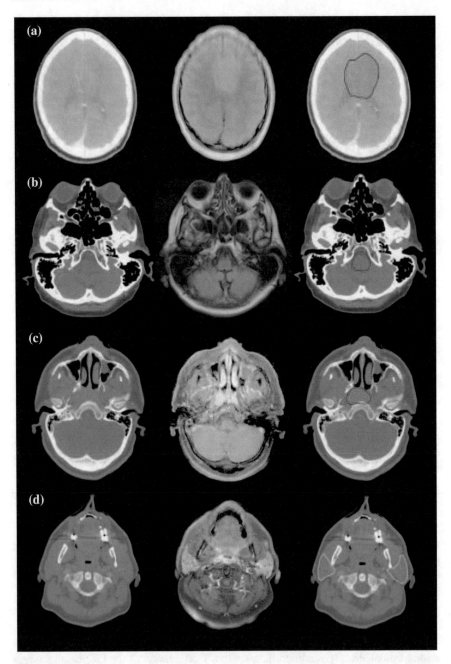

Fig. 4 Examples of the use of MR images for supplementing CT simulation images for radiation therapy treatment planning. **a** Glioblastoma. **b** Brainstem. **c** Nasopharynx. **d** Parotid glands. The first column is the CT simulation, the second the MR scan, and the third shows the superposition of the segmented structure on the CT simulation. Images from Devic (2012)

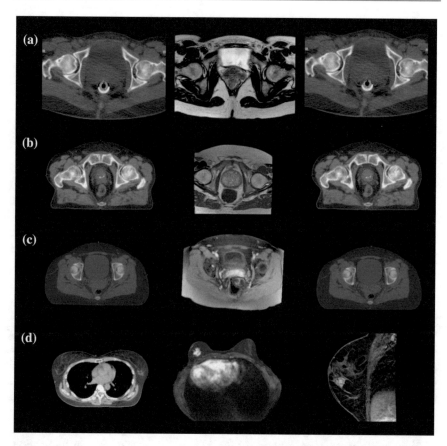

Fig. 5 Examples of the use of MR images for supplementing CT simulation images for radiation therapy treatment planning. **a** Rectal. **b** Prostate. **c** GYN. **d** Breast. The first column is the CT simulation, the second the MR scan, and the third shows the superposition of the segmented structure on the CT simulation. Images from Devic (2012)

90 cm diameter bores. This contrasts with MRI scanners, which have bores only as large as 75 cm diameter. This constrains somewhat either the treatment position or the correspondence between the treatment and scanned positions.

MR scanners employ RF sensing coils. The signal intensity falls off rapidly with increasing distance between the RF sensing coils and the imaged tumor or organ. Therefore, most RF coils are in direct or immediate contact with the patient. Rigid coil systems such as head coils interfere with head immobilization systems, while flexible coils placed on the skin can distort the skin and deform the tumor and normal organ geometry. Figure 6 shows an example of an MR simulator patient with the necessary immobilization hardware and imaging coils.

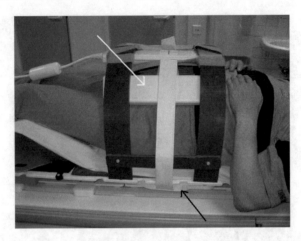

Fig. 6 Photograph of MR simulation patient showing immobilization system and suspended radiofrequency coils. Image from Kapanen et al. (2013)

The spatial integrity of CT is outstanding. The images are reconstructed from transmitted radiation beamlets whose geometry is defined by the relative positions of the X-ray source and the detector. With MR imaging, on the other hand, the tissue locations are determined by the acquisition sequence. Positions may be determined by the relationship between a magnetic field gradient and applied RF frequency, or from a relationship between received RF frequency or phase and magnetic field gradient. In general, it is the absolute magnetic field that determines localization, and main magnetic field homogeneity and gradient field accuracy determine spatial accuracy. Main magnetic field homogeneity is typically specified within a spherical volume centered at the MR system center. Within this region, spatial accuracy will have a tighter specification than beyond the region. CT, on the other hand, is accurate within a cylindrical volume that encompasses the projected X-rays. This difference in accuracy specification, as well as the loss of the direct geometric relationship between the equipment hardware and the image voxel positions means that MR image quality assurance needs to include spatial accuracy evaluation.

Various methods for conducting quality assurance on MR simulators have been proposed. Kapanean et al. (2013) described the process of commissioning an MR-only simulation and treatment planning for prostate cancer. They employed a 70 cm diameter GE 1.5T MR scanner that had an indexed flat couch top and positioning lasers. Paulson et al. (2015) described the quality assurance procedures required for MR simulation. They employed a 3.0T Siemens MR Scanner with a 70 cm diameter bore. They described the patient-specific quality assurance techniques to assure fidelity and utility of the MR images (Table 1) as well as routine quality assurance procedures (Table 2). There have not yet been widely accepted protocols for patient-specific or routine quality assurance, but the American Association of Physicists in Medicine has a task group entitled "Use of MRI Data in

Table 1 Patient-specific quality assurance processes recommended by Paulson et al. (2015)

Sim setup	Sim exam	Dosimetry
• Target volumes centered within bore (to extent possible) during CT sim • Headphones molded into alpha cradles/vac-locs for abdomen MRI simulation exams • Immobilization devices fit within MRI bore template	• Coverage sufficient (10 cm past markers for sarcoma) • Images screened for artifacts • 3D distortion correction applied to all images • Off-resonance correction applied (if necessary) • Subtractions performed • Reformats of coronal and sagittal slices to axial slices performed • Functional/physiological data integrity verified • Functional/physiological parameter maps generated	• Distortion-corrected MR images loaded and labeled according to MR Sim Reference Guide (Table II) • CT-MR image registration accuracy verified

Table 2 Routine quality assurance processes recommended by Paulson et al. (2015)

Weekly QA (MRI technologists)	Monthly QA (therapy physicists)	Annual QA (MRI physicists)
• Transmitter gain constancy • Center frequency constancy • Signal-to-noise ratio constancy • Slice thickness accuracy • Slice position accuracy	• Patient safety (monitors, intercom, panic ball, emergency offs, and signage) • Patient comfort (bore lights, and bore fan) • Percent signal ghosting • Percent image uniformity • High/low contrast constancy • Laser alignment • Couch position accuracy • Image artifacts	• RF coil integrity check • B0 constancy • B1 + constancy • Gradient linearity constancy

Treatment Planning and Stereotactic Procedures—Spatial Accuracy and Quality Control Procedures" that is developing quality assurance recommendations.

MRI voxel intensities are related to the RF signal strength acquired during the imaging sequence. Therefore, the voxel values for a specific piece of tissue will depend strongly on the sequence, coil design and coil position. Image guided radiation therapy couples the images used for treatment planning with those acquired during setup. Universally, setup images of internal tissues are acquired using kilovoltage X-rays. Transmission X-ray images such as radiographs display the integral attenuation coefficients of the tissues and hardware lying between the source and detector. Cone-beam CT is employed to acquire 3D images, and each voxel represents the linear attenuation coefficient of the tissue, albeit with decreased quantitative accuracy relative to diagnostic CT scans. When radiographic images are acquired to position the patient, they are compared against images created by projecting rays through the CT simulation scan and predicting the radiographs.

These are termed digitally reconstructed radiographs. When radiographs are used for positioning, comparing the radiographs to digitally reconstructed radiographs is straightforward. The tissues that provide image contrast are bone, soft tissues, lungs, and air cavities, by virtue of their differing physical density and atomic number. With MR simulation, projection through the MR image will not provide a useful DRR. The proposed method for dealing with this is to use MR images to create a synthetic CT.

The principle challenge of using MR images to create kV X-ray DRRs is the lack of a functional relationship between the linear attenuation coefficient and MR image intensity. This is due mostly to the fact that air and bone both provide low MR signals for most sequences, air due to the lack of protons, and bone due to the rapid loss of magnetization of protons in solid materials.

The use of CT scans for both dose calculation and for the generation of patient positioning reference images is fortuitous and discussions about the generation of synthetic CT scans almost always convolves the two applications of CT. There is no reason why this needs to be so for MR simulation, an electron density map could be generated separately from an image used to generate reference setup images. This is true because the requirements for generating the two image datasets vary greatly and creating a single dataset that would fulfill both requirements adds unnecessary challenges to the MR simulation workflow. The electron density map used for treatment planning does not need voxel-by voxel spatial integrity. Rather, it needs to be accurate on average so that the photon attenuation and scatter properties are accurately computed. Megavoltage X-rays are relatively insensitive to electron density calculation errors, especially on the voxel level. The reference setup image dataset, on the other hand has to embody the spatial contrast behavior present in a CT scan. For example, the position of a bony edge needs to be correctly positioned (and distinguished from the edge of an air cavity). However, the voxel values themselves do not need to strictly speaking be accurate. When the image dataset is compared against a cone-beam CT or projections are used to create DRRs that are compared against radiographs, it is the bony (and less so air cavity) localization that needs to be accurate for the human or computerized registration to identify the patient's position. Unfortunately, most publications have not made this distinction, so separating published approaches to separately overcoming these challenges is difficult.

There are two proposed methods for creating synthetic CT scans from MR images, including segmenting images and assigning CT numbers, and acquiring a series of MR images and computing the CT numbers.

Segmenting Approaches

Much of the early MR simulation work concerned the generation of electron density maps and the subsequent dose calculation accuracy. Prabhakar et al. (2007) evaluated the use of MR alone for 3D treatment planning in brain tumors. They evaluated treatment plans from 25 brain tumor patients scanned with a CT and 1.5T MRI scanner. The treatment plans comparing the use of CT with and without heterogeneity correction and the MR with a bulk density assignment showed no statistically significant difference in coverage. Ramsey and Oliver (1998) as early as 1998 developed a method for calculating dose distributions and generating DRRs using only one T1 MRI image dataset. They assumed a linear relationship between the MR voxel value and physical density to generate the synthetic CT. This provided the ability to differentiate between the skull and the brain, but not air cavities. They evaluated their technique using archived MR patient images and a RANDO phantom, generating DRRs and irradiating TLD chips in the phantom (comparing to homogeneous dose calculations) to evaluate dosimetric accuracy of their method. The MR plan underestimated dose by less than 2% of a CT-based plan for a single photon beam passing through the cranium. When the dose passed through air cavities, the dose discrepancy increased to 2–4%.

Like the head, the pelvis contains relatively homogeneous density tissues, exclusive of the pelvis and femurs. Evaluations of prostate treatment plans with a single water-equivalent density have shown differences as small as 1% (Petersch et al. 2004) and greater than 2% (Chen et al. 2004a, b; Lee et al. 2003). Assigning separate densities to bone and soft tissue have provided doses within 2% of the dose calculated using CT (Lee et al. 2003; Karlsson et al. 2009). Lambert et al. (2011) evaluated the dose distribution accuracy of prostate treatment plans, comparing bulk density assignment (soft tissue and bones separately assigned) with full heterogeneity assignments for 39 patients that had both CT and MRI images. They created three treatment plans using the CT simulation, one with the full heterogeneity, one with densities assigned to bone and water to other tissues, and one with just water density, and two plans based on MR images with the same bulk density assignments as the CT scans. They found that the tumor doses were equivalent between the MR and CT bulk density plans, with minor variations assumed to come from differences in external patient contours. Point doses differed by $-1.4 \pm 1.7\%$ and $-2.6 \pm 1.7\%$ for the CT and MR uniform density plans compared against the CT simulation based plans, respectively, and $0.1 \pm 1.2\%$ and $-1.3 \pm 1.6\%$ for the CT and MR bone/soft tissue bulk density assigned plans compared against the CT simulation based plans, respectively.

Given that there are more than two tissue classes in the brain and pelvis, investigators have shown that contouring more classes of tissues improves the dosimetric accuracy to within 1% for intracranial targets (Jonsson et al. 2010; Kristensen et al. 2008) and between 1 and 2% for prostate (Chen et al. 2004a, b; Lee et al. 2003; Jonsson et al. 2010; Eilertsen et al. 2008). While the accuracy of bulk density assignments have been established, they have not become a popular treatment planning approach because of the effort required and the limited benefit of not acquiring a CT simulation in addition to the MR simulation.

Semi-automated and Automated Approaches

A relatively manual approach was proposed by Kim et al. (2015) to generate simulated CT scans. They used three typical MR sequences: a 3D T1 weighted fast field echo sequence, a 3D T2-weighted turbo spin echo sequence, and a 3D balanced turbo field echo sequence. To provide high-intensity values in bone, an inverse intensity volumetric image was derived by subtracting weighted intensity values from the 95th percentile intensity value. Bony anatomy was contoured using the T2-weighted images. Air was assigned a single density value, but other tissues were assigned an intensity based on a weighted sum of the acquired and derived MR image voxel values. The registered CT scans were used to train the weights. The technique produced synthetic CT scans that had HU errors of only 2.0 ± 8.0 HU and 11.9 ± 46.7 HU for soft tissue and femoral bones, respectively. The impact on treatment plans of using the synthetic CT were negligible except for differences associated with variations in organ positions between the MR and CT simulation sessions. Kim et al. conducted a qualitative assessment of synthetic DRRs and found them to be similar to the CT-sim generated DRRs.

Huan et al. (2014) evaluated a method for creating DRRs by segmenting airways from MR simulation images. They concentrated on the skull to create both simulated CT scans and simulated DRRs. They judged that inaccuracies in airway segmentation would impact DRR generation accuracy less than inaccuracies in bone segmentation. Airways were manually contoured on transverse scans at 6 anatomic levels to create an air mask. Compact bone, spongy bone, and soft tissue masks were then automatically generated using the MR voxel values and the air mask. The MR intensities within the masks were used to create the simulated CT scans and corresponding DRRs. They evaluated this process for 20 stereotactic radiosurgery patients. They evaluated their process for 20 patients undergoing stereotactic radiosurgery in the brain. The maximum geometric difference between MR-based and CT-based DRRS of the skull was less than 2 mm.

The biggest challenge for automating synthetic CT generation is the fact that for most MR sequences, neither high density bony tissues nor low density tissues emit RF signals, so both of these tissue types show up as black in MR images. The reason that MR images have poor signal in bone is that the coupling between protons and the rest of bony anatomy leads to very rapid realignment of the proton magnetic moments after excitation. Ultrashort echo time (UTE) imaging is one method to acquire signal from solid tissues (Robson et al. 2003).

Yang et al. (2016) employed UTE sequences, employing nonselective radiofrequency excitation pulses and asymmetrical readouts to sample the k-space using a 3D radial trajectory. Two echoes were employed, one at TE = 0.07 ms and one at TE = 4.28 ms from each excitation with a readout bandwidth of 511 Hz pixel^{-1}. Figure 7 shows an example from that work. Yang et al. also determined the accuracy of using the synthetic DRR versus the clinical DRR for patient setup and showed that the correspondence was within 1 mm. Their goal was to produce DRRs for positioning, not synthetic CT scans for treatment planning, so they did not evaluate the accuracy of the HU values.

Zheng et al. (2015) had a similar effort to generate synthetic CT scans from MR images. They evaluated 10 patients scanned used a 1.0T open magnet system, employing Dixon and inverted UTE images. Air was automatically segmented using unwrapped UTE phase maps rather than the intensity maps of previous investigators. The synthetic CT scans were computed using weighted sums of the T2, FLAIR,

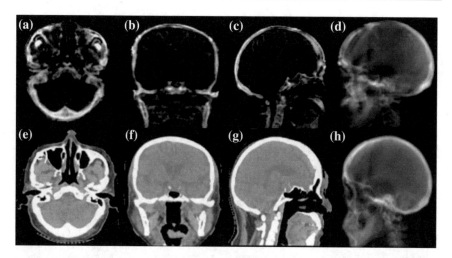

Fig. 7 **a–c** UTE-MRI-based bone images. **d** UTE-MRI DRR generated from a left lateral beam. **e–g** Corresponding CT images. **h** Corresponding DRR. Image from Yang et al. (2016)

UTE1, and bone-enhanced images. The bone-enhanced images were generated by inverting the UTE magnitude image from the first echo by subtracting the magnitude image from its maximum intensity value. Water/fat maps were generated from the 2-point Dixon method with unrestricted choice of echo times. They validated the segmentation by calculating segmentation errors and Dice similarity indices against the CT simulation. They evaluated the quality of the synthetic HU values by comparing against the CT simulation. The Dice similarity indices were 0.87 ± 0.04. The mean absolute errors of the HU values were 147.5 ± 8.3 HU with the largest errors occurring at bone-air interfaces. Treatment plans showed excellent agreement between the synthetic CT and CT simulation, with 99.4% passing with gamma criteria of 2% and 2 mm. Figure 8 shows examples of the intermediate images as well as the resulting segmentation image from their example.

At a recent conference entitled "4th MR in RT Symposium", held on June 18–19, 2016 at the University of Michigan, there were a number of presentations on the state of the art in MR imaging techniques to replace CT's role in generating electron density maps and in generating DRRs. Liu et al. (2016) used a single MR scan to provide tissue classification for the female pelvis and classify tissues for electron density measurements without an atlas or ultra-short TE imaging. They employed a T1_VIBE_Dixon sequence which yielded 3 images of differing contrast, so called in-phase T1-weighted, fat, and water weighted. In the pelvis, the main challenge was distinguishing between bone and air. A bone shape model was used to generate a crude bone mask. Air voxels outside the mask were identified as air, then a 5-class fuzzy c-means classification (bone, muscle, fat, marrow, and intra-pelvic soft tissue) was performed on the MR data with a regularization term that assigned voxels outside the bone mask to have zero membership in the bone class. Nominal attenuations were employed along with the classification probabilities to generate

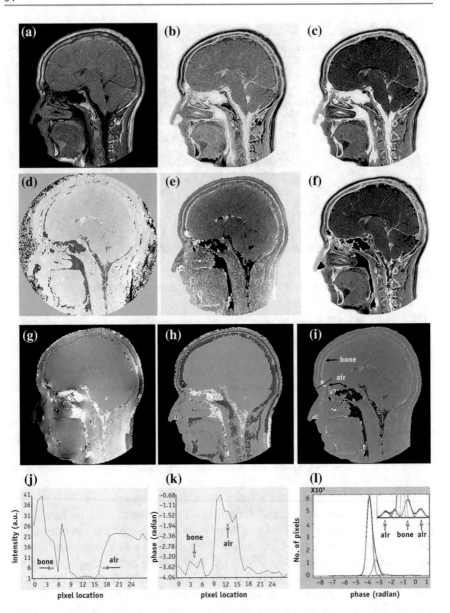

Fig. 8 From Zheng et al. (2015). Images showing process of generating pseudo CT from MR images. **a** UTE image at echo time TE = 0.144 ms. **b** Inverted UTE magnitude image. **c** Bone enhanced image. **d** Original UTE phase. **e** Unwrapped UTE phase. **f** Final bone enhanced image with air masks. **g** Susceptibility induced phase map at TE1. **h** Chemical shift—related phase at TE1. **i** Phase zero map obtained by subtracting images (**g**) and (**f**) from (**e**). **j** Signal intensity profile along line in (**a**). **k** Signal intensity profile along line in (**i**). **l** Histogram of phase zero and the fitting of the histogram with a 6-kernel Gaussian Mixture Model (*upper right corner*) using the expectation maximization algorithm. *Arrows* show separation of air kernels from bone and other tissue kernels

the simulated CT scans. Treatment plans were conducted on the simulated CT scans and the dose distributions compared to the actual CT scans. The mean absolute errors in HU assignments were relatively small (less than 20 HU for muscle, fat, and intra-pelvic soft tissues), 137 for bony tissues less than 850 HU and 189 for higher HU. The DVHs were clinically identical for the CT and synthetic CT plans.

Price et al. (2016), employed UTE images for assessing the generation of DRRs for brain cancer positioning. They compared both MV and kV planar imaging and CBCT imaging to their synthetic CT scans. The synthetic and actual DRRs agreed to within 1 mm.

3   MR + RT

The AAPM published the Task Group 104 report entitled "The role of in-room kV X-ray imaging for patient setup and target localization". The report was intended to provide information for the existing systems and advice for commissioning and routine quality assurance. The report addressed two gantry-mounted X-ray based imaging systems, the Elekta Synergy and the Varian On-Board Imager. Both systems were capable of producing radiographs and cone-beam CT image datasets. Aside from earlier work with ultrasound imaging, these devices were the first mass-produced imaging systems that yielded three-dimensional in-room images used for patient positioning. Prior to that time, clinicians had only two-dimensional projection images to work with.

The first description of the on-board CBCT concept was provided by Jaffray et al. (1999). They described a system of a kV X-ray source and a detector attached to the linear accelerator gantry. The source and detector would acquire planar images while the gantry rotated and the images used to reconstruct a 3D CBCT image. The earliest work was done using a phosphorescent plate viewed through a mirror by a camera. The system provided relatively poor CT images of phantoms, due in part to sensitivity variations in the camera and mechanical distortion of the system during rotation. The feasibility of CBCT increased markedly with the advent of large solid-state detectors. By 2008, the quality of CBCT images was improving to the point that they were being considered for clinical applications (Yin et al. 2008). Interestingly, the AAPM TG 104 report showed only a screen-grab of a CBCT from one vendor in an image describing workflow. That image, although relatively small, showed clear artifacts making it inferior to conventional CT.

The quality of CBCT rapidly improved and its clinical acceptance increased in parallel. Linear accelerators with CBCT technology are now the standard of care, and CBCT can be used to position all patients that cannot employ radiographic positioning for bony or marker-based alignment. Still, while CBCT has improved, it still suffers from the same limitations as helical CT, namely that the images are created by the linear attenuation coefficient differences between tissues.

MRI has no such limitation. Tissue conspicuity varies widely for different MR sequences. Modern MR scanners acquire stellar images in very short times, with high spatial resolution, low noise, and with few artifacts. This has been due to improvements in field homogeneity, gradient slewing rates, radiofrequency system design, coil design, pulse sequence design, and image reconstruction techniques. Therefore, one has to wonder; given the vastly superior imaging offered by MRI, why have MRI scanners not been coupled to linear accelerators in radiation therapy suites?

MR images measure the magnetization of tissue protons as they precess within the patient. The signals are so small, that MR scanners have to be completely surrounded by conducting metal (typically copper). Small cracks or holes in the copper allow RF signals to enter and reduce the quality of the signals used to create the images. Linear accelerators employ high power radiofrequency fields to accelerate electrons, which are then either delivered directly to the patient, or converted to high-energy bremsstrahlung X-rays by having the electrons strike a stopping target. The isolation of the MR scanner from the RF linear accelerator noise is a major hurdle in the design of combined MR and linear accelerators.

The linear accelerators themselves utilize specific magnetic fields for their operation, or need low magnetic fields to operate. The magnetic field of an MR scanner can be relatively huge and impede linear accelerator operations.

The radiofrequency energy needed to accelerate the electrons is created in a magnetron. A magnetron utilizes emitted electrons moving in a magnetic field to create radiofrequency energy. If the magnetron is placed in a magnetic field, it will fail to properly function. Similarly, the port circulator, a device that deviates radiofrequency waves such that waves reflected in the linear accelerator are steered to a water dump, will not work correctly when placed in an external field. The linear accelerator itself accelerates electrons, which would not travel a straight path if the linear accelerator were in an external magnetic field. Finally, the RF energy would precess when traveling in an external magnetic field. The RF is transported in waveguides that require the RF field polarization to be constant throughout transport, so the RF transmission efficiency would degrade if the RF polarization were allowed to precess.

As was previously mentioned, the challenges of overcoming the incompatibility between a linear accelerator and MR unit have discouraged the development of these systems.

3.1 ViewRay MRIdian

In 2003, Dr. James Dempsey, Ph.D., then an assistant professor at the University of Florida realized that the state of the art radiation therapy treatment modality, namely intensity modulated radiation therapy (IMRT), could be produced using a Cobalt source. Cobalt had been employed in the United States as a teletherapy source until the 1980s, when linear accelerators developed more features. During that time, it was assumed that the proper beam energy needed to treat a patient increased as the tumor depth increased, owning to the increased penetration of the higher energy X-rays. When IMRT was developed, clinics realized that IMRT dose optimization reduced the penetration advantage of higher energy beams, and the lower average secondary electron energy led to sharper penumbra, which allowed the IMRT dose optimization systems to create more conformal treatment plans. Still, it was generally thought that Cobalt energies (approximately equivalent to 3 MV) were insufficient to create clinically useful treatment plans. Given that Cobalt was a radioactive material, it needed sufficient activity to produce a useful teletherapy beam, so the source was typically a 2.0 cm diameter cylinder. This translated to a geometric penumbra of a few millimeters, while the geometric penumbra of higher energy X-rays was so small (typically 1 mm), it could almost be ignored.

Dr. Dempsey showed that IMRT treatment plans could be created using Cobalt sources, and that the treatment plans were not substantially less conformal than those created for typical linear accelerators. Still, there was no compelling reason to change, the dose rate for a single Cobalt source was inadequate for practical IMRT, and linear accelerators were more flexible.

Dr. Dempsey capitalized on the fact that IMRT could be delivered using Cobalt and that this eliminated the challenges of combining a linear accelerator with an MR scanner. He founded the company ViewRay in 2004 and sold his first system to Washington University in 2010. The system utilized three Cobalt sources to provide a total of 550 cGy per minute at isocenter with new sources. While this was not stellar performance, it was clinically acceptable, since a large fraction of any treatment timeslot did not utilize beam. Figure 9 shows a schematic and photograph of the system.

The ViewRay system utilized a split-bore, superconducting magnet with a magnetic field strength of 0.345T. The MR acquisition and reconstruction system was built by Siemens. The decision to use such a low field was predicated on two factors; first low field MR scanners typically exhibit less geometric distortion than higher field magnets, and second that the magnetic field perturbs the secondary electrons created during X-ray dose deposition.

Distortion is possible with any MR system, and for radiation therapy must be contained and controlled to within clinical tolerances. While such tolerances have not been established for MR + RT systems, typical spatial accuracy specifications would be 1 mm and 2 mm for stereotactic and no-stereotactic treatments, respectively. Sources of distortion include main magnetic field inhomogeneity, gradient inhomogeneity, susceptibility variations in tissues, and chemical shift. The magnetic field homogeneity can be controlled through design specific factors, and yields millimeter spatial accuracy for a 20–40 cm diameter sphere for typical magnets. Susceptibility and chemical shift artifacts are functions of the magnetic field strength; the greater the magnetic field strength, the greater the artifacts, leading to organ boundaries appearing offset from where they actually are. ViewRay had determined that with 0.345T fields such artifacts would be clincally negligible.

The perturbation of secondary electrons is also a function of magnetic field strength. The Lorentz force causes the secondary electrons tracks to be perturbed. In homogeneous tissues, this causes the lateral beam penumbrae to be asymmetrical,

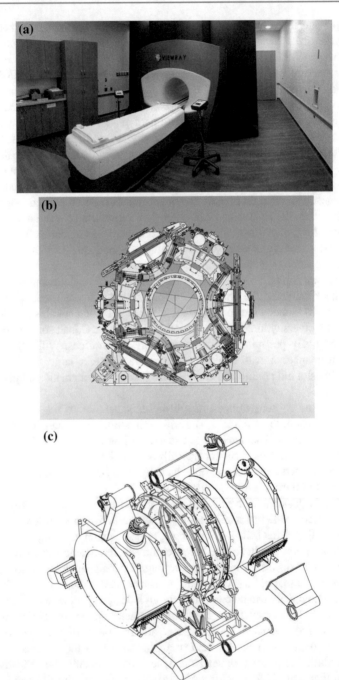

Fig. 9 **a** Photograph of the ViewRay MRIdian system installed at UCLA. **b** Schematic of the system in the transverse orientation, showing the three shields and two of the radiation beams. **c** Break apart view of ViewRay dewars and gantry ring

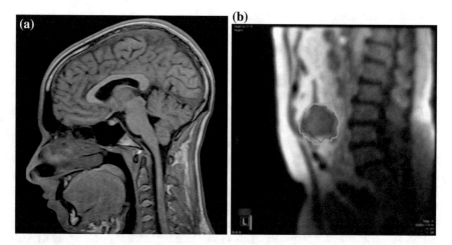

Fig. 10 a ViewRay setup image. **b** Gating image of abdominal tumor. This image is a single frame from a 4 frame per second

skewing to one direction as the average electron track is distorted by the magnetic field. This effect can be modeled in the treatment planning system and does not appear to cause significant dose degradation, due in part to its limited impact away from the beam penumbrae, and its consistent behavior. There are greater issues in heterogeneous tissues, specifically at interfaces between normal and low density tissues, such as lungs, or in air cavities and beam exits. In these cases, the radius of curvature of the secondary electron track can be sufficiently large in the low density media to allow the electrons to return to the exit of the high density media and re-irradiate the exit surface. This can cause large dose hot spots at the exit, and correspondingly large cold spots if the beam renters soft tissue. While these hot and cold spots can be predicted, they are sufficiently large that they may be clinically relevant.

The ViewRay imaging system provides real-time cine planar imaging, with one sagittal plane at 4 frames per second or 3 orthogonal frames at one frame per second. They provide high spatial resolution 3D imaging for patient setup purposes utilizing a TRUFE imaging sequence. This sequence yields hybrid T1 and T2 contrast. They have a 50 cm diameter spherical field of view with an imaging accuracy specification that meets all IEC, AAPM, ACR, and NEMA specifications, and can move the patient couch vertically 20 cm and laterally up to 14 cm to reposition the patient prior to treatment.

The system allows the user to identify and track the target or a surrogate during treatment. The system gates the cobalt beam by examining the tracked structure and determining if the structure is within the gating window. The user is allowed to specify the fraction of the structure within the window to gate the beam on. Figure 10 shows examples of the setup imaging and gating imaging.

Linear Accelerator + MR Units

The ViewRay MRIdian system was the first clinically used combined MR and radiation therapy system, in part due to ViewRay's decision to use Cobalt as the radiation beam source. Other groups, including ViewRay, have developed prototypes that integrate linear accelerators and MR images. All of these have had to manage the natural incompatibility of linear accelerators and magnetic resonance imagers.

MR imagers require extremely low background RF noise. This means that the RF noise from the linear accelerator hardware needs to be contained within the individual components. Just as the RF noise outside the MRI room is blocked by a Faraday Cage, typically a copper enclosure, the RF noise in the linear accelerator can be isolated by enclosing the RF components that have RF leakage using Copper. While that will theoretically enclose the RF, the Copper does not readily absorb RF, but instead reflects RF. This means that the intensity of internal RF will climb until it reaches equilibrium until the absorption and leakage equals the added RF. The RF intensity may be so large that even slight leakage will be sufficient to disturb the MR scanning signal. ViewRay managed this challenge by enclosing the RF enclosures with carbon fiber, a material used to isolate stealth aircraft from radar. Figure 11 shows a photograph of one of the Copper enclosures and the internal carbon fiber.

The other challenge of integrating a linear accelerator with an MRI is the isolation of the magnetic field sensitive components of the linear accelerator from the magnetic field. This is typically managed by moving the sensitive components away from the magnet (reducing the field in which the components lie) and shielding those components. The Elekta system utilized a 145 cm source to isocenter distance in part to reduce the magnetic field at the linear accelerator. They utilized local shielding to isolate the linear accelerator from the magnetic field.

ViewRay needed to use a reduced source-to-isocenter distance to manage clearance with the MR components. They wanted to maintain the same MR

Fig. 11 Carbon Fiber encased copper enclosure used to isolate RF leaking linear accelerator components

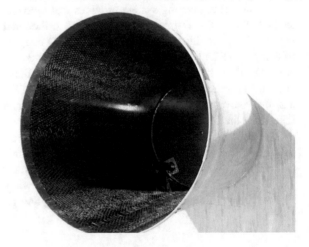

(a)   **(b)**

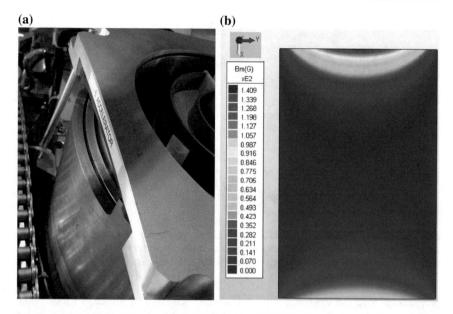

Fig. 12 **a** Photograph of the passive magnetic field shields, showing two of the concentric steel shells used to reduce the magnetic fields in which the sensitive components experience to below 40 Gauss. **b** Map of the magnetic field in a plane passing through the center of the shells, showing the reduced magnetic field

footprint when transitioning between Cobalt and Linear accelerator and allow users to upgrade between the two systems. They needed to reduce the magnetic fields from 3450 Gauss to 40 Gauss only a few centimeters from the homogeneous field region. They elected to use passive steel shielding, but steel shields magnetic fields by creating surface magnetization. Once the material thickness gets to approximately 1 cm, the additional shielding offered by thickening the material decrease greatly. Therefore, they elected to design the shielding as concentric cylindrical shells, providing a reduced magnetic field region inside the shells. Figure 12 shows the steel shells and the corresponding magnetic fields.

The linear accelerator itself needed to be within a field of less than 1 Gauss, so additional mu-metal shielding was employed.

3.2 Commercial Units

3.2.1 ViewRay

ViewRay utilizes the same MR unit as their Cobalt-based MRIdian system. They use a split-field 0.345T superconducting magnet and a Siemens radiofrequency and image processing system. They will employ a 6 MV linear accelerator matched to a doubly divergent double stacked MLC. Each leaf will subtend 8.0 mm at isocenter, so the step size between neighboring leaves will be 4.0 mm (Fig. 13). The beam is

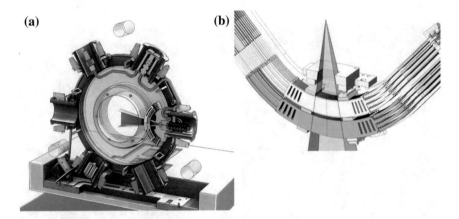

Fig. 13 **a** Schematic of new design of ViewRay linear accelerator components. There are 6 bays where magnetic field sensitive electronics can be placed. Those locations that have such electronics have the cylindrical magnetic shielding. **b** Doubly focused double stacked MLC design

perpendicular to the magnetic field orientation. The design employs a Helmholtz coil design that allows the radiation beam to pass through a minimum of material, namely the whole body coil and gradient coils.

3.2.2 Phillips/Elekta

Elekta is a radiation therapy company with a long track record of manufacturing radiation therapy linear accelerators. Phillips is an imaging company that produces MRI units. They partnered into developing a MR + RT system that has been installed in a number of centers worldwide. The original paper describing their system was published in 2008 by Lagendijk et al. (2008). They showed a very basic outline of the system (Fig. 14).

They utilize a more traditional MR imaging system coupled with a 6 MV linear accelerator. The beam passes through the MR dewars but not the main magnetic coil, which is split similarly to the ViewRay system, or the gradient coils, which are also split. The beam passes through an equivalent of 11 cm of Aluminum, hardening the beam somewhat to an equivalent of approximately 7 MV. They utilize a 1.5T cylindrical superconducting magnet. The magnetic field at the linear accelerator was reduced by modifying the active magnetic shielding of the MRI. They employed the aluminum cryostat wall as part of the Faraday cage that isolates the RF sensitive electronics from the linear accelerator. This places the linear accelerator and its components outside the Faraday Cage and means that both ends of the bore of the magnet will be placed in a wall that contains part of the Faraday Cage.

3.2.3 MagneTx

The Cross-Cancer Institute designed an experimental system consisting of a 0.2T MRI an integrated 6 MV linear accelerator. Fallone et al. (2009) showed that this system could simultaneously image and produce beam. This unit employed passive

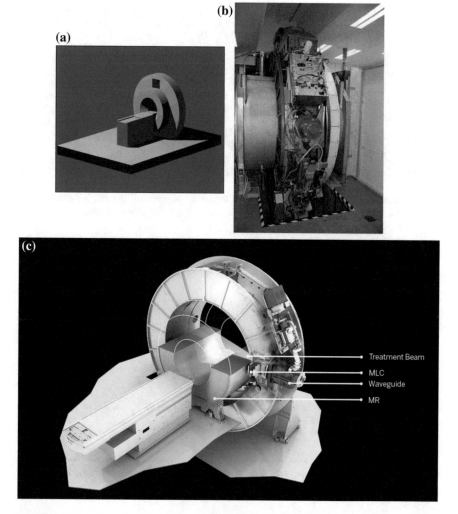

Fig. 14 a Early schematic (Lagendijk et al. 2008) and **b** later prototype (Lagendijk et al. 2014) of the Elekta Philips system. **c** Schematic of the clinical system (from website)

shielding of the linear accelerator. Cross-Cancer Institute is developing a prototype human system that utilizes a 0.5 MRI and a 6 MV linear accelerator. Figure 15 shows their prototype unit. Unlike the other systems, the MR is a parallel plane system and the X-ray beam is parallel to the main magnetic field. The system utilizes high temperature superconductors, avoiding the need for liquid helium, and the magnet can be rapidly cycled on and off. The linear accelerator and MR gantry rotate to provide different beam entry angles. The coaxial geometry provides the benefit that the Lorenz force does not distort the radiation dose as it does with perpendicularly aligned systems.

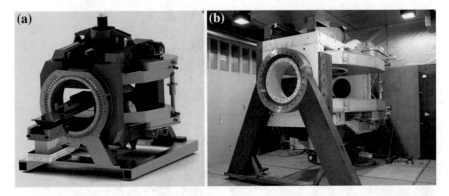

Fig. 15 Cross Cancer Center MR Linac. **a** 3D rendering of proposed system. **b** Prototype unit.
Images from http://www.mp.med.ualberta.ca/linac-mr/photo_gallery.html#phase-2

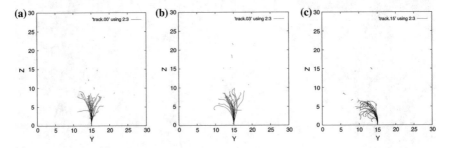

Fig. 16 Monte Carlo calculations of secondary electron tracks as a function of magnetic field
strength. **a** 0T, **b** 0.35T, **c** 1.5T

4 Clinical Challenges of MR + RT: Lorenz Force and Radiation Dosimetry

In the absence of magnetic fields, secondary electrons travel in a symmetric pattern
about the photon beam direction. They scatter and disperse as they leave the
interaction point, causing blurring of the dose distributions. The magnitude of this
blurring is proportional to the photon beam energy, so 18 MV photon beams have
more blurring than 6 MV photon beams because of the greater range of their
secondary electrons. For systems that have perpendicular orientations between the
main magnetic field and the oncoming X-rays, the Lorenz force will attempt to steer
the electrons in a circle. However, their continued interactions will perturb an
otherwise circular orbit (Fig. 16). This causes open field radiation doses to have
perturbed penumbrae. While the penumbrae may appear to be skewed, they can be
accurately calculated, for example, by including the Lorenz force in a Monte Carlo
dose calculation.

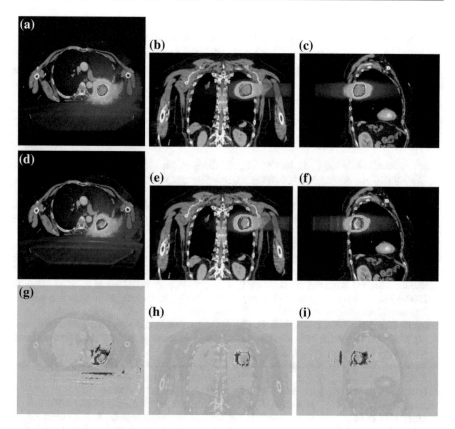

Fig. 17 Lung dose distributions without and with a uniform 1.5T magnetic field. **a–c** No magnetic field. **d–f** With 1.5T magnetic field. **g–i** Dose difference, 1.5T field–0T field dose distributions. From Yang et al. (2015)

The impact of this perturbation on the dose distribution within air cavities is profound. Yang et al. (2015), examined dose distribution perturbations in the pelvis, head and neck, and lung for magnetic field strengths of 0.35T, 0.7T, 1.0T, 1.5T, and 3.0T. They showed that the dose to the pelvis and head-and-neck exhibited dose distributions that were almost identical with and without the magnetic field. This was not true for the lung cancer case. Figure 17 compares the dose distributions with and without a 1.5T magnetic field. The dose distributions are clearly different, caused primarily by the change in secondary electron transport in the heterogeneity boundaries near the tumor. While fluence modulation may mitigate some of the dose heterogeneity, the mitigation fluences will be coupled to the room coordinates, while the tumor may move due to breathing or patient setup errors. Therefore, the mitigation fluence modulation may be misplaced relative to the magnetic-field generated dose heterogeneity.

Similar results were found by Prior et al. (2016). They examined the dose distributions for pancreas and prostate patient treatment plans with no magnetic field and in the presence of a 1.5T magnetic field (axis perpendicular to the X-ray beams) and found that the target dose was within 3%, while the normal structure doses were within 5%.

References

Chen LL, Price RA, Wang L, Li JS, Qin LH, McNeeley S, Ma CMC, Freedman GM, Pollack A (2004a) MRI-based treatment planning for radiotherapy: dosimetric verification for prostate IMRT. Int J Radiat Oncol Biol Phys 60:636–647

Chen L, Price RA, Nguyen TB, Wang L, Li JS, Qin L, Ding M, Palacio E, Ma CM, Pollack A (2004b) Dosimetric evaluation of MRI-based treatment planning for prostate cancer. Phys Med Biol 49:5157–5170

Devic S (2012) MRI simulation for radiotherapy treatment planning. Med Phys 39:6701–6711

Eilertsen K, Vestad LNTA, Geier O, Skretting A (2008) A simulation of MRI based dose calculations on the basis of radiotherapy planning CT images. Acta Oncol 47:1294–1302

Fallone BG, Murray B, Rathee S, Stanescu T, Steciw S, Vidakovic S, Blosser E, Tymofichuk D (2009) First MR images obtained during megavoltage photon irradiation from a prototype integrated linac-MR system. Med Phys 36:2084–2088

Huan Y, Caldwell C, Balogh J, Mah K (2014) Toward magnetic resonance-only simulation: segmentation of bone in MR for radiation therapy verification of the head. Int J Radiat Oncol Biol Phys 89:649–657

Jaffray DA, Drake DG, Moreau M, Martinez AA, Wong JW (1999) A radiographic and tomographic imaging system integrated into a medical linear accelerator for localization of bone and soft-tissue targets. Int J Radiat Oncol Biol Phys 45:773–789

Jonsson JH, Karlsson MG, Karlsson M, Nyholm T (2010) Treatment planning using MRI data: an analysis of the dose calculation accuracy for different treatment regions. Radiat Oncol 5:62

Kapanen M, Collan J, Beule A, Seppala T, Saarilahti K, Tenhunen M (2013) Commissioning of MRI-only based treatment planning procedure for external beam radiotherapy of prostate. Magn Reson Med 70:127–135

Karlsson M, Karlsson MG, Nyholm T, Amies C, Zackrisson B (2009) Dedicated magnetic resonance imaging in the radiotherapy clinic. Int J Radiat Oncol Biol Phys 74:644–651

Kim J, Glide-Hurst C, Doemer A, Wen N, Movsas B, Chetty IJ (2015) Implementation of a novel algorithm for generating synthetic CT images from magnetic resonance imaging data sets for prostate cancer radiation therapy. Int J Radiat Oncol Biol Phys 91:39–47

Kristensen BH, Laursen FJ, Logager V, Geertsen PF, Krarup-Hansen A (2008) Dosimetric and geometric evaluation of an open low-field magnetic resonance simulator for radiotherapy treatment planning of brain tumours. Radiother Oncol 87:100–109

Lagendijk JJW, Raaymakers BW, Raaijmakers AJE, Overweg J, Brown KJ, Kerkhof EM, van der Put RW, Hardemark B, van Vutpen M, van der Heide UA (2008) MRI/linac integration. Radiother Oncol 86:25–29

Lagendijk JJW, Raaymakers BW, Van den Berg CAT, Moerland MA, Philippens ME, van Vulpen M (2014) MR guidance in radiotherapy. Phys Med Biol 59:R349–R369

Lambert J, Greer PB, Menk F, Patterson J, Parker J, Dahl K, Gupta S, Capp A, Wratten C, Tang C, Kumar M, Dowling J, Hauville S, Hughes C, Fisher K, Lau P, Denham JW, Salvado O (2011) MRI-guided prostate radiation therapy planning: investigation of dosimetric accuracy of MRI-based dose planning. Radiother Oncol 98:330–334

Lee YK, Bollet M, Charles-Edwards G, Flower MA, Leach MO, McNair H, Moore E, Rowbottom C, Webb S (2003) Radiotherapy treatment planning of prostate cancer using magnetic resonance imaging alone. Radiother Oncol 66:203–216

Liu L, Cao Y, Fessler JA, Jolly S, Balter JM (2016) A female pelvic bone shape model for air/bone separation in support of synthetic CT generation for radiation therapy. Phys Med Biol 61:169–182

Paulson ES, Erickson B, Schultz C, Li XA (2015) Comprehensive MRI simulation methodology using a dedicated MRI scanner in radiation oncology for external beam radiation treatment planning. Med Phys 42:28–39

Petersch B, Bogner J, Fransson A, Lorang T, Potter R (2004) Effects of geometric distortion in 0.2 T MRI on radiotherapy treatment planning of prostate cancer. Radiother Oncol 71:55–64

Prabhakar R, Julka PK, Ganesh T, Munshi A, Joshi RC, Rath GK (2007) Feasibility of using MRI alone for 3D radiation treatment planning in brain tumors. Jpn J Clin Oncol 37:405–411

Price RG, Kim JP, Zheng W, Chetty IJ, Glide-Hurst C (2016) Image guided radiation therapy using synthetic computed tomography images in brain cancer. Int J Radiat Oncol Biol Phys 95:1281–1289

Prior P, Chen X, Botros M, Paulson ES, Lawton C, Erickson B, Li XA (2016) MRI-based IMRT planning for MR-linac: comparison between CT- and MRI-based plans for pancreatic and prostate cancers. Phys Med Biol 61:3819–3842

Ramsey CR, Oliver AL (1998) Magnetic resonance imaging based digitally reconstructed radiographs, virtual simulation, and three-dimensional treatment planning for brain neoplasms. Med Phys 25:1928–1934

Robson MD, Gatehouse PD, Bydder M, Bydder GM (2003) Magnetic resonance: an introduction to ultrashort TE (UTE) imaging. J Comput Assist Tomogr 27:825–846

Schmidt MA, Payne GS (2015) Radiotherapy planning using MRI. Phys Med Biol 60:R323–R361

Yang YM, Geurts M, Smilowitz JB, Sterpin E, Bednarz BP (2015) Monte Carlo simulations of patient dose perturbations in rotational-type radiotherapy due to a transverse magnetic field: a tomotherapy investigation. Med Phys 42:715–725

Yang Y, Cao M, Kaprealian T, Sheng K, Gao Y, Han F, Gomez C, Santhanam A, Tenn S, Agazaryan N, Low DA, Hu P (2016) Accuracy of UTE-MRI-based patient setup for brain cancer radiation therapy. Med Phys 43:262–267

Yin FF, Wang Z, Yoo S, Wu QJ, Kirkpatrick J, Larrier N, Meyer J, Willett CG, Marks LB (2008) Integration of cone-beam CT in stereotactic body radiation therapy. Technol Cancer Res Treat 7:133–139

Zheng W, Kim JP, Kadbi M, Movsas B, Chetty IJ, Glide-Hurst CK (2015) magnetic resonance-based automatic air segmentation for generation of synthetic computed tomography scans in the head region. Int J Radiat Oncol Biol Phys 93:497–506

Oncologic Applications of Magnetic Resonance Guided Focused Ultrasound

Dario B. Rodrigues, Paul R. Stauffer, John Eisenbrey, Valeria Beckhoff and Mark D. Hurwitz

Abstract

Focused ultrasound (FUS) is a noninvasive thermal therapy that utilizes energy generated from ultrasound waves to ablate a small target area. The ability of FUS to heat tumors to ablative temperatures in a very precise manner, thereby sparing surrounding tissues, has been equated to surgery with the advantages of reduced tissue trauma and recovery time. FUS may also be used to induce moderate temperature hyperthermia to enhance effects of radiation, chemotherapy, and potentially immunotherapy. The combination of magnetic resonance guidance with FUS (MRgFUS) provides the ability to plan, monitor, and steer treatments in near real-time, further contributing to the safety and effectiveness profile of FUS. Regulatory clearance for noninvasive palliative treatment of bone metastases has been realized. Additional palliative and curative treatments for a wide range of oncologic conditions including prostate, breast, gynecologic, gastrointestinal and brain cancers, and soft tissue tumors are in active

D.B. Rodrigues · P.R. Stauffer · M.D. Hurwitz (✉)
Thermal Oncology Program, Department of Radiation Oncology, Thomas Jefferson University, Philadelphia, PA 19107, USA
e-mail: mark.hurwitz@jefferson.edu

D.B. Rodrigues
e-mail: dario.rodrigues@jefferson.edu

P.R. Stauffer
e-mail: paul.stauffer@jefferson.edu

J. Eisenbrey
Department of Radiology, Thomas Jefferson University, Philadelphia, PA 19107, USA
e-mail: john.eisenbrey@jefferson.edu

V. Beckhoff
Department of Biomedical Engineering, Drexel University, Philadelphia, PA 19104, USA
e-mail: vb349@drexel.edu

© Springer International Publishing AG 2017
J.Y.C. Wong et al. (eds.), *Advances in Radiation Oncology*,
Cancer Treatment and Research 172, DOI 10.1007/978-3-319-53235-6_4

development. This chapter provides an overview of MRgFUS including biological effects and physical parameters description. A comprehensive review of all currently approved and evolving oncological applications of MRgFUS then follows. Finally, an overview is provided of wide ranging leading edge research helping to define future applications for the field including the role of MRgFUS in multimodality cancer therapy.

Keywords

Focused ultrasound · MR guidance · Thermal ablation · Bone metastases · Prostate cancer · Breast cancer · Soft tissue sarcoma · Brain cancer · Liver cancer · Pancreatic cancer · Colorectal cancer

Abbreviations

AE	Adverse events
AVM	Arteriovenous malformation
BBB	Blood brain barrier
BPI	Brief pain inventory
BPI-QoL	Brief pain inventory-Quality of life
CE	European conformity
CR	Complete response
CT	Computed tomography
DCE-MRI	Dynamic contrast-enhanced magnetic resonance imaging
DNA	Deoxyribonucleic acid
ECD	Endorectal cooling device
FDA	Food and drug administration
FUS	Focused ultrasound
HCC	Hepatocellular carcinoma
HIFU	High-intensity focused ultrasound
IBMCWP	International bone metastasis consensus working party
IIEF	International index of erectile function
IPSS	International prostate symptom score
MDA	MD Anderson criteria
MR	Magnetic resonance
MRgFUS	Magnetic resonance guided focused ultrasound
MR-HIFU	Magnetic resonance high-intensity focused ultrasound
MRT	MR thermometry
NPV	Non-perfused volume
NR	No response
NRS	Numerical rating scale
OMED	Changes in analgesic intake
OR	Overall response
PD	Progressive disease
PP	Pain progression

PR	Partial response
PSA	Prostate specific antigen
QLQ-BM22	European Organization for Research and Treatment of Cancer—Quality of life questionnaire for patients with bone metastases
QoL	Quality of life
RF	Radio frequency
RR	Recurrence
UA	Ultrasound applicator
USgFUS	Ultrasound guided focused ultrasound
VAS	Visual analog scale

1 Introduction

Thermal medicine is an emerging field that is based upon therapeutic manipulation of temperature. Thermal therapy may be performed with very cold temperatures—cryotherapy (<-40 °C), or with one of three distinct protocols of elevated temperature: fever-range hyperthermia around 39–41 °C lasting several hours; moderate hyperthermia around 41–45 °C for 30–60 min; and high-temperature thermal ablation, usually 50–85 °C with heat typically applied to each area of the target for several seconds (Stauffer 2005). The biologic effects expected from these different temperature ranges vary widely. At fever-range temperatures, blood perfusion, permeability of tumor microvasculature, and cellular metabolic rate are increased, potentially enhancing drug uptake and local activity as well as stimulation of immune response (Xu et al. 2007; Dewhirst et al. 2012). At moderately higher temperatures of 41–45 °C, the primary goal is to enhance other forms of therapy such as radiation or chemotherapy through a number of overlapping effects on cells, vasculature and tumor physiology. Since higher perfusion improves tissue oxygenation and pH, this increases sensitivity to radiation (Vujaskovic et al. 2000), while the elevated temperature inhibits repair of sub-lethal radiation damage. The radiobiology of heat combinations with radiation are described in detail in numerous publications (Dewhirst et al. 2012, 2005; Sneed et al. 2010; Hall and Giaccia 2006). Combined with chemotherapy, moderate hyperthermia increases cellular metabolism and nutrient consumption, thus enhancing cellular uptake of locally concentrated drug (Dahl 1995; Hahn 1979). In addition to enhancing the local toxicity of systemically administered chemotherapeutics, local hyperthermia has been shown to increase the extravasation of drug out of leaky tumor microvasculature and thereby increase local concentration of bioavailable drug around tumor cells (Dewhirst et al. 2012). This effect may be magnified using nanoparticle drug carriers such as temperature sensitive liposomes that release drug rapidly within the transit time through a heated tumor, potentially increasing total drug delivery by 20–30 fold (Kong et al. 2000). For temperatures above 48 °C, the effects on tissue are more direct, with protein denaturation, coagulation and tissue necrosis following immediately after the heat insult. Besides thermal ablation, mechanical effects such as cavitation and radiation forces may also induce damage (Hectors et al. 2016).

Thermal Oncology concerns the treatment of cancer with heat or cold. Optimum selection of one of the thermal treatment protocols defined above depends on location and extent of the tumor target. For large or irregularly shaped tumors extending out into surrounding host tissues, it may be most appropriate to apply moderate hyperthermia to a large region that encompasses all imageable tumor including a margin, and rely on synergism of heat with radiation and/or chemotherapy to accomplish differential tumor kill over a course of fractionated treatments. For a well-circumscribed lesion in a region of non-critical tissue with some biological reserve (i.e. liver, muscle, fat), an aggressive heating approach may be more appropriate that can ablate the entire tumor target with only a thin rim of surrounding margin. In such cases, focal ablation can accomplish effective thermal surgery in a single treatment session. For this strategy, a high degree of control of power deposition is required to produce ablative temperatures within the target while avoiding overheating of surrounding critical normal tissues.

Numerous reviews clearly describe the capabilities and limitations of available electromagnetic and ultrasonic heating technologies (Stauffer 2005; Diederich and Hynynen 1999; Hynynen 1990; Hynynen and McDannold 2004; Lee 1995; Van Rhoon 2013). Generally, the long wavelength associated with radiofrequency and microwave heating devices prohibits a tight focus in tissue in lieu of a regional concentration of heat. On the contrary, typical clinical ultrasound systems have large multi-transducer arrays on the surface and are able to produce a 1–2 mm diameter by 3–7 mm long focal region at depth in the body. Each focused ultrasound exposure is known as sonication. The high intensity focus quickly ablates tissue (<10–20 s) so that the focal point can be shifted and the process iterated to produce overlapping ablation zones that eventually combine into one large ablated tissue volume (Fig. 1). Because heating only occurs where the ultrasound waves converge, the surrounding tissue remains unaffected. This procedure is known as high-intensity focused ultrasound (HIFU) ablation or simply focused ultrasound (FUS) ablation.

The ability to target tissues deep within the human body depends on the frequency and intensity of the ultrasound wave and the tissue properties through which the wave must travel. Lower frequency acoustic waves are better suited to penetrate deep into tissue, but may require more energy to cause thermal tissue ablation; while higher frequency waves cause heating more easily, but tend to get absorbed more readily and therefore cannot penetrate into deep tissues. Such parameters can be manipulated during FUS treatment to maximize energy delivery to the targeted tissue. Another consideration for planning FUS treatment is the scattering of ultrasound waves when travelling through different mediums. Most human tissues, with the exception of bone and fat, have the same acoustic properties as water: for this reason liquid gel is used to couple extracorporeal ultrasound transducers to

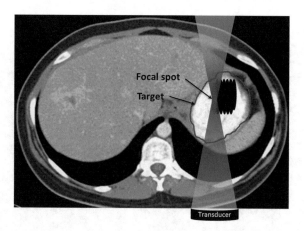

Fig. 1 Schematic of a FUS procedure, a method of focusing sound waves to create heat at a focal spot at depth in the body. The tissue temperature at the focal spot is elevated to nearly 85 °C in a matter of seconds, resulting in tissue destruction, while the tissue outside the heat focus remains unharmed

human skin. Similarly, bone absorbs a high amount of ultrasound energy, which can lead to unwanted heating along the bone surface while missing the target tissue (Avedian et al. 2011). These factors must be accounted for when planning and implementing FUS treatment.

Because thermal ablation of human soft tissue produces an immediate radical change in tissue properties from the host tissue, the ablation volume can be visualized during treatment via non-invasive imaging. Dependent on location in the body, the most commonly used approaches are ultrasound and magnetic resonance imaging (Copelan et al. 2015). Real time monitoring of lesion formation provides immediate feedback to control movement of the ultrasound focus for successive ablation events and also offers non-invasive verification of the cumulative extent of necrosis. Initially, ultrasound was the primary method for image guided ablation. Due to advances in quality and availability of high resolution MR systems, recent clinical work is shifting quickly to 1.5 and 3 T magnets for higher resolution definition of anatomy, metabolic status, and tissue temperature for real-time guidance of ablation procedures (Copelan et al. 2015; Woodrum et al. 2015; Kim 2015). Images of treatment planning and real-time temperature guidance are provided in Fig. 2.

Given the wide-ranging applicability of FUS, numerous extracorporeal and intracorporeal devices (e.g. transrectal, transurethral, intravascular, interstitial, etc.) have been designed to optimize application-specific treatment delivery. Today, custom tailored tools for specific organs or clinical situations are available for brain, breast, prostate, abdominal organs, and bone. These approaches take advantage of unique devices in order to achieve the best comfort and positioning of the patient as well as to obtain an effective FUS. At present, three MR-guided systems are available:

(a)

(b)

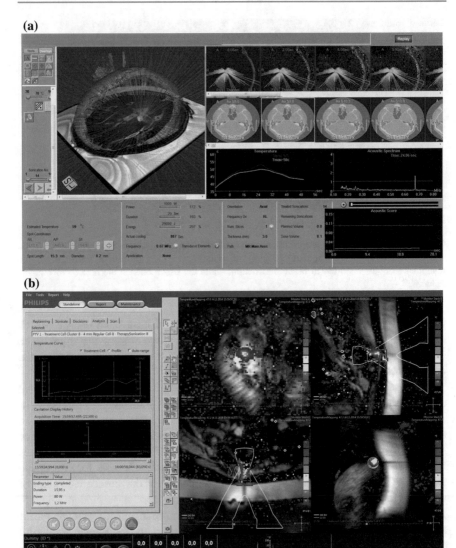

Fig. 2 Examples of treatment planning/guidance systems for MRgFUS. **a** Treatment planning/ guidance for the Exablate Neuro system. Planning screens allow the operator to set treatment parameters, monitor beam path of the transducer array, thermal lesion location, time/temperature graphs, and ultrasound frequency spectrum (Image courtesy of the INSIGHTEC Ltd.) **b** Treatment guidance for the Sonalleve MR-HIFU system demonstrating the "Therapy Wizard" on the *left* and monitoring slices in the imaging panel. This system allows the operator to monitor real-time temperature rise at the target, as well as in near-field and far-field regions (Image courtesy of Philips)

Table 1 Summary of ongoing clinical trials on MR-guided FUS for oncological applications

Trial	Site	Patients	Device	Phase	Countries (centers)	Primary outcome
NCT00981578	Bone metastases	50	ExAblate	Phase I	United States (5)	Safety
NCT01091883	Bone metastases	60	ExAblate	Phase III	Israel (1)	Safety
NCT01586273	Bone metastases	64	Sonalleve	Phase II	Korea (1), The Netherlands (1), UK (1)	Pain palliation
NCT01693770	Bone metastases	18	ExAblate	Phase I/II	Italy (1)	Safety and pain palliation
NCT01833806	Bone metastases	70	ExAblate	Phase IV	United States (7)	Pain palliation
NCT01834937	Bone metastases	50	ExAblate	Phase IV	United States (4)	Safety
NCT01964677	Bone metastases	12	Sonalleve	Phase II	United Kingdom (1)	Pain palliation
NCT02616016	Bone metastases	10	Sonalleve	Phase II	Canada (1)	Pain palliation
NCT02718404	Bone metastases	41	Sonalleve	Phase II	Italy (1)	Pain palliation
NCT01620359	Breast	200	ExAblate	Phase II	Germany (1)	Safety and efficacy
NCT02407613	Breast	10	Sonalleve	Phase I/II	Netherlands (1)	Efficacy
NCT01226576	Prostate	80	ExAblate	Phase II	Canada (1), Israel (1), Italy (1), Singapore (1), UK (1)	Safety and efficacy
NCT01657942	Prostate	40	ExAblate	Phase I	United States (6)	Safety and efficacy
NCT01686958	Prostate	30	TULSA-PRO	Phase I	United States (1), Canada (1), Germany (1)	Safety
NCT00147056	Brain	10	ExAblate neuro	Phase I	United States (2)	Safety
NCT01473485	Brain	10	ExAblate neuro	Phase I	Canada (1)	Safety
NCT01698437	Brain	10	ExAblate neuro	Phase I	Switzerland (1)	Safety
NCT02343991	Brain	10	ExAblate neuro	Phase I	Canada (1)	Safety
NCT02181075	Liver	28	Sonalleve	Phase I	UK (1)	Feasibility
NCT01786850	Pancreas	–	ExAblate	Phase II	Italy (1)	Efficacy

(continued)

Table 1 (continued)

Trial	Site	Patients	Device	Phase	Countries (centers)	Primary outcome
NCT01965002	Soft Tissue	30	ExAblate	Phase I/II	United States (1)	Safety
NCT02076906	Solid tumors	14	Sonalleve	Phase I	United States (1)	Safety
NCT02536183	Solid tumors	34	Sonalleve	Phase I	United States (1)	Safety
NCT02557854	Solid tumors	14	Sonalleve	Phase I	United States (1)	Safety
NCT02714621	Gynae metastases	35	Sonalleve	Phase II	UK (1)	Pain palliation
NCT02528175	Rectum	20	Sonalleve	Phase I	Canada (1)	Safety

- The Exablate MRgFUS system (INSIGHTEC Ltd., Haifa, Israel), which received the CE Mark and US Food and Drug Administration (FDA) approval for treatment of fibroids in 2002 and 2004, and palliative treatment of bone metastases in 2007 and 2012, respectively. Clinical studies are currently ongoing in prostate (phase I/II), breast (phase II), brain (phase I), soft tissue (phase I/II) and pancreas (phase II).
- The Sonalleve MR-HIFU system (Koninklijke Philips Electronics N.V., Eindhoven, The Netherlands), received CE Mark for the palliative treatment of bone metastases in 2011. FDA studies for palliative treatment of bone metastases from breast cancer are in phase II/III clinical trials. Clinical studies are currently ongoing in breast (phase I/II), liver (phase I), soft tissue (phase I), rectum (phase II) and gynae metastases (phase I).
- The TULSA-PRO system (Profound Medical Inc., Toronto ON, Canada) received the CE Mark for treatment of prostate cancer in 2016.

The following sections review the results of ongoing clinical trials (Table 1) in the primary clinical sites of application while describing existing equipment systems for MR-guided FUS (MRgFUS), also known as MR-HIFU. The majority of MRgFUS procedures aim for ablation or thermal surgery, however ultrasound transducers can operate at a lower intensity to produce therapeutic hyperthermia (40–45 °C) in the target, which is an adjuvant technique to enhance the therapeutic response of radiation and/or chemotherapy (De Haas-Kock et al. 2009). The chapter ends with an overview of ongoing research that will help define future applications for the field.

2 Clinical Applications of MRgFUS

2.1 Bone Metastases

Bone metastases are the most common source of pain in cancer patients (Berenson et al. 2006). Autopsy studies have shown that up to 85% of patients with breast, prostate and lung cancer have bone metastases at the time of death, where breast and prostate cancer patients often have survival measured in years. Based on strong clinical evidence from phase I, II and III clinical trials, MRgFUS has received both CE and FDA approvals for management of bone metastases-related pain. The therapeutic goals of such clinical studies included pain palliation, tumor reduction, prevention of impending pathologic fractures, and/or tumor decompression (Rodrigues et al. 2015). The denervation of the periosteum, which contains pain-reporting nerve fibers, is considered a major factor in pain palliation perception (Catane et al. 2007). This explains the rapid relief following FUS treatment which is characterized by significantly higher power deposition in the periosteum and bone relative to surrounding soft tissues. Tumor debulking caused by thermal ablation also plays a role since it diminishes the pressure on the adjacent tissue (Napoli et al. 2013; Hurwitz et al. 2014).

Several hundred patients have been treated who have exhausted, declined, or are unsuitable for other pain palliation methods. The success of the treatment can be evaluated based on changes in pain and quality of life scores, as well as decrease in pain medication usage. These include the Brief Pain Inventory (BPI), a validated 11-point scale for the evaluation of pain (0 = no pain, 10 = unbearable pain) in cancer patients (Cleeland and Ryan 1994), which has two different names: numerical rating scale (NRS) and visual analog scale (VAS). Quality of Life (QoL) is considered an important secondary endpoint in the majority of clinical studies that address painful bone metastases, and is equally evaluated in a 11-point scale (Rosenthal and Callstrom 2012) using tools such as the Brief Pain Inventory (BPI-QoL) (Cleeland and Ryan 1994) or QLQ-BM22, a questionnaire developed by the European Organization for Research and Treatment of Cancer (Chow et al. 2009). The majority of studies associated response with a ≥ 2-point decrease in pain at the treated site without increase in analgesic intake. Finally, the MD Anderson (MDA) criteria has been used to evaluate treatment efficacy via local tumor control (Costelloe et al. 2010). Quantitatively, these criteria define partial response (PR) as a decrease of $\geq 50\%$ in the sum of the perpendicular measurements of a lesion, and progressive disease (PD) as an increase of $\geq 25\%$ in this sum. A secondary measure is change in tumor size.

Liberman et al. in (2009) published the first multicenter clinical study on the use of MRgFUS for pain palliation of bone metastases. This report incorporated previously reported results (Catane et al. 2007) and (Gianfelice et al. 2008), and comprised of 31 patients with 32 bone lesions. Three-month follow-up was available for 25 out of 31 patients. A significant reduction in pain (>2 points) was reported by 72% of patients, with 36% reporting a VAS score of 0. The average

VAS score decreased from 5.9 prior to treatment to 1.8 at the three-month follow-up, with 52% of patients reporting substantial pain relief within three days. 24% of patients had no response and one patient experienced worsened pain levels. A reduction in opioid usage was reported in 67% of patients with recorded medication data. No major complications were noted.

In 2013, Napoli et al. reported a prospective, single-arm research study with 18 patients treated with MRgFUS for painful bone metastases (Napoli et al. 2013). The pain severity score changed significantly from a baseline average of 7.1–1.1 at three-month follow-up. A score of 0 for pain severity, without medication intake, was reported by 72% of patients at final follow-up, consistent with a complete response to treatment. Computed tomography (CT) examinations demonstrated increased bone density with restoration of cortical borders in five patients (28%). According to the MDA criteria (Costelloe et al. 2010), a complete response to treatment was observed in two patients (11%), a partial response in four patients (22%), stable disease in 10 patients (56%) and progressive disease in two patients (11%). No treatment-related adverse events were recorded during the study.

The results of a multicenter phase III clinical trial on bone tumors were published by Hurwitz et al. (2014). 147 patients with metastatic bone pain, refractory to other pain interventions often including radiation, were randomized to MRgFUS treatment or placebo treatment. Patients randomized to placebo underwent the same procedure as those receiving MRgFUS treatment but without energy deposition. The pain response rates three months after treatment were 64% in the MRgFUS treated arm versus 20% in the placebo arm. Complete pain relief was observed in 23% of treated patients, compared to 6% of patients who received placebo treatment. Approximately two-thirds of responders experienced significant pain relief—as defined by a decrease in worst NRS score of 2 points or more—within three days of treatment, establishing the ability of MRgFUS to induce fast pain response. This response was accompanied by a similarly rapid improvement in patient function scores. The most common complication was pain during MRgFUS treatment (32%) and major complications occurred in 3% of treated patients: two patients had pathological fractures and one patient had third-degree skin burn. However, one fracture was outside the treated area, and the skin burn was due to a violation of the inclusion criteria protocol. Furthermore, the majority of adverse events (60%) were transient and resolved on the treatment day and 51 patients (46%) had no adverse events.

The phase III trial as reported by Hurwitz et al. was subject to a retrospective analysis of the safety of combination MRgFUS with active systemic chemotherapy (Meyer et al. 2014). Chemotherapy data were available for 104 patients and patients were followed for three months. Ninety patients were treated without chemotherapy, and 14 were treated with chemotherapy. There was no significant difference between the response rates of the chemotherapy group (71%) and the non-chemotherapy group (68%) with $p = 0.78$. The overall adverse event rates were 57% for chemotherapy patients and 45% for non-chemotherapy patients ($p = 0.38$), whereas the sonication pain was 50% and 28% for the same groups ($p = 0.11$), respectively. Remaining adverse event rates were not significantly different ($p = 0.17$).

Several single-arm trials have since been published supporting the safety and efficacy demonstrated in the phase III clinical trial. A prospective multicenter study with 72 patients was performed to evaluate the efficacy of MRgFUS for pain palliation of bone metastasis in patients who had exhausted radiotherapy or refused other therapeutic options (Zaccagna et al. 2014). Thirty four patients (47%) reported complete response to treatment and discontinued medications. Twenty nine patients (40%) experienced a pain score reduction >2 points, consistent with partial response. The remaining 9 patients (13%) had recurrence after treatment. Significant differences between baseline (VAS = 6) and follow-up (VAS = 2) average values and medication intake were observed. Similarly, a significant difference was found for QLQ-BM22 between baseline and follow-up. No treatment-related adverse events were recorded. Bazzocchi et al. (2015) evaluated the clinical outcome of 64 patients (90 lesions) with painful bone metastases that were treated with MRgFUS. The treated lesions ranged between 1 and 14 cm. On a lesion-based approach, average VAS score at baseline was 5.3 decreasing to 2.7 at one month, and to 1.8 after 12 months. Two treatment-related adverse events (3%) were reported: a single case of small skin burn and one case of prostate inflammation in a patient treated to the ischiopubic ramus. More recently, Gu et al. treated 23 patients with painful bone metastases with NRS ≥ 4 and that have not received radiotherapy or chemotherapy for pain palliation at least two weeks prior to MRgFUS treatment (Gu et al. 2015). Adverse events included pain in therapeutic area (13%), which relieved spontaneous within one week and numbness in lower limb (4%) that relieved after physiotherapy. Before treatment the average NRS was 6.0, which decreased to 3.7 and 2.2 at the one-week and three-month follow up, respectively. In the same timeframe, the average BPI-QoL score decreased from 39 to 27 and 21; and the QLQ-BM22 score decreased from 52 to 44 and 39, respectively. The clinical benefits of pain palliation and patient's quality of life improved and were sustained after treatment at least to three months.

Further studies have introduced innovative approaches to treatment delivery. In 2014, Huisman and colleagues reported the first experience with volumetric MRgFUS for palliative treatment of painful bone metastases in 11 patients, a technique intended to reduce treatment time (Huisman et al. 2014). Three days after treatment, the pain score NRS decreased significantly from baseline median of 8 to 6 correlating with a response in six patients (55%). At one-month follow-up, which was available for nine patients, there was no pain recurrence, pain scores decreased significantly compared to baseline, and six patients (67%) obtained pain response. No treatment-related major complications were observed. More recently, Joo et al. (2015) evaluated the safety and effectiveness of a novel MRgFUS Conformal Bone System for the palliation of painful bone metastases. As opposed to table mounted systems, this applicator can be positioned on the target area with the patient in any position thereby optimizing patient comfort. Six painful metastatic bone lesions in five patients were treated and all patients showed significant pain relief within two weeks. Two patients experienced complete pain reduction that lasted for one year. The size of the enhancing soft tissue mass in metastatic lesions decreased, and new bone formation was seen on follow-up images (Fig. 3). No severe adverse events occurred.

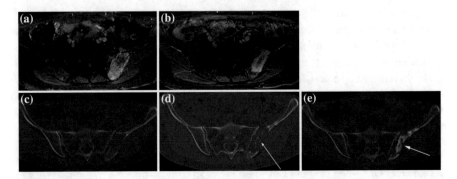

Fig. 3 Patient imaging before and after MRgFUS treatment for bone metastases. Comparison of **a** DCE-MRI before treatment and **b** at 90 days after treatment—note the decrease in size of the enhancing mass. Comparison of **c** CT before treatment and **d** at 90 days after treatment—note the new bone formation (*arrow*). **e** Further new bone formation (*arrow*) was seen on CT at one year post-treatment. Adapted with permission from Joo et al. (2015)

In summary, MRgFUS provides fast and durable relief of painful bone metastases as well as improved function in patients who failed or who are not candidates for radiation (Table 2). Given the impact of these clinically significant results, coupled with a favorable side effect profile, MRgFUS can now be considered a viable treatment option for painful bone metastases. Further studies are underway to assess the role of MRgFUS as a first-line therapy for patients with bone metastases (Table 1).

2.2 Breast Cancer

The first feasibility studies for use of MRgFUS in treatment of breast cancer date back over 15 years. Initial rates of complete or near complete ablation were 20–50%, but with ongoing refinement of the technique, more impressive results are now being reported. The first case report of MRgFUS for treatment of breast cancer was reported by Huber and colleagues (2001). The investigators described their experience with a patient who underwent MRgFUS five days prior to breast conservation surgery. Gianfelice and colleagues were the first to report on the accuracy of MRgFUS for treatment of a series of breast cancer patients, according to a treat-and-resect protocol. Twelve patients with invasive breast cancer were treated with two MRgFUS systems prior to surgery (Gianfelice et al. 2003). Histopathological analysis of resected tumor revealed a mean of 88% of cancer tissue necrosed in nine patients treated with the second generation system. However, residual tumor was noted at the periphery of the tumor in all patients, indicating the need for larger ablation margins in the range of 5 mm around the MR defined tumor. The complete list of studies can be found in Table 3.

Noting the importance of defining treatment effect with imaging, these investigators subsequently assessed the value of DCE-MRI parameters to monitor residual

Table 2 Clinical studies of MR-guided FUS for treatment of bone tumors

Study	Patients	Endpoints	FUS + MR	Follow-up	Assessment	Outcome (w = weeks, m = months)
Liberman et al. (2009)	31	Safety Palliation	Exablate 2000 1.5T MR	6 months	IBMCWP Imaging	72% OR, 36% CR, 36% PR, 24% NR and 4% PP at 3 m VAS: 5.9 (3.5–8.5) → 1.8 (0–8) at 3 m No AE reported
Napoli et al. (2013)	18	Palliation Tumor control	Exablate 2100 3T MR	3 months	IBMCWP MDA BPI Imaging	89% OR, 72% CR, 17% PR and 11% PP at 3 m VAS: 7.1 (4–10) → 2.5 (0–5) at 1 m → 1.0 (0–3) at 3 m No AE reported
Hurwitz et al. (2014)	112	Palliation Safety QoL	Exablate 2000 MR unknown	3 months	IBMCWP BPI Imaging	64% OR, 23% CR at 3 m NRS reduced 3.6 ± 3.1 points at 3 m Major AE: 2% fracture, <1% 3rd degree skin burn, neuropathy Minor AE: 32% pain, 2% fatigue, skin burn, <1% blood in urine, fever, myositis, numbness, skin rash
Huisman et al. (2014)	11	Safety Palliation	Philips Sonalleve 1.5T MR	1 month	IBMCWP OMED	67% OR, 11% CR and 56% PR at 1 m (n = 9) VAS: 8 (6–10) → 4 (0–7) at 1 m (n = 9) Minor AE: 9% pain, skin burn
Zaccagna et al. (2014)	72	Palliation QoL	Exablate 2100 MR unknown	6 months	IBMCWP QLQ-BM22 Imaging	47% CR, 40% PR, 13% PP at 6 m VAS: 6 (5–8) → 2 (0–3) at 6 m No AE reported
Bazzocchi et al. (2015)	64	Safety Palliation	Exablate 2100 1.5 MR	12 months	IBMCWP VAS	71% OR, 19% CR, 52%PR, 14% NR and 14% PP at 12 m VAS: 5.3 ± 2.7 → 2.7 ± 2.3 (1 m), 1.8 ± 2.1 (12 m) Minor AE: <2% skin burn, prostate inflammation
Joo et al. (2015)	5	Safety Palliation	Exablate 2100 3T MR	1 year	VAS Imaging	33% CR (12 m), 50% PR and 17% PP at 2 m VAS: 5.9 ± 1.9 → 2.1 ± 2.9 at 1 m Minor AE: 20% pain, 20% skin burn

(continued)

Table 2 (continued)

Study	Patients	Endpoints	FUS + MR	Follow-up	Assessment	Outcome (w = weeks, m = months)
Gu et al. (2015)	23	Safety Palliation	Exablate 2100 1.5T	3 months	NRS BPI-QoL QLQ-BM22	NRS: $6.0 \pm 1.5 \rightarrow 3.7 \pm 1.7$ (1w), 3.1 ± 2.0 (1 m), 2.2 ± 1.0 (3 m) BPI: $39 \pm 16 \rightarrow 27 \pm 18$ (1w), 26 ± 18 (1 m), 21 ± 18 (3 m) QLQ: $52 \pm 13 \rightarrow 44 \pm 12$ (1w), 42 ± 12 (1 m), 39 ± 12 (3 m) Minor AE: 13% pain, 4% numbness

AE Adverse event; *BPI-QoL* Brief pain inventory-quality of life; *CR* Complete response; *IBMCWP guidelines* International bone metastasis consensus working party; *MDA criteria* MD Anderson criteria; *MR* Magnetic resonance; *NR* No response; *NRS* Numeric rating scale (0–10); *OMED* Changes in analgesic intake; *OR* Overall response; *PR* Partial response; *PP* Pain progression; *QLQ-BM22* European Organization for Research and Treatment of Cancer-Quality of Life Questionnaire for patients with Bone Metastases; *VAS* Visual analogue scale (0–10)

Table 3 Clinical studies of MR-guided FUS for treatment of breast tumors

Study	Patients	Endpoints	FUS + MR	Follow-up	Assessment	Outcome
Huber et al. (2001)	1	Feasibility safety efficacy	Custom FUS 1.5T MR	5 days	Imaging Immuno-histochemistry	Lethal and sub lethal tumor damage Minor AE: mild pressure
Gianfelice et al. (2003)	12	Safety efficacy	Exablate 2000 (models 1 and 2) 1.5T MR	3–14 days	Imaging Histopathology	Model 1 (3/12): 100% PR (10–86% residual tumor) Model 2 (9/12): 22% CR and 78% PR (2–40% residual tumor) Minor AE: 100% pain, 17% skin burn
Gianfelice et al. (2003)	24	Feasibility safety efficacy	Exablate 2000 1.5 T MR	6 months	Imaging Histopathology	79% OR 21% NR or RR Minor AE: 100% pain, 4.2% skin burn
Gianfelice et al. (2003)	17	Safety efficacy	Exablate 2000 1.5T MR	3–14 days	Histopathology Imaging	23.5% CR 53% PR (< 10% residual cancer volume) 23.5% PR (30–75% residual cancer volume) No AE reported
Zippel et al. (2005)	10	Feasibility safety efficacy	Exablate 2000 MR Unknown	7–10 days	Histopathology	20% CR 20% PR (microscopic foci of residual tumor) 30% PR (10% residual tumor) 30% PR (10–30% residual tumor) Minor AE: pain, 10% skin burn
Khiat et al. (2006)	25	Efficacy	Exablate 2000 1.5T MR	3–14 days	Histopathology Imaging	27% CR 42% PR (<10% residual tumor) 27% PR (20–90% residual tumor)
Furusawa et al. (2006)	28	Safety efficacy	Exablate 2000 1.5T MR	2 weeks	Histopathology Imaging	54% CR, 46% PR Major AE: 4% 3rd degree burn Minor AE: 14% pain, 4% allergic reaction

(continued)

Table 3 (continued)

Study	Patients	Endpoints	FUS + MR	Follow-up	Assessment	Outcome
Furusawa et al. (2007)	21	Safety efficacy	Exablate 2000 1.5T MR	3–26 months	Histopathology Imaging	95% CR, 5% RR Minor AE: 10% skin burns
Napoli et al. (2013)	10	Efficacy	Exablate 2100 3T MR	21 days	Histopathology Imaging	90% CR 10% PR (15% residual tumor)
Merckel et al. (2016)	10	Safety efficacy	Philips Sonalleve 1.5T MR	2–10 days	Histopathology Imaging	60% PR, 30% NR and 10% data not available Minor AE: 20% nausea and vomiting, 20% pain

AE Adverse event; *CR* Complete response; *MR* Magnetic resonance; *NR* No response; *OR* Overall response; *PR* Partial response; *RR* Recurrence umor following MRgFUS treatment of breast tumors. DCE-MRI data were acquired before and after the MRgFUS treatment of 17 patients with breast tumors <3.5 cm. Tumors were surgically resected and the presence of residual tumor was determined by histopathological analysis. The percentage of residual tumor was correlated with three DCE-MRI parameters measured at the maximally enhancing site of each tumor. Notably, complete necrosis or less than 10% residual tumor was observed in 76% lesions at the time of surgery including 23% with complete response. Allowing for a seven day post-treatment delay, a good correlation was found between the DCE-MRI parameters and the percentage of residual viable tumor determined by histopathology. The authors concluded the results suggest that parameters from DCE-MRI data can provide a reliable non-invasive method for assessing residual tumor following MRgFUS treatment of breast tumors (Gianfelice et al. 2003).

In a follow-up report on 24 women with a single biopsy proven breast carcinoma who were not surgical candidates, MRgFUS was used as an adjunct to tamoxifen. Biopsy was performed after six month follow-up and retreatment with MRgFUS was performed if residual tumor was present, in which case a second biopsy was performed one month later. Treatment was well tolerated with only one second-degree skin burn associated with treatment. Overall, 79% had negative biopsy results after one or two treatment sessions. The presence of enhancement or lack thereof on follow-up MR imaging appeared to correlate well with biopsy findings (Gianfelice et al. 2003). Zippel et al. reported the results of a phase I trial with use of the same MRgFUS system with similar results (Zippel and Papa 2005). They treated 10 patients followed by lumpectomy one week later with complete necrosis noted in two patients. Khiat et al. (2006) further assessed tumor eradication and the effect of post-treatment delay for evaluation of MR images on the presence of residual cancer. Twenty-five patients with 26 tumors underwent histopatholog-ical analyses following MRgFUS showed no residual cancer in eight lesions (31%) and <10% residual cancer in 11 lesions (42%). They too recommended an interval of approximately seven days to determine the effectiveness of MRgFUS. More recently Napoli have reported a complete response rate of 90% and partial response rate of 10% in 10 patients treated with a 3 T system (Napoli et al. 2013), with a successful example shown in Fig. 4.

In follow-up to an initial feasibility report (Furusawa et al. 2006), Furusawa and colleagues published their experience with 21 cases of biopsy-proven invasive and noninvasive ductal carcinoma of the breast treated by MRgFUS. Median tumor size was 15 mm ranging from 5 to 50 mm. Seventeen patients received a single treat-ment and four patients were treated twice. With median follow-up of 14 months, one patient experienced local recurrence, with the remaining patients demonstrating no evidence of radiographic recurrence. Treatment was well tolerated, with skin burns in two patients (Furusawa et al. 2007). Furusawa subsequently has reported an update on an expanded cohort of 87 patients treated since 2005. The main inclusion criteria were biopsy-proven breast cancer up to 15 mm in size and well-demarcated mass seen in DCE-MRI. Postoperative needle biopsy was per-formed again within three weeks after ablation. The median age was 56 years and

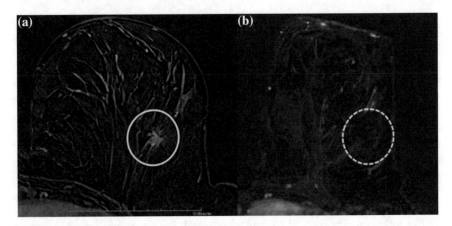

Fig. 4 Patient with breast cancer. **a** Gadolinium-enhanced T1 gradient recalled echo fat-saturated axial image shows the malignant highly vascular nodule. **b** After MRgFUS treatment, no residual enhancement of ablated lesion is detectable. Reprinted with permission from Napoli et al. (2013)

the average tumor size was 11 mm. With a median follow-up period of 68 months, no severe adverse events were noted. Local recurrence developed seven years after the initial treatment in only one invasive breast cancer case. There were no distant recurrences noted (Furusawa et al. 2015).

MRgFUS appears to be a promising method for replacing some surgical breast procedures with potential cosmetic benefits in very carefully selected patients. Two phase I/II clinical trials are current accruing patients for further confirmation of safety and effectiveness of this noninvasive procedure (Table 1).

2.3 Prostate Cancer

The most extensive clinical use of FUS has been for prostate cancer. Techniques include transrectal and transurethral approaches, with either whole gland or focal ablation. Of the tens of thousands of patients treated to date, almost all have been treated using ultrasound guidance, with regulatory approvals achieved in Europe, Asia, and recently in the United States. Although only a small fraction of prostate patients have been treated with MR guidance (Table 4), MR offers significant advantages over ultrasound guidance. These advantages include much better defined targeting with DCE-MRI and real-time temperature guidance to ensure adequate tumor ablation while protecting critical normal tissues such as urethra, bladder neck, rectum, and neurovascular bundles.

To date, five preliminary feasibility studies of MRgFUS for treatment of prostate cancer have been published, all involving eight or fewer patients treated with transurethral (Siddiqui et al. 2010; Chopra et al. 2012) or transrectal approach (Lindner et al. 2012; Napoli et al. 2013; Ghai et al. 2015). Taken together, these studies have demonstrated the ability of MRgFUS to effectively treat the intended

Table 4 Clinical studies of MR-guided FUS for prostate tumors

Study	Patients	Endpoints	FUS + MR	Follow-up	Assessment	Outcome (m = months)
Chopra et al. (2012)	8	Feasibility Safety	Custom FUS Transurethral 1.5T MR	4 months	Histopathology PSA screening	PSA: 2.7–13.1 ng/ml → 0–0.06 ng/ml Minor AE (n = 1): small bruise from pressure
Lindner et al. (2012)	1	Feasibility Safety	Exablate 2100 Transrectal 1.5T MR	1 month	Imaging IIEF, IPSS	Effective devascularization with persistent non-perfusion at the site of ablation at 1 m No AE reported
Napoli et al. (2013)	5	Feasibility Safety	Exablate 2100 Transrectal 3T MR	7–14 days	Histopathology	100% CR in the treated area, but all patients presented tumor outside the treated area No AE reported
Ghai et al. (2015)	4	Feasibility Safety efficacy	Exablate 2100 Transrectal 1.5T MR	6 months	Histopathology Imaging	75% CR and 25% PR in the treated areas Minor AE (n = 1): mild proctalgia
Chin et al. (2016)	30	Feasibility Safety efficacy	TULSA-PRO Transurethral 3T MR	12 months	Histopathology PSA IIEF, IPSS	14% CR, 55% PR, 31% NR or RR PSA 5.8 → 0.8 ng/ml (median, 12 m) Major AE: 3% epididymitis Minor AE: 50% hematuria, 33% urinary tract infections, 27% acute urinary retention, 17% pain and discomfort
Yuh et al. (2016)	3	Feasibility Safety Efficacy	Exablate 2100 Transrectal 3T MR	18 months	Histopathology PSA IIEF, IPSS Biopsy	Biopsy (6 m): 2 negative and 1 positive PSA: 1 decreased and 2 stable Minor AE (n = 1): hematuria from Foley trauma

AE Adverse event; *CR* Complete response; *IIEF* International index of erectile function; *IPSS* International prostate symptom score; *MR* Magnetic resonance; *NR* No response; *PR* Partial response; *PSA* Prostate specific antigen; *RR* Recurrence

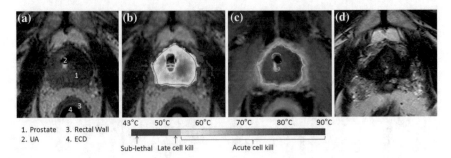

Fig. 5 Example MRI findings through the prostate mid-gland. **a** Treatment planning transverse MR image, showing the TULSA-PRO device in a patient: transurethral Ultrasound Applicator (UA) and Endorectal Cooling Device (ECD). **b** Maximum temperature measured during ultrasound treatment using real-time MR thermometry; the acute cell kill target temperature (≥ 55 °C) was shaped accurately and precisely to the treatment plan (*black contour*). **c** DCE-MRI image acquired immediately after treatment, demonstrating the hypointense region of non-perfused prostate tissue concordant with the acute ablative temperatures on MR thermometry. **d** Corresponding location in the prostate at 12-month follow-up, showing 85% reduced prostate volume. Image courtesy of Profound Medical Inc

targeted areas with few or no adverse effects. More recently, Chin et al. reported a series of 30 patients treated with a 3T MR guided transurethral system (Fig. 5). At the 12-months follow-up, a 14% complete and 55% partial response rates were noted with median PSA declining from 5.8 ng/ml pre-treatment to 0.8 ng/ml at 12 months. Urinary IPSS score improved slightly from 8 to 5 over the same period with no change in sexual function as measured by the IIEF. One major adverse event (epididymitis) was noted with all other toxicities scored as minor including 50% hematuria, 33% urinary tract infections, and 27% acute urinary retention (Chin et al. 2016).

At present, two phase I and one multi-institutional phase II study have been opened to assess the use of MRgFUS partial gland ablation in subjects with low or low-intermediate risk prostate cancer (Table 1). In the latter (NCT01226576), 80 patients with cT1c and cT2a, N0, M0, PSA ≤ 10 ng/ml and Gleason score 6 or 7 who may currently be on watchful waiting or active surveillance and not in need of imminent radical therapy are eligible. Up to two cancerous lesions may be identified for MRgFUS ablation in the prostate with each tumor not exceeding more than 10 mm in maximal linear dimension.

2.4 Brain Cancer

MRgFUS has great potential for treating brain tumors, because the technique could be used to ablate targeted tissue without injuring the normal brain. The main challenge for FUS in the brain is the high energy absorption in bone, which leads to excessive heating in the skull and adjacent brain parenchyma (Kobus and McDannold 2015). In addition, local variations in the skull thickness acts as defocusing lens (Hynynen 2010). Despite these challenges, several advances have now accelerated the development of transcranial MRgFUS. First, it was discovered that a relatively sharp focus can be produced through intact skull using a low frequency phased array (Sun and Hynynen 1998; Hynynen and Jolesz 1998) coupled with software that compensates for skull-induced distortions of FUS (Aubry et al. 2003). The skull heating problem can be overcome using a phased array applicator with large surface areas that spread the ultrasound energy over much of the skull (Sun and Hynynen 1999; Clement et al. 2000). Second, modern medical imaging can provide enough information to allow precise focusing non-invasively (Clement and Hynynen 2002; Pernot et al. 2003). The development of sophisticated MR imaging sequences permit high-resolution visualization of brain targets, as well as real-time tissue temperature maps, thus allowing real-time monitoring and guidance for FUS (McDannold and Jolesz 2000; Hynynen et al. 2000; Ishihara et al. 1995; Odeen et al. 2014).

In 2006, Ram and colleagues reported a phase I clinical study to treat three patients with recurrent glioblastoma multiforme (Ram et al. 2006). Prior to MRgFUS treatment, patients underwent a standard craniotomy over the tumor area to create the bony window necessary for penetration of the ultrasound waves. Histological analysis in one patient showed sharp delineation between viable tumor and thermocoagulated tumor at the treated site. One patient made an uneventful recovery, but nine months later showed evidence of tumor progression and died of her disease 10 months after the MRgFUS treatment. The remaining two patients were still alive after 33 and 38 months. Two adverse events were reported, a mild left hemiparesis that developed three days after treatment in one patient and mild transient worsening of preexisting dysphasia in another patient.

McDannold et al. (2010) published their experience with a dedicated MRgFUS system for brain applications (512 elements, 670 kHz) in three patients with high-grade glioma. All patients underwent the procedure under conscious sedation and tolerated the procedure well. Their results suggest that it is feasible to heat tumors in the brain without overheating the tissue at the brain surface and without performing a craniotomy. However, the targetable regions may be limited to deep and central locations in the brain. Nonetheless, these are precisely the locations where surgery is challenging or not an option. After this experience several technical adjustments were implemented (Lipsman et al. 2014), leading to an improved system with a conformal hemispherical shape (Fig. 6). This system has now been used to treat more than 200 patients with a range of neurological disorders through precise thermal ablation. No severe adverse events have been observed and the device has received regulatory approvals for treatment of movement disorders (essential tremor and Parkinson's tremor) and neuropathic pain in several countries (Foley et al. 2015).

Motivated by the excellent results in non-oncological applications, Coluccia and colleagues reported a case report to demonstrate feasibility and safety in a patient with recurrent glioblastoma (Coluccia et al. 2014). The patient received local anesthesia for the positioning of a stereotactic frame. Post-operative MR images showed well circumscribed areas of non-enhancing volumes at the location of

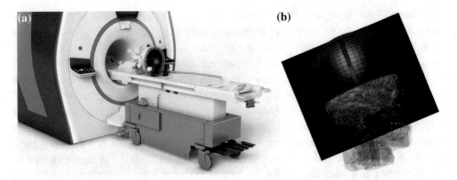

Fig. 6 a Commercially available transcranial MRgFUS system, which integrates a 650 kHz hemispheric array with 1024 ultrasound transducers into a clinical MRI system. The patient's head is fixed to the system in a stereotactic frame and a diaphragm placed around the patient's scalp before filling the transducer with degassed water to allow ultrasound waves to propagate into the head (Courtesy of INSIGHTEC Ltd.). **b** Treatment planning is based on initial MRI scans, with modelling to plan the dynamic scanning of heat focus for contiguous heating of large tissue volumes (Courtesy of IT'IS Foundation, Zürich, Switzerland)

sonicated tumor tissue. No adverse events were reported. While the total ablation volume is substantial (0.7 cc), it is still relatively small, i.e., 10% of the enhancing tumor volume (6.5 cc), and not sufficient for significant cytoreduction as is the key for sustained tumor control. Nonetheless, this result demonstrated, for the first time, the feasibility of using noninvasive transcranial MRgFUS to safely ablate brain tumor tissue.

2.5 Liver Cancer

Invasive thermal ablations with radio frequency (RF) or laser-probes have been shown to increase local tumor control and survival in patients with primary or metastatic liver tumors (Lin 2009). The use of FUS to ablate tumors deep in the liver offers the first completely noninvasive alternative to these techniques and it has been widely tested with US imaging guidance (USgFUS), mostly in China (Wu 2006; Wu et al. 2004). In a clinical trial with 55 patients with large (average 8 cm) hepatocellular carcinoma (HCC), Wu et al. demonstrated a complete ablation rate up to 69% without major complications, overall survival rates of 62% at 12 months and 35% at 18 months (Wu et al. 2004). Leslie et al. (2008) reported a phase II efficacy trial that showed USgFUS to be feasible. Using USgFUS, Xu et al. (2011) reported a two-year survival rate of 80% in patients with stage Ib HCC, 51% in stage IIa, and 47% in stage IIIa. In patients with unresectable HCC receiving USgFUS, it was demonstrated one- and three-year survival rates of 88% and 62%, respectively (Ng et al. 2011). Chan and colleagues evaluated the feasibility of USgFUS and patient survival in 27 patients with recurrent HCC (average tumor size of 1.8 cm) after first-line therapy with either hepatectomy or RF ablation at a median follow-up of 28 months. Complete tumor ablation was obtained in 85% of the patients. The three-year overall survival rate was 70% (Chan et al. 2013).

The principal feasibility of USgFUS ablation has been proven and extensively validated for parenchymal abdominal organs; introduction of MR-guidance in this field should thus be considered a natural evolution of this modality. There are only occasional reports of MRgFUS ablation in abdominal organs, mostly on animal models of liver tissue (Kopelman et al. 2006; Courivaud et al. 2014), with clinical trials in humans still ongoing (Table 1). Human treatments have been implemented so far with suspended respiration, which requires intubation and anesthesia. This respiratory gating approach overcomes liver motion during MR temperature measurement and also allows accurate targeting (Okada et al. 2006; Tokuda et al. 2008). More recently, real-time liver motion compensation has been developed and tested both in animal models (Quesson et al. 2011; Zachiu et al. 2015; Wijlemans et al. 2015; Holbrook et al. 2014) and in healthy volunteers (Napoli et al. 2013), potentially providing a chance for more accurate MRI guidance of liver ablation. Another difficulty in using FUS for abdominal targets is the presence of intervening anatomy such as ribs and bowel, which limit the acoustic window. To overcome this problem, sonications are delivered only between the ribs (Quesson et al. 2010; Zhou 2011).

So far, only single case reports were documented on the use of MRgFUS for treatment of liver cancer for a patient with HCC that refused RF ablation (Okada et al. 2006). The tumor measured about 15 mm in diameter and was located in the lateral segment of the liver, where there was no rib or bowel loop in the path of the ultrasound beam. Using respiratory gating, the tumor was completely ablated. In 2013, Napoli et al. performed a successful MRgFUS ablation in one patient with unifocal HCC, who was not eligible for other treatment options (Napoli et al. 2013). Post-treatment follow-up revealed a decrease of α-fetoprotein compared to baseline levels. Treatment efficacy was evaluated with DCE-MRI, revealing an extensive decrease of contrast uptake from tumor after MRgFUS ablation compared to baseline examination, correlating with significant reduction of symptom severity. More recently, Anzidei et al. (2014) presented a study designed to evaluate the feasibility and safety of MRgFUS for treatment of solid tumors in the upper abdomen, including one patient with HCC. Treatment response was evaluated by assessing the non-perfused volume (NPV) of ablated tissue at MR and the degree of pain severity. Immediately after treatment and at one-month follow-up, the lesion showed complete ablation (100% NPV); six-month follow-up images showed a small focus of recurrent tumor tissue along the lateral edge of the ablation zone, with a NPV of 85%. Histological analysis after liver transplantation showed fibrosis in the ablated area with minimal local tumor recurrence.

In summary, MRgFUS for liver lesions is still at an early stage due to the limited therapeutic window through the ribcage and complications from respiratory motion. Nonetheless, the aforementioned case studies indicate that MRgFUS for liver ablation is feasible. The integration of recent technology will allow the use of a higher number of phased-array elements and MRI-based tracking and gating, which will permit the acoustic beams to be synchronized with the moving organ to allow treatment of freely breathing patients.

2.6 Pancreatic Cancer

Anzidei and colleagues have reported the results of a pilot study with six patients assessing feasibility, safety, pain palliation, and potential for local tumor control with MRgFUS for pancreatic cancer (Anzidei et al. 2014). Outcome assessments with a follow-up between three and six months were based on imaging for response, yielding a 83% complete and 17% partial response rates. The VAS scale was used to assess pain and it decreased from an average of 7.3 pre-treatment to 3.8 one month post-treatment, which was consistent with a clinically meaningful improvement in pain. More recently, Jove-Vidal and colleagues reported encouraging results with USgFUS in 45 patients with unresected tumors treated between 2008 and 2015 with 83% overall response rate as assessed at eight weeks, with an encouraging median survival of 16 months and overall survival of 34% at five-year follow-up. The toxicity profile included the following major complications: severe pancreatitis (4%), third-degree skin burn that required plastic surgery (4%), and duodenal perforation (2%). These early results with USgFUS await validation including with use of MR-guided techniques (Vidal-Jove et al. 2016).

2.7 Soft Tissue Tumors

MRgFUS clinical studies for soft-tissue tumors are limited. In 2015, Ghanouni and colleagues reported a clinical study with seven patients with desmoid tumors, two patients with arteriovenous malformation (AVM) and one patient with a sarcoma in the thigh (Ghanouni et al. 2015). The average NPV for desmoid tumors (42–1010 cc) was 58%, whereas the sarcoma (20 cc) was 97%. Five of the desmoid tumor patients were included in a subsequent multicenter trial with 15 patients (Ghanouni et al. 2016). The median viable targeted tumor volume decreased 63%, corresponding to a decrease from 105 to 54 ml in volume. Pain response was also assessed, with a significant pain reduction (NRS) from 6 to 1 after MRgFUS treatment. Only minor complications were observed. The authors concluded that MRgFUS may safely and effectively treat extra-abdominal desmoid tumors.

Further studies are required to assess the role of MRgFUS as first-line therapy in patients with soft tissue tumors. There are currently three clinical trials open for accrual, including a phase I/II study to determine the safety and efficacy of MRgFUS in the treatment of soft tissue tumors of the extremities (NCT01965002) and a phase I study to determine if MRgFUS is safe and feasible for treatment of children with refractory or relapsed solid tumors (NCT02076906). The last clinical study is a multimodality approach that aims to determine whether Doxil (liposomal doxorubicin) given prior to MRgFUS hyperthermia is safe for the treatment of pediatric and young adult patients with recurrent and refractory solid tumors (NCT02557854). A preliminary report of this trial included seven tumors in six patients with osteosarcoma (n = 3), Ewing sarcoma (n = 3) and neurofibrosarcoma (n = 1). The MR thermometry (MRT) quality results of lower extremities was sufficient to control MRgFUS hyperthermia, but motion compensation or breath may be required to achieve reliable MRT in pelvic and abdominal tumors in pediatric patients (Laetsch et al. 2016).

2.8 Cervical Cancer

The first MRgFUS application to receive clinical certification was the treatment of uterine fibroids that received CE Mark in 2002 and FDA approval in 2004 (Dick and Gedroyc 2010). Despite the success in treating these benign neoplasms of the uterus (Clark et al. 2014), only one clinical case of treating cervical carcinoma with MRgFUS has been reported. Machtinger et al. (2008) presented a case report for pain relief in a 29-year-old patient suffering from recurrent cervical carcinoma. This patient failed traditional treatments and underwent two MRgFUS treatments two weeks apart, resulting in a substantial decrease in pelvic pain. No adverse events were reported during the procedure or during the follow-up. The patient remained free of pain for four months after treatment. A 35 patient pilot study started in 2016 to determine whether or not it is feasible to use MRgFUS to treat symptomatic pain and bleeding from recurrent gynecological malignancies with an acceptable safety profile (NCT02714621).

2.9 Colorectal Cancer

The colon and rectum sites are particularly difficult to heat with noninvasive focused ultrasound due to the shadowing effect of the sacral bone. In 2004, researchers in China published a study suggesting that USgFUS ablation combined with radiation could be safe and effective in patients with rectal carcinoma (Jun-Qun et al. 2004). Later, in 2011, researchers in London reported a single case of advanced, recurrent rectal carcinoma treated with transrectal focused ultrasound (Monzon et al. 2011). These limited clinical results have been supplemented with promising preclinical studies. A recent preclinical study showed that FUS along with gold nanoparticles and pulsed light, could shrink tumors (Sazgarnia et al. 2013), and another preclinical study suggested that FUS can enhance the targeted delivery of chemotherapy (Park et al. 2013).

Clearly, recurrent rectal cancer is a vexing clinical problem and current retreatment protocols have limited efficacy (Ahmed et al. 2014). With this in mind, a clinical trial was designed to test the hypothesis that MRgFUS hyperthermia is technically feasible and can be safely used in combination with concurrent reirradiation and chemotherapy for the treatment of recurrent rectal cancer without increased side-effects (NCT02528175). The first report from this trial includes a patient with rectal recurrence in the pelvic sidewall. During MRgFUS, the patient was under conscious sedation, and provided verbal feedback to the physician to decide when to pause the treatment. The patient did not report pain, and has no adverse effects after 90 days of follow-up. Therapeutic temperatures were achieved with no treatment-related toxicity (Chu et al. 2016).

2.10   Emerging Clinical Applications of MRgFUS

MRgFUS treatment of renal disease must overcome many similar challenges as reported for treatment of liver cancer due to their similar location in the ribcage (Quesson et al. 2011). For this reason, the clinical trial NCT01197820 addressed the technical feasibility of MRgFUS for treatment of both liver and kidney with a focus on challenges related to organ motion. The safety and feasibility of USgFUS was previously established in 2003 (Wu et al. 2003) and later in 2005 (Illing et al. 2005), but the ablation of liver tumors was achieved more consistently than for kidney tumors: 100% versus 67%, assessed radiologically. The primary reason relates to higher blood perfusion in kidneys, which carries away heat more efficiently than in liver (Quesson et al. 2011). A recent preclinical study reported the use of MRgFUS to create renal lesions on six mechanically-ventilated pigs (Saeed et al. 2016). Histopathology examinations and DCE-MRI showed presence of coagulative necrosis, interstitial hemorrhage and vascular damage in the renal target lesions. The authors suggested that in order to address the high blood perfusion in kidneys, the MRgFUS could be used to mediate vascular occlusion prior to targeting the tumor.

One of the most recent target applications for MRgFUS is head and neck cancer. Although there are no current clinical results, Lee and colleagues published the clinical protocol of a pilot study to assess safety, toxicity and feasibility of MRgFUS in the head and neck region (Lee et al. 2016). This prospective trial plans to recruit 10 patients to undergo MRgFUS prior to palliative radiotherapy. The authors hypothesize that treatment will cause de-vascularization and necrosis of the targeted lesion by heating the tissue to 55–90 °C during approximately 30 s. Also, a margin of 1 cm will be left between the ablation zone and neighboring critical structures. Serious adverse events and toxicity will be evaluated at 1, 7, 14, 30, 90 days follow-up, and post-MR imaging will be performed. In addition, clinical studies are under consideration to examine the use of MRgFUS to enhance standard chemo-radiotherapy treatments of locally advanced, unresectable head and neck tumors.

Pre-clinical work has been completed or is ongoing for several additional clinical applications. Because of diaphragm movement and air content of ventilated lungs, lung tumors have never been treated with FUS (Wolfram et al. 2014). However, Lesser et al. proposed flooding one lung to produce a suitable acoustic pathway to treat lung tumors with MRgFUS. This approach was investigated in in vivo pig models and in ex vivo human tissues (Wolfram et al. 2014; Lesser et al. 2016). In other site, Karakitosis et al. presented a feasibility study to induce thermal ablation in the vertebral body and intervertebral discs using MRgFUS. The study demonstrated that the heating pattern could induce thermal ablation in the target, with no damage in adjacent critical structures such as nerves (Karakitsios et al. 2016). The feasibility of esophageal thermal ablation using intraluminal MRgFUS has also been demonstrated in a preclinical setting (Melodelima et al. 2005).

3 Future Directions

Increasing clinical interest in MRgFUS has fueled continued development of the modality for a variety of clinical applications. Future directions within the field are expected to utilize ongoing research in both the MR and ultrasound fields to further leverage current advancements. These advancements are in various stages of development or early clinical adoption and are expected to benefit the field of MRgFUS for oncological applications.

3.1 Targeted Drug Delivery

A variety of applications using MRgFUS for targeted drug delivery have recently been presented in the literature. The applications generally focus on areas that are amenable to both MR and US imaging, and that have also presented historical challenges for delivery of therapeutics. One such area is the localized delivery of therapeutic agents across the blood brain barrier (BBB). Delivery of therapeutics from the vasculature to brain extracellular fluid is greatly limited by the presence of tight junctions, which restrict passage of molecules larger than 400 Da or those that form greater than eight hydrogen bonds with water. These exclusions rule out direct passage of over 99% of therapeutic drugs (Pardridge 2005). However, as ultrasound waves propagate through tissue, they interact with dissolved gases in a process known as cavitation, leading to the formation of gas-filled microbubbles that has been shown to temporarily increase BBB permeability (De Smet et al. 2013; Liu et al. 2012; Diaz et al. 2014; Nance et al. 2014; Marquet et al. 2011). Using this approach, Nance et al. (2014) demonstrated in rats that MRgFUS enables delivery of 60 nm nanoparticles across the BBB when disrupted by microbubble cavitation, making localized delivery of drugs to the brain feasible. This approach has also been demonstrated in non-human primates (Marquet et al. 2011), and a first-in-humans clinical trial is currently underway for the delivery of doxorubicin to solid brain tumors (NCT02343991). In addition, it has been shown in a preclinical setting (via both MRI and histological analyses) that the BBB reverts to its original structure without permanent damage within four hours after the end of the sonication (Tung et al. 2011).

Targeted drug delivery can be achieved using MRgFUS by encapsulating the drug of choice within either a temperature or acoustic pressure sensitive carrier. These carriers can be injected systemically, but release their contents only when triggered within the targeted area. Temperature-sensitive liposomes have been fabricated to deliver anticancer drugs at moderate temperatures (Ponce et al. 2006; Escoffre et al. 2013; Zagar et al. 2014). After systemic injection, these liposomes aggregate within the tumor space either as a function of the enhanced permeation and retention effect, or through passive targeting with the conjugation of tumor-specific peptides on the surface of the carrier (Ponce et al. 2006). Localized hyperthermia using MRgFUS can then be used to generate localized release of the chemotherapeutics. Similarly, drugs can be conjugated or encapsulated within ultrasound-sensitive microbubbles or nanoemulsions, and their localized release triggered with focused ultrasound (Rapoport et al. 2013; Eisenbrey et al. 2010, 2015). These results have demonstrated significant advantages in preclinical cancer models (Cochran et al. 2011; Zhu et al. 2016), and eventual clinical trials are expected.

Similar approaches using the combination of MRgFUS and microbubble cavitation have been used in gene transfection applications. Gene therapy translation has generally suffered from low overall delivery and transfection efficiencies (Al-Dosari and Gao 2009). Using the bioeffects described above, different groups have shown improved delivery and transfection efficiencies using the combination MRgFUS and microbubble cavitation. This work is currently in preclinical stages and covers a wide range of applications including improved gene transfection in the spinal cord (Weber-Adrian et al. 2015), treatment of cardiovascular disease (Chen et al. 2013), and solid tumors (Carson et al. 2011). These encouraging results are expected to translate to pilot clinical trials in the near future.

3.2   Image Optimization

3.2.1   Image Fusion

As imaging modalities, the inherent strengths and limitations of MR and ultrasound make them natural adjuncts in diagnostic imaging. MR suffers from relatively low temporal resolution making guidance difficult in soft tissues prone to respiratory motion such as the liver and kidneys (Napoli et al. 2013). USgFUS for liver and renal tumors is more prevalent in the literature in part due to the favorable cost and ability of ultrasound image guidance to effectively deal with organ motion (Schlesinger et al. 2013). However, hepatic lesions visible on MR may not be seen on ultrasound imaging, particularly lesions less than 2 cm and those closer to the diaphragm (Lee et al. 2010), limiting the ability to ablate these masses with USgFUS. Image fusion systems may be an alternative to these limitations. These systems use co-registration of MR or CT image stacks with real-time ultrasound data using magnetic sensors attached to the ultrasound transducer and a stationary reference center stationed near the patient (Ewertsen et al. 2013). Electromagnetic needle tracking systems can also be implemented for MR/US fusion guided procedures and have been used for a variety of interventions including liver and kidney mass biopsy and ablation and targeted prostate biopsy (Ewertsen et al. 2013). These approaches have improved confidence in targeting technically challenging lesions

(Kang and Rhim 2015) and should be applicable to FUS therapies in the future. As an alternative, but similar approach, MR compatible ultrasound transducers have also been developed enabling real-time MR/US hybrid guidance (Petrusca et al. 2013). This approach would benefit from the inclusion of both the real-time motion compensation of ultrasound guidance and MR-thermometry treatment monitoring.

3.2.2 Synergistic MR and US Contrast Agents

Multimodality contrast agents are expected to be useful for MRgFUS. These agents will enable better image guidance and monitoring by improving visualization of targeted regions on both modalities. Additionally, inclusion of ultrasound contrast agents or nanoemulsions have been shown to lower cavitation thresholds in FUS, thereby selectively sensitizing areas of interest to tissue heating (Kopechek et al. 2014; Farny et al. 2010). Multimodality contrast agents for ultrasound and MR imaging have been developed consisting of microbubbles with either iron oxide or gadolinium in the shell (Teraphongphom et al. 2015). More recently, these particles have been modified to include doxorubicin for potential targeted cancer therapy (Teraphongphom 2016). An example of this work is provided in Fig. 7, showing attachment of iron oxide nanoparticles conjugated to a poly-lactic acid microbubble on transmission electron microscopy, and these same multi-modality agents on fluorescence microscopy showing the presence of doxorubicin (in red) within the shell of the microbubble. While these particles are still in early preclinical studies, their potential clinical impact may be significant in that they combine both the therapeutic and imaging benefits described above.

3.3 Multimodality MRgFUS Treatments

Perhaps the greatest benefits of MRgFUS in oncology remain to be realized through its integration in multimodality oncologic care. Many cancer patients are treated with combinations of surgery, radiation, and chemotherapy; yet there is a paucity of research exploring the integration of ablative therapies such as MRgFUS with other anti-cancer therapies. Beyond the utility of MRgFUS for targeted drug delivery and opening the blood brain barrier, MRgFUS may also augment effects of standard approaches to chemotherapy through enhanced effects mediated at the heated—but non-ablated—rim of tissue adjacent to the ablation zone. Moderate temperature elevation in this tumor margin should significantly enhance the effects of radio-therapy, including complementary tumor cell killing based on stage of the cell cycle, pH, degree of hypoxia, and repair inhibition of radiation induced DNA damage (Hurwitz and Stauffer 2014). Benefits seen in randomized studies com-bining hyperthermia and radiation or chemotherapy for many tumor types point to the promise of similar benefits with thermal therapy induced with MRgFUS (Hurwitz and Stauffer 2014). Likewise, hyperthermia has been shown in preclinical models to have multiple anti-tumor effects mediated through augmentation of immune response across the cancer-immunity cycle (Toraya-Brown and Fiering 2014). Tumor antigen spillage with MRgFUS ablation is one of many ways this

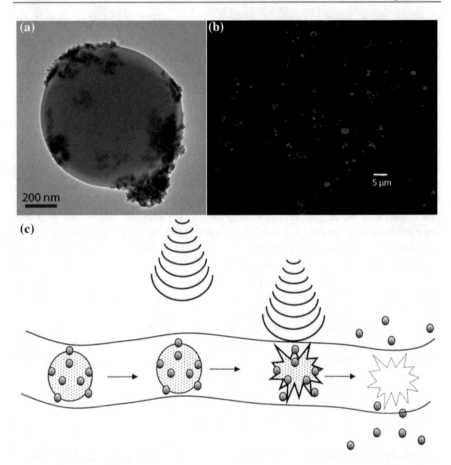

Fig. 7 Poly-lactic acid ultrasound contrast agents loaded with iron oxide nanoparticles which are visible on transmission electron microscopy (**a**) and doxorubicin which is visible on fluorescence microscopy (**b**) for targeted drug delivery with MRgFUS (Courtesy of Dr. Nutte Teraphongphom). **c** Schematic representation of substance delivery using ultrasound-targeted microbubble destruction. An ultrasound contrast agent with an attached or incorporated bioactive substance is administered into the vasculature and will distribute throughout the capillaries. Ultrasound can then destroy microbubbles in the target region, thus releasing the transported substance into the surrounding tissue [Reprinted with permission (Bekeredjian et al. 2005)]

modality may work across the therapeutic temperature profile to make immunotherapy more effective. In addition, the aforementioned mechanical effects combined with thermal effects can induce vasoconstriction or even hemostasis. This strategy is being considered as a noninvasive method to cut off the blood supply to tumors, effectively starving them of vital nutrients and making them more vulnerable to other treatments (Goertz 2015).

Finally, new techniques are in development that should shorten treatment time. Strategies to accomplish this important goal include the injection of microbubbles to increase the absorption of acoustic energy, optimized scanning algorithms, and also the use of spiral sonications; all techniques that should reduce the time of MRgFUS treatments.

4 Concluding Remarks

Without doubt, the next decade will see rapid advances in both clinical and technological application of MR-guided focused ultrasound. As results from preclinical models translate to clinical trials, clinicians will have a powerful new tool for expand treatment capabilities for their cancer patients who may not want or cannot tolerate an operation. MRgFUS may also serve as a powerful adjuvant or enhancer to other treatments, including gene therapy, radiation therapy, chemotherapy, and immunotherapy. Larger studies with longer follow-up will help characterize the long-term clinical and radiological effects, allowing better comparisons with approved modalities. Despite impressive temperature (0.1 °C) and spatial (1 mm diameter) accuracy, the most dramatic advances for MRgFUS will be technical. Currently, the typical procedure length for MRgFUS is of the order of 2–4 h. With evolving software, off-line analysis of tumor anatomy and its surroundings, as well as experience, procedure length will be significantly shortened. In summary, MRgFUS is a rapidly emerging technology offering a non-invasive treatment option either as monotherapy or in combination with other anti-neoplastic modalities.

References

Ahmed S, Johnson K, Ahmed O, Iqbal N (2014) Advances in the management of colorectal cancer: from biology to treatment. Int J Colorectal Dis 29(9):1031–1042. doi:10.1007/s00384-014-1928-5

Al-Dosari MS, Gao X (2009) Nonviral gene delivery: principle, limitations, and recent progress. AAPS J 11(4):671–681. doi:10.1208/s12248-009-9143-y

Anzidei M, Napoli A, Sandolo F, Marincola BC, Di Martino M, Berloco P, Bosco S, Bezzi M, Catalano C (2014a) Magnetic resonance-guided focused ultrasound ablation in abdominal moving organs: a feasibility study in selected cases of pancreatic and liver cancer. Cardiovasc Intervent Radiol 37(6):1611–1617. doi:10.1007/s00270-014-0861-x

Anzidei M, Marincola BC, Bezzi M, Brachetti G, Nudo F, Cortesi E, Berloco P, Catalano C, Napoli A (2014b) Magnetic resonance-guided high-intensity focused ultrasound treatment of locally advanced pancreatic adenocarcinoma: preliminary experience for pain palliation and local tumor control. Invest Radiol 49(12):759–765. doi:10.1097/RLI.0000000000000080

Aubry JF, Tanter M, Pernot M, Thomas JL, Fink M (2003) Experimental demonstration of noninvasive transskull adaptive focusing based on prior computed tomography scans. J Acoust Soc Am 113(1):84–93. doi:10.1121/1.1529663

Avedian RS, Gold G, Ghanouni P, Pauly KB (2011) Magnetic resonance guided high-intensity focused ultrasound ablation of musculoskeletal tumors. Curr Orthop Pract 22(4):303–308. doi:10.1097/BCO.0b013e318220dad5

Bazzocchi A, Facchini G, Spinnato P, Donatiello S, Diano D, Rimondi E, Battaglia M, Albisinni U (2015) Palliation of painful bone metastases: the "Rizzoli" experience. In: Annual congress of the European society of musculoskeletal radiology, York, UK, 18–20 June 2015. pp P-0136. doi:10.1594/essr2015/P-0136

Bekeredjian R, Grayburn PA, Shohet RV (2005) Use of ultrasound contrast agents for gene or drug delivery in cardiovascular medicine. J Am Coll Cardiol 45(3):329–335. doi:10.1016/j.jacc.2004.08.067

Berenson JR, Rajdev L, Broder M (2006) Cancer biology and therapy. J Am Coll Radiol 5 (9):1078–1081. doi:10.4161/cbt.5.9.3306

Carson AR, McTiernan CF, Lavery L, Hodnick A, Grata M, Leng XP, Wang JJ, Chen XC, Modzelewski RA, Villanueva FS (2011) Gene therapy of carcinoma using ultrasound-targeted microbubble destruction. Ultrasound Med Biol 37(3):393–402. doi:10.1016/j.ultrasmedbio.2010.11.011

Catane R, Beck A, Inbar Y, Rabin T, Shabshin N, Hengst S, Pfeffer RM, Hanannel A, Dogadkin O, Liberman B, Kopelman D (2007) MR-guided focused ultrasound surgery (MRgFUS) for the palliation of pain in patients with bone metastases - preliminary clinical experience. Ann Oncol 18(1):163–167. doi:10.1093/annonc/mdl335

Chan AC, Cheung TT, Fan ST, Chok KS, Chan SC, Poon RT, Lo CM (2013) Survival analysis of high-intensity focused ultrasound therapy versus radiofrequency ablation in the treatment of recurrent hepatocellular carcinoma. Ann Surg 257(4):686–692. doi:10.1097/SLA.0b013e3182822c02

Chen ZY, Lin Y, Yang F, Jiang L, Ge S (2013) Gene therapy for cardiovascular disease mediated by ultrasound and microbubbles. Cardiovasc Ultrasound 11:11. doi:10.1186/1476-7120-11-11

Chin JL, Billia M, Relle J, Roethke MC, Popeneciu IV, Kuru TH, Hatiboglu G, Mueller-Wolf MB, Motsch J, Romagnoli C, Kassam Z, Harle CC, Hafron J, Nandalur KR, Chronik BA, Burtnyk M, Schlemmer HP, Pahernik S (2016) Magnetic resonance imaging-guided transurethral ultrasound ablation of prostate tissue in patients with localized prostate cancer: a prospective phase 1 clinical trial. Eur Urol S0302-2838 (15):01238-01235. doi:10.1016/j.eururo.2015.12.029

Chopra R, Colquhoun A, Burtnyk M, N'Djin WA, Kobelevskiy I, Boyes A, Siddiqui K, Foster H, Sugar L, Haider MA, Bronskill M, Klotz L (2012) MR imaging-controlled transurethral ultrasound therapy for conformal treatment of prostate tissue: initial feasibility in humans. Radiology 265(1):303–313. doi:10.1148/radiol.12112263

Chow E, Hird A, Velikova G, Johnson C, Dewolf L, Bezjak A, Wu J, Shafiq J, Sezer O, Kardamakis D, van der Linden Y, Ma B, Castro M, Foro Arnalot P, Ahmedzai S, Clemons M, Hoskin P, Yee A, Brundaye M, Bottomley A, Grp EQL (2009) The European organisation for research and treatment of cancer quality of life questionnaire for patients with bone metastases: the EORTC QLQ-BM22. Eur J Cancer 45(7):1146–1152. doi:10.1016/j.ejca.2008.11.013

Chu W, Staruch R, Pichardo S, Huang Y, Mougenot C, Tillander M, Köhler M, Ylihautala M, McGuffin M, Czarnota G, Hynynen K (2016) MR-HIFU mild hyperthermia for locally recurrent rectal cancer: temperature mapping and heating quality in first patient. In: 12th International congress of hyperthermic oncology (ICHO 2016), New Orleans, LA, 11–15 April 2016, p 144

Clark NA, Mumford SL, Segars JH (2014) Reproductive impact of MRI-guided focused ultrasound surgery for fibroids: a systematic review of the evidence. Curr Opin Obstet Gynecol 26(3):151–161. doi:10.1097/GCO.0000000000000070

Cleeland CS, Ryan KM (1994) Pain assessment: global use of the brief pain inventory. Ann Acad Med Singapore 23(2):129–138

Clement GT, Hynynen K (2002) A non-invasive method for focusing ultrasound through the human skull. Phys Med Biol 47(8):1219–1236. doi:10.1088/0031-9155/47/8/301

Clement GT, Sun J, Giesecke T, Hynynen K (2000) A hemisphere array for non-invasive ultrasound brain therapy and surgery. Phys Med Biol 45(12):3707–3719. doi:10.1088/0031-9155/45/12/314

Cochran MC, Eisenbrey JR, Soulen MC, Schultz SM, Ouma RO, White SB, Furth EE, Wheatley MA (2011) Disposition of ultrasound sensitive polymeric drug carrier in a rat hepatocellular carcinoma model. Acad Radiol 18(11):1341–1348. doi:10.1016/j.acra.2011. 06.013

Coluccia D, Fandino J, Schwyzer L, O'Gorman R, Remonda L, Anon J, Martin E, Werner B (2014) First noninvasive thermal ablation of a brain tumor with MR-guided focused ultrasound. J Ther Ultrasound 2:17. doi:10.1186/2050-5736-2-17

Copelan A, Hartman J, Chehab M, Venkatesan AM (2015) High-Intensity focused ultrasound: current status for image-guided therapy. Semin Intervent Radiol 32(4):398–415. doi:10.1055/s-0035-1564793

Costelloe CM, Chuang HH, Madewell JE, Ueno NT (2010) Cancer response criteria and bone metastases: RECIST 1.1, MDA and PERCIST. J Cancer 1:80–92

Courivaud F, Kazaryan AM, Lund A, Orszagh VC, Svindland A, Marangos IP, Halvorsen PS, Jebsen P, Fosse E, Hol PK, Edwin B (2014) Thermal fixation of swine liver tissue after magnetic resonance-guided high-intensity focused ultrasound ablation. Ultrasound Med Biol 40(7):1564–1577. doi:10.1016/j.ultrasmedbio.2014.02.007

Dahl O (1995) Interaction of heat and drugs in vitro and in vivo. In: Seegenschmiedt MH, Fessenden P, Vernon CC (eds) Thermoradiotherapy and thermochemotherapy: volume 1, biology, physiology and physics. Springer-Verlag, Berlin, pp 103–121

De Haas-Kock DFM, Buijsen J, Pijls-Johannesma M, Lutgens L, Lammering G, van Mastrigt GAPG, De Ruysscher DKM, Lambin P, van der Zee J (2009) Concomitant hyperthermia and radiation therapy for treating locally advanced rectal cancer. Cochrane Database Syst Rev (3):CD006269. doi:10.1002/14651858.CD006269.pub2

De Smet M, Hijnen NM, Langereis S, Elevelt A, Heijman E, Dubois L, Lambin P, Grull H (2013) Magnetic resonance guided high-intensity focused ultrasound mediated hyperthermia improves the intratumoral distribution of temperature-sensitive liposomal doxorubicin. Invest Radiol 48 (6):395–405. doi:10.1097/RLI.0b013e3182806940

Dewhirst MW, Vujaskovic Z, Jones E, Thrall D (2005) Re-setting the biologic rationale for thermal therapy. Int J Hyperthermia 21(8):779–790. doi:10.1080/02656730500271668

Dewhirst MW, Das SK, Stauffer PR, Craciunescu OA, Vujaskovic Z, Thrall D (2012) Hyperthermia. In: Gunderson LL, Tepper JE (eds) Clinical radiation oncology, 3rd edn. Elsevier, Philladelphia, pp 385–403

Diaz RJ, McVeigh PZ, O'Reilly MA, Burrell K, Bebenek M, Smith C, Etame AB, Zadeh G, Hynynen K, Wilson BC, Rutka JT (2014) Focused ultrasound delivery of Raman nanoparticles across the blood-brain barrier: potential for targeting experimental brain tumors. Nanomedicine 10(5):1075–1087. doi:10.1016/j.nano.2013.12.006

Dick EA, Gedroyc WM (2010) ExAblate magnetic resonance-guided focused ultrasound system in multiple body applications. Expert Rev Med Devices 7(5):589–597. doi:10.1586/erd.10.38

Diederich CJ, Hynynen K (1999) Ultrasound technology for hyperthermia. Ultrasound Med Biol 25(6):871–887. doi:10.1016/S0301-5629(99)00048-4

Eisenbrey JR, Burstein OM, Kambhampati R, Forsberg F, Liu JB, Wheatley MA (2010) Development and optimization of a doxorubicin loaded poly(lactic acid) contrast agent for ultrasound directed drug delivery. J Control Release 143(1):38–44. doi:10.1016/j.jconrel.2009. 12.021

Eisenbrey JR, Albala L, Kramer MR, Daroshefski N, Brown D, Liu JB, Stanczak M, O'Kane P, Forsberg F, Wheatley MA (2015) Development of an ultrasound sensitive oxygen carrier for oxygen delivery to hypoxic tissue. Int J Pharm 478(1):361–367. doi:10.1016/j.ijpharm.2014. 11.023

Escoffre JM, Novell A, de Smet M, Bouakaz A (2013) Focused ultrasound mediated drug delivery from temperature-sensitive liposomes: in-vitro characterization and validation. Phys Med Biol 58(22):8135–8151. doi:10.1088/0031-9155/58/22/8135

Ewertsen C, Saftoiu A, Gruionu LG, Karstrup S, Nielsen MB (2013) Real-time image fusion involving diagnostic ultrasound. AJR Am J Roentgenol 200(3):W249–W255. doi:10.2214/AJR.12.8904

Farny CH, Holt RG, Roy RA (2010) The correlation between bubble-enhanced HIFU heating and cavitation power. IEEE Trans Biomed Eng 57(1):175–184. doi:10.1109/Tbme.2009.2028133

Foley J, Kassell N, LeBlang S, Weber P, Snell JEM, Paeng DK (2015) Moore D workshop summary. In: Focused ultrasound for glioblastoma workshop, Charlottesville, VA, 9–10 Nov 2015. Focused Ultrasound Foundation, pp 4–6

Furusawa H, Namba K, Thomsen S, Akiyama F, Bendet A, Tanaka C, Yasuda Y, Nakahara H (2006) Magnetic resonance-guided focused ultrasound surgery of breast cancer: reliability and effectiveness. J Am Coll Surg 203(1):54–63. doi:10.1016/j.jamcollsurg.2006.04.002

Furusawa H, Namba K, Nakahara H, Tanaka C, Yasuda Y, Hirabara E, Imahariyama M, Komaki K (2007) The evolving non-surgical ablation of breast cancer: MR guided focused ultrasound (MRgFUS). Breast Cancer 14(1):55–58. doi:10.2325/jbcs.14.55

Furusawa H, Shidooka J, Inomata M, Hirabara E, Nakahara H, Ymaguchi Y (2015) MRgFUS of small breast cancer: what should be learned from a case of local recurrence. J Ther Ultrasound 3(Suppl 1):O75–O75. doi:10.1186/2050-5736-3-S1-O75

Ghai S, Louis AS, Van Vliet M, Lindner U, Haider MA, Hlasny E, Spensieri P, Van Der Kwast TH, McCluskey SA, Kucharczyk W, Trachtenberg J (2015) Real-time MRI-guided focused ultrasound for focal therapy of locally confined low-risk prostate cancer: feasibility and preliminary outcomes. AJR Am J Roentgenol 205(2):W177–W184. doi:10.2214/AJR.14.13098

Ghanouni P, Pauly KB, Bitton R, Avedian R, Bucknor M, Gold G (2015) MR guided focused ultrasound treatment of soft tissue tumors of the extremities—preliminary experience. J Ther Ultrasound 3(Suppl 1):O69–O69. doi:10.1186/2050-5736-3-S1-O69

Ghanouni P, Dobrotwir A, Bazzocchi A, Bucknor M, Bitton R, Rosenberg J, Telischak K, Busacca M, Ferrari S, Albisinni U, Walters S, Gold G, Ganjoo K, Napoli A, Pauly KB, Avedian R (2016) Magnetic resonance-guided focused ultrasound treatment of extra-abdominal desmoid tumors: a retrospective multicenter study. Eur Radiol In press. doi:10.1007/s00330-016-4376-5

Gianfelice D, Khiat A, Amara M, Belblidia A, Boulanger Y (2003a) MR imaging-guided focused US ablation of breast cancer: histopathologic assessment of effectiveness—initial experience. Radiology 227(3):849–855. doi:10.1148/radiol.2281012163

Gianfelice D, Khiat A, Amara M, Belblidia A, Boulanger Y (2003b) MR imaging-guided focused ultrasound surgery of breast cancer: correlation of dynamic contrast-enhanced MRI with histopathologic findings. Breast Cancer Res Treat 82(2):93–101. doi:10.1023/B:BREA.0000003956.11376.5b

Gianfelice D, Khiat A, Boulanger Y, Amara M, Belblidia A (2003c) Feasibility of magnetic resonance imaging-guided focused ultrasound surgery as an adjunct to tamoxifen therapy in high-risk surgical patients with breast carcinoma. J Vasc Interv Radiol 14(10):1275–1282. doi:10.1097/01.RVL.0000092900.73329.A2

Gianfelice D, Gupta C, Kucharczyk W, Bret P, Havill D, Clemons M (2008) Palliative treatment of painful bone metastases with MR imaging-guided focused ultrasound. Radiology 249(1):355–363. doi:10.1148/radiol.2491071523

Goertz DE (2015) An overview of the influence of therapeutic ultrasound exposures on the vasculature: high intensity ultrasound and microbubble-mediated bioeffects. Int J Hyperth 31(2):134–144. doi:10.3109/02656736.2015.1009179

Gu J, Wang H, Tang N, Hua Y, Yang H, Qiu Y, Ge R, Zhou Y, Wang W, Zhang G (2015) Magnetic resonance guided focused ultrasound surgery for pain palliation of bone metastases: early experience of clinical application in China. Zhonghua Yi Xue Za Zhi 95(41):3328–3332

Hahn GM (1979) Potential for therapy of drugs and hyperthermia. Cancer Res 39:2264–2268

Hall EJ, Giaccia AJ (2006) Radiobiology for the radiologist, 6th edn. Lippincott Williams & Wilkins, Philadelphia

Hectors SJ, Jacobs I, Moonen CT, Strijkers GJ, Nicolay K (2016) MRI methods for the evaluation of high intensity focused ultrasound tumor treatment: current status and future needs. Magn Reson Med 75(1):302–317. doi:10.1002/mrm.25758

Holbrook AB, Ghanouni P, Santos JM, Dumoulin C, Medan Y, Pauly KB (2014) Respiration based steering for high intensity focused ultrasound liver ablation. Magn Reson Med 71 (2):797–806. doi:10.1002/mrm.24695

Huber PE, Jenne JW, Rastert R, Simiantonakis I, Sinn HP, Strittmatter HJ, von Fournier D, Wannenmacher MF, Debus J (2001) A new noninvasive approach in breast cancer therapy using magnetic resonance imaging-guided focused ultrasound surgery. Cancer Res 61 (23):8441–8447

Huisman M, Lam MK, Bartels LW, Nijenhuis RJ, Moonen CT, Knuttel FM, Verkooijen HM, van Vulpen M, van den Bosch MA (2014) Feasibility of volumetric MRI-guided high intensity focused ultrasound (MR-HIFU) for painful bone metastases. J Ther Ultrasound 2:16. doi:10. 1186/2050-5736-2-16

Hurwitz M, Stauffer P (2014) Hyperthermia, radiation and chemotherapy: the role of heat in multidisciplinary cancer care. Semin Oncol 41(6):714–729. doi:10.1053/j.seminoncol.2014.09. 014

Hurwitz MD, Ghanouni P, Kanaev SV, Iozeffi D, Gianfelice D, Fennessy FM, Kuten A, Meyer JE, LeBlang SD, Roberts A, Choi J, Larner JM, Napoli A, Turkevich VG, Inbar Y, Tempany CM, Pfeffer RM (2014) Magnetic resonance-guided focused ultrasound for patients with painful bone metastases: phase III trial results. J Natl Cancer Inst 106 (5). doi:10.1093/jnci/dju082

Hynynen K (1990) Biophysics and technology of ultrasound hyperthermia. In: Gautherie M (ed) Methods of external hyperthermia heating. Clinical thermology, subseries thermotherapy. Springer, Berlin, Heidelberg, pp 61–115

Hynynen K (2010) MRI-guided focused ultrasound treatments. Ultra 50(2):221–229. doi:10.1016/ j.ultras.2009.08.015

Hynynen K, Jolesz FA (1998) Demonstration of potential noninvasive ultrasound brain therapy through an intact skull. Ultrasound Med Biol 24(2):275–283. doi:10.1016/S0301-5629(97) 00269-X

Hynynen K, McDannold N (2004) MRI guided and monitored focused ultrasound thermal ablation methods: a review of progress. Int J Hyperthermia 20(7):725–737. doi:10.1080/ 02656730410001716597

Hynynen K, McDannold N, Mulkern RV, Jolesz FA (2000) Temperature monitoring in fat with MRI. Magn Reson Med 43(6):901–904. doi:10.1002/1522-2594(200006)43:6<901:AID-MRM18>3.0.CO;2-A

Illing RO, Kennedy JE, Wu F, ter Haar GR, Protheroe AS, Friend PJ, Gleeson FV, Cranston DW, Phillips RR, Middleton MR (2005) The safety and feasibility of extracorporeal high-intensity focused ultrasound (HIFU) for the treatment of liver and kidney tumours in a Western population. Br J Cancer 93(8):890–895. doi:10.1038/sj.bjc.6602803

Ishihara Y, Calderon A, Watanabe H, Okamoto K, Suzuki Y, Kuroda K, Suzuki Y (1995) A precise and fast temperature mapping using water proton chemical shift. Magn Reson Med 34 (6):814–823. doi:10.1002/mrm.1910340606

Joo B, Park MS, Lee SH, Choi HJ, Lim ST, Rha SY, Rachmilevitch I, Lee YH, Suh JS (2015) Pain palliation in patients with bone metastases using magnetic resonance-guided focused ultrasound with conformal bone system: a preliminary report. Yonsei Med J 56(2):503–509. doi:10.3349/ymj.2015.56.2.503

Jun-Qun Z, Guo-Min W, Bo Y, Gong-Xian W, Shen-Xu H (2004) Short-term results of 89 cases of rectal carcinoma treated with high-intensity focused ultrasound and low-dose radiotherapy. Ultrasound Med Biol 30(1):57–60. doi:10.1016/j.ultrasmedbio.2003.08.014

Kang TW, Rhim H (2015) Recent advances in tumor ablation for hepatocellular carcinoma. Liver Cancer 4(3):176–187. doi:10.1159/000367740

Karakitsios I, Mihcin S, Saliev T, Melzer A (2016) Feasibility study of pre-clinical thiel embalmed human cadaver for MR-guided focused ultrasound of the spine. Minim Invasive Ther Allied Technol 25(3):154–161. doi:10.3109/13645706.2016.1150297

Khiat A, Gianfelice D, Amara M, Boulanger Y (2006) Influence of post-treatment delay on the evaluation of the response to focused ultrasound surgery of breast cancer by dynamic contrast enhanced MRI. Br J Radiol 79(940):308–314. doi:10.1259/bjr/23046051

Kim YS (2015) Advances in MR image-guided high-intensity focused ultrasound therapy. Int J Hyperth 31(3):225–232. doi:10.3109/02656736.2014.976773

Kobus T, McDannold N (2015) Update on clinical magnetic resonance-guided focused ultrasound applications. Magn Reson Imaging Clin N Am 23(4):657–667. doi:10.1016/j.mric.2015.05.013

Kong G, Anyarambhatla G, Petros WP, Braun RD, Colvin OM, Needham D, Dewhirst MW (2000) Efficacy of liposomes and hyperthermia in a human tumor xenograft model: importance of triggered drug release. Cancer Res 60(24):6950–6957

Kopechek JA, Park EJ, Zhang YZ, Vykhodtseva NI, McDannold NJ, Porter TM (2014) Cavitation-enhanced MR-guided focused ultrasound ablation of rabbit tumors in vivo using phase shift nanoemulsions. Phys Med Biol 59(13):3465–3481. doi:10.1088/0031-9155/59/13/3465

Kopelman D, Inbar Y, Hanannel A, Freundlich D, Castel D, Perel A, Greenfeld A, Salamon T, Sareli M, Valeanu A, Papa M (2006) Magnetic resonance-guided focused ultrasound surgery (MRgFUS): ablation of liver tissue in a porcine model. Eur J Radiol 59(2):157–162. doi:10.1016/j.ejrad.2006.04.008

Laetsch T, Staruch R, Koral K, Chopra R (2016) Prospective imaging study of magnetic resonance thermometry quality in pediatric solid tumors. In: 12th international congress of hyperthermic oncology (ICHO 2016), New Orleans, LA, 11–15 April 2016, p 144

Lee ER (1995) Electromagnetic superficial heating technology. In: Seegenschmiedt MH, Fessenden P, Vernon CC (eds) Thermoradiotherapy and thermochemotherapy, vol 1, chapter 10. Springer, Berlin, Heidelberg, pp 193–217

Lee MW, Kim YJ, Park HS, Yu NC, Jung SI, Ko SY, Jeon HJ (2010) Targeted sonography for small hepatocellular carcinoma discovered by CT or MRI: factors affecting sonographic detection. AJR Am J Roentgenol 194(5):W396–W400. doi:10.2214/AJR.09.3171

Lee J, Farha G, Poon I, Karam I, Higgins K, Pichardo S, Hynynen K, Enepekides D (2016) Magnetic resonance-guided high-intensity focused ultrasound combined with radiotherapy for palliation of head and neck cancer-a pilot study. J Ther Ultrasound 4:12. doi:10.1186/s40349-016-0055-x

Leslie TA, Kennedy JE, Illing RO, Ter Haar GR, Wu F, Phillips RR, Friend PJ, Roberts IS, Cranston DW, Middleton MR (2008) High-intensity focused ultrasound ablation of liver tumours: can radiological assessment predict the histological response? Br J Radiol 81 (967):564–571. doi:10.1259/bjr/27118953

Lesser TG, Schubert H, Gullmar D, Reichenbach JR, Wolfram F (2016) One-lung flooding reduces the ipsilateral diaphragm motion during mechanical ventilation. Eur J Med Res 21 (1):9. doi:10.1186/s40001-016-0205-1

Liberman B, Gianfelice D, Inbar Y, Beck A, Rabin T, Shabshin N, Chander G, Hengst S, Pfeffer R, Chechick A, Hanannel A, Dogadkin O, Catane R (2009) Pain palliation in patients with bone metastases using MR-guided focused ultrasound surgery: a multicenter study. Ann Surg Oncol 16(1):140–146. doi:10.1245/s10434-008-0011-2

Lin SM (2009) Recent advances in radiofrequency ablation in the treatment of hepatocellular carcinoma and metastatic liver cancers. Chang Gung Med J 32(1):22–32

Lindner U, Ghai S, Spensieri P, Hlasny E, Van Der Kwast TH, McCluskey SA, Haider MA, Kucharczyk W, Trachtenberg J (2012) Focal magnetic resonance guided focused ultrasound for prostate cancer: initial North American experience. Can Urol Assoc J 6(6):E283–E286. doi:10.5489/cuaj.12218

Lipsman N, Mainprize TG, Schwartz ML, Hynynen K, Lozano AM (2014) Intracranial applications of magnetic resonance-guided focused ultrasound. Neurother: J Am Soc Exp NeuroTher 11(3):593–605. doi:10.1007/s13311-014-0281-2

Liu HL, Yang HW, Hua MY, Wei KC (2012) Enhanced therapeutic agent delivery through magnetic resonance imaging-monitored focused ultrasound blood-brain barrier disruption for brain tumor treatment: an overview of the current preclinical status. Neurosurg Focus 32(1). doi:10.3171/2011.10.Focus11238

Machtinger R, Inbar Y, Ben-Baruch G, Korach J, Rabinovici J (2008) MRgFUS for pain relief as palliative treatment in recurrent cervical carcinoma: a case report. Gynecol Oncol 108(1):241–243. doi:10.1016/j.ygyno.2007.08.079

Marquet F, Tung YS, Teichert T, Ferrera VP, Konofagou EE (2011) Noninvasive, transient and selective blood-brain barrier opening in non-human primates in vivo. PLoS ONE 6(7):e22598. doi:10.1371/journal.pone.0022598

McDannold NJ, Jolesz FA (2000) Magnetic resonance image-guided thermal ablations. Top Magn Reson Imaging 11(3):191–202. doi:10.1097/00002142-200006000-00005

McDannold N, Clement GT, Black P, Jolesz F, Hynynen K (2010) Transcranial magnetic resonance imaging- guided focused ultrasound surgery of brain tumors: initial findings in 3 patients. Neurosurgery 66(2):323–332; discussion 332. doi:10.1227/01.NEU.0000360379.95800.2F

Melodelima D, Salomir R, Chapelon JY, Theillere Y, Moonen C, Cathignol D (2005) Intraluminal high intensity ultrasound treatment in the esophagus under fast MR temperature mapping: in vivo studies. Magn Reson Med 54(4):975–982. doi:10.1002/mrm.20638

Merckel LG, Knuttel FM, Deckers R, van Dalen T, Schubert G, Peters NH, Weits T, van Diest PJ, Mali WP, Vaessen PH, van Gorp JM, Moonen CT, Bartels LW, van den Bosch MA (2016) First clinical experience with a dedicated MRI-guided high-intensity focused ultrasound system for breast cancer ablation. Eur Radiol In Press. doi:10.1007/s00330-016-4222-9

Meyer J, Pfeffer R, Kanaev S, Iozeffi D, Gianfelice D, Ghanouni P, Militianu D, Hurwitz M (2014) MR-guided focused ultrasound for painful bone metastases: safety when combined with chemotherapy. In: 4th International focused ultrasound symposium, Bethesda, 12–16 Oct 2014. pp 50–BM

Monzon L, Wasan H, Leen E, Ahmed H, Dawson PM, Harvey C, Muhamed A, Hand J, Price P, Abel PD (2011) Transrectal high-intensity focused ultrasonography is feasible as a new therapeutic option for advanced recurrent rectal cancer: report on the first case worldwide. Ann R Coll Surg Engl 93(6):e119–e121. doi:10.1308/147870811X592458

Nance E, Timbie K, Miller GW, Song J, Louttit C, Klibanov AL, Shih TY, Swaminathan G, Tamargo RJ, Woodworth GF, Hanes J, Price RJ (2014) Non-invasive delivery of stealth, brain-penetrating nanoparticles across the blood—brain barrier using MRI-guided focused ultrasound. J Control Release 189:123–132. doi:10.1016/j.jconrel.2014.06.031

Napoli A, Anzidei M, Marincola BC, Brachetti G, Ciolina F, Cartocci G, Marsecano C, Zaccagna F, Marchetti L, Cortesi E, Catalano C (2013a) Primary pain palliation and local tumor control in bone metastases treated with magnetic resonance-guided focused ultrasound. Invest Radiol 48(6):351–358. doi:10.1097/RLI.0b013e318285bbab

Napoli A, Anzidei M, Ciolina F, Marotta E, Cavallo Marincola B, Brachetti G, Di Mare L, Cartocci G, Boni F, Noce V, Bertaccini L, Catalano C (2013b) MR-guided high-intensity focused ultrasound: current status of an emerging technology. Cardiovasc Intervent Radiol 36 (5):1190–1203. doi:10.1007/s00270-013-0592-4

Napoli A, Anzidei M, De Nunzio C, Cartocci G, Panebianco V, De Dominicis C, Catalano C, Petrucci F, Leonardo C (2013c) Real-time magnetic resonance-guided high-intensity focused ultrasound focal therapy for localised prostate cancer: preliminary experience. Eur Urol 63 (2):395–398. doi:10.1016/j.eururo.2012.11.002

Ng KK, Poon RT, Chan SC, Chok KS, Cheung TT, Tung H, Chu F, Tso WK, Yu WC, Lo CM, Fan ST (2011) High-intensity focused ultrasound for hepatocellular carcinoma: a single-center experience. Ann Surg 253(5):981–987. doi:10.1097/SLA.0b013e3182128a8b

Odeen H, de Bever J, Almquist S, Farrer A, Todd N, Payne A, Snell JW, Christensen DA, Parker DL (2014) Treatment envelope evaluation in transcranial magnetic resonance-guided focused ultrasound utilizing 3D MR thermometry. J Ther Ultrasound 2:19. doi:10.1186/2050-5736-2-19

Okada A, Murakami T, Mikami K, Onishi H, Tanigawa N, Marukawa T, Nakamura H (2006) A case of hepatocellular carcinoma treated by MR-guided focused ultrasound ablation with respiratory gating. Magn Reson Med Sci 5(3):167–171. doi:10.2463/mrms.5.167

Pardridge WM (2005) The blood-brain barrier: bottleneck in brain drug development. NeuroRx 2 (1):3–14. doi:10.1602/neurorx.2.1.3

Park MJ, Kim YS, Yang J, Sun WC, Park H, Chae SY, Namgung MS, Choi KS (2013) Pulsed high-intensity focused ultrasound therapy enhances targeted delivery of cetuximab to colon cancer xenograft model in mice. Ultrasound Med Biol 39(2):292–299. doi:10.1016/j.ultrasmedbio.2012.10.008

Pernot M, Aubry JF, Tanter M, Thomas JL, Fink M (2003) High power transcranial beam steering for ultrasonic brain therapy. Phys Med Biol 48(16):2577–2589. doi:10.1088/0031-9155/48/16/301

Petrusca L, Cattin P, De Luca V, Preiswerk F, Celicanin Z, Auboiroux V, Viallon M, Arnold P, Santini F, Terraz S, Scheffler K, Becker CD, Salomir R (2013) Hybrid ultrasound/magnetic resonance simultaneous acquisition and image fusion for motion monitoring in the upper abdomen. Invest Radiol 48(5):333–340. doi:10.1097/RLI.0b013e31828236c3

Ponce AM, Vujaskovic Z, Yuan F, Needham D, Dewhirst MW (2006) Hyperthermia mediated liposomal drug delivery. Int J Hyperth 22(3):205–213. doi:10.1080/02656730600582956

Quesson B, Merle M, Kohler MO, Mougenot C, Roujol S, de Senneville BD, Moonen CT (2010) A method for MRI guidance of intercostal high intensity focused ultrasound ablation in the liver. Med Phys 37(6):2533–2540. doi:10.1118/1.3413996

Quesson B, Laurent C, Maclair G, de Senneville BD, Mougenot C, Ries M, Carteret T, Rullier A, Moonen CT (2011) Real-time volumetric MRI thermometry of focused ultrasound ablation in vivo: a feasibility study in pig liver and kidney. NMR Biomed 24(2):145–153. doi:10.1002/nbm.1563

Ram Z, Cohen ZR, Harnof S, Tal S, Faibel M, Nass D, Maier SE, Hadani M, Mardor Y (2006) Magnetic resonance imaging-guided, high-intensity focused ultrasound for brain tumor therapy. Neurosurgery 59(5):949–955; discussion 955–946. doi:10.1227/01.NEU.0000254439.02736.D8

Rapoport N, Payne A, Dillon C, Shea J, Scaife C, Gupta R (2013) Focused ultrasound-mediated drug delivery to pancreatic cancer in a mouse model. J Ther Ultrasound 1:11. doi:10.1186/2050-5736-1-11

Rodrigues DB, Stauffer PR, Vrba D, Hurwitz MD (2015) Focused ultrasound for treatment of bone tumours. Int J Hyperth 31(3):260–271. doi:10.3109/02656736.2015.1006690

Rosenthal D, Callstrom MR (2012) Critical review and state of the art in interventional oncology: benign and metastatic disease involving bone. Radiology 262(3):765–780. doi:10.1148/radiol.11101384

Saeed M, Krug R, Do L, Hetts SW, Wilson MW (2016) Renal ablation using magnetic resonance-guided high intensity focused ultrasound: Magnetic resonance imaging and histopathology assessment. World J Radiol 8(3):298–307. doi:10.4329/wjr.v8.i3.298

Sazgarnia A, Shanei A, Taheri AR, Meibodi NT, Eshghi H, Attaran N, Shanei MM (2013) Therapeutic effects of acoustic cavitation in the presence of gold nanoparticles on a colon tumor model. J Ultrasound Med 32(3):475–483

Schlesinger D, Benedict S, Diederich C, Gedroyc W, Klibanov A, Larner J (2013) MR-guided focused ultrasound surgery, present and future. Med Phys 40(8):080901. doi:10.1118/1.4811136

Siddiqui K, Chopra R, Vedula S, Sugar L, Haider M, Boyes A, Musquera M, Bronskill M, Klotz L (2010) MRI-guided transurethral ultrasound therapy of the prostate gland using real-time thermal mapping: initial studies. Urology 76(6):1506–1511. doi:10.1016/j.urology.2010.04.046

Sneed PK, Stauffer PR, Li G, Sun X, Myerson R (2010) Hyperthermia. In: Phillips T, Hoppe R, Roach M (eds) Textbook of radiation oncology, 3rd edn. Elsevier, Philadelphia, pp 1564–1593

Stauffer PR (2005) Evolving technology for thermal therapy of cancer. Int J Hyperth 21(8):731–744. doi:10.1080/02656730500331868

Sun J, Hynynen K (1998) Focusing of therapeutic ultrasound through a human skull: a numerical study. J Acoust Soc Am 104(3 Pt 1):1705–1715. doi:10.1121/1.424383

Sun J, Hynynen K (1999) The potential of transskull ultrasound therapy and surgery using the maximum available skull surface area. J Acoust Soc Am 105(4):2519–2527. doi:10.1121/1.426863

Teraphongphom N (2016) Theranostic nanoparticle and drug loaded contrast agents and their biomedical applications. PhD thesis, Drexel University, Philadelphia

Teraphongphom N, Chhour P, Eisenbrey JR, Naha PC, Witschey WRT, Opasanont B, Jablonowski L, Cormode DP, Wheatley MA (2015) Nanoparticle loaded polymeric microbubbles as contrast agents for multimodal imaging. Langmuir 31(43):11858–11867. doi:10.1021/acs.langmuir.5b03473

Tokuda J, Morikawa S, Haque HA, Tsukamoto T, Matsumiya K, Liao H, Masamune K, Dohi T (2008) Adaptive 4D MR imaging using navigator-based respiratory signal for MRI-guided therapy. Magn Reson Med 59(5):1051–1061. doi:10.1002/mrm.21436

Toraya-Brown S, Fiering S (2014) Local tumour hyperthermia as immunotherapy for metastatic cancer. Int J Hyperth 30(8):531–539. doi:10.3109/02656736.2014.968640

Tung YS, Vlachos F, Feshitan JA, Borden MA, Konofagou EE (2011) The mechanism of interaction between focused ultrasound and microbubbles in blood-brain barrier opening in mice. J Acoust Soc Am 130(5):3059–3067. doi:10.1121/1.3646905

Van Rhoon GC (2013) External electromagnetic methods and devices. In: Moros EG (ed) Physics of thermal therapy: fundamentals and clincial applications. Taylor and Francis, Boca Ratan, pp 139–158

Vidal-Jove J, Eres N, Perich E, Jaen A, del Castillo MA (2016) Interventional oncology: role of focused ultrasound (USgHIFU) in pancreatic cancer. Five years experience and tumor ablation considerations in the Western stage. In: 12th International congress of hyperthermic oncology (ICHO 2016), New Orleans, LA, 11–15 April 2016. p 210

Vujaskovic Z, Poulson JM, Gaskin AA, Thrall DE, Page RL, Charles HC, MacFall JR, Brizel DM, Meyer RE, Prescott DM, Samulski TV, Dewhirst MW (2000) Temperature-dependent changes in physiologic parameters of spontaneous canine soft tissue sarcomas after combined radiotherapy and hyperthermia treatment. Int J Radiat Oncol Biol Phys 46(1):179–185. doi:10.1016/S0360-3016(99)00362-4

Weber-Adrian D, Thevenot E, O'Reilly MA, Oakden W, Akens MK, Ellens N, Markham-Coultes K, Burgess A, Finkelstein J, Yee AJM, Whyne CM, Foust KD, Kaspar BK, Stanisz GJ, Chopra R, Hynynen K, Aubert I (2015) Gene delivery to the spinal cord using MRI-guided focused ultrasound. Gene Ther 22(7):568–577. doi:10.1038/gt.2015.25

Wijlemans JW, de Greef M, Schubert G, Bartels LW, Moonen CT, van den Bosch MA, Ries M (2015) A clinically feasible treatment protocol for magnetic resonance-guided high-intensity focused ultrasound ablation in the liver. Invest Radiol 50(1):24–31. doi:10.1097/RLI.0000000000000091

Wolfram F, Boltze C, Schubert H, Bischoff S, Lesser TG (2014) Effect of lung flooding and high-intensity focused ultrasound on lung tumours: an experimental study in an ex vivo human cancer model and simulated in vivo tumours in pigs. Eur J Med Res 19:1. doi:10.1186/2047-783X-19-1

Woodrum DA, Kawashima A, Gorny KR, Mynderse LA (2015) Magnetic resonance-guided thermal therapy for localized and recurrent prostate cancer. Magn Reson Imaging Clin N Am 23(4):607–619. doi:10.1016/j.mric.2015.05.014

Wu F (2006) Extracorporeal high intensity focused ultrasound in the treatment of patients with solid malignancy. Minim Invasive Ther Allied Technol 15(1):26–35. doi:10.1080/13645700500470124

Wu F, Wang ZB, Chen WZ, Bai J, Zhu H, Qiao TY (2003) Preliminary experience using high intensity focused ultrasound for the treatment of patients with advanced stage renal malignancy. J Urol 170(6 Pt 1):2237–2240. doi:10.1097/01.ju.0000097123.34790.70

Wu F, Wang ZB, Chen WZ, Zhu H, Bai J, Zou JZ, Li KQ, Jin CB, Xie FL, Su HB (2004) Extracorporeal high intensity focused ultrasound ablation in the treatment of patients with large hepatocellular carcinoma. Ann Surg Oncol 11(12):1061–1069. doi:10.1245/ASO.2004.02.026

Xu Y, Choi J, Hylander B, Sen A, Evans SS, Kraybill WG, Repasky EA (2007) Fever-range whole body hyperthermia increases the number of perfused tumor blood vessels and therapeutic efficacy of liposomally encapsulated doxorubicin. Int J Hyperth 23(6):513–527. doi:10.1080/02656730701666112

Xu G, Luo G, He L, Li J, Shan H, Zhang R, Li Y, Gao X, Lin S, Wang G (2011) Follow-up of high-intensity focused ultrasound treatment for patients with hepatocellular carcinoma. Ultrasound Med Biol 37(12):1993–1999. doi:10.1016/j.ultrasmedbio.2011.08.011

Yuh B, Liu A, Beatty R, Jung A, Wong JY (2016) Focal therapy using magnetic resonance image-guided focused ultrasound in patients with localized prostate cancer. J Ther Ultrasound 4:8. doi:10.1186/s40349-016-0054-y

Zaccagna F, Giulia B, Bazzocchi A, Spinnato P, Albisinni U, Napoli A, Catalano C (2014) Palliative treatment of painful bone metastases with MR imaging–guided focused ultrasound surgery: a two-centre study. In: 4th international focused ultrasound symposium, Bethesda, 12–16 Oct 2014. pp 51–BM

Zachiu C, Papadakis N, Ries M, Moonen C, Denis de Senneville B (2015) An improved optical flow tracking technique for real-time MR-guided beam therapies in moving organs. Phys Med Biol 60(23):9003–9029. doi:10.1088/0031-9155/60/23/9003

Zagar TM, Vujaskovic Z, Formenti S, Rugo H, Muggia F, O'Connor B, Myerson R, Stauffer P, Hsu IC, Diederich C, Straube W, Boss MK, Boico A, Craciunescu O, Maccarini P, Needham D, Borys N, Blackwell KL, Dewhirst MW (2014) Two phase I dose-escalation/pharmacokinetics studies of low temperature liposomal doxorubicin (LTLD) and mild local hyperthermia in heavily pretreated patients with local regionally recurrent breast cancer. Int J Hyperth 30 (5):285–294. doi:10.3109/02656736.2014.936049

Zhou YF (2011) High intensity focused ultrasound in clinical tumor ablation. World J Clin Oncol 2(1):8–27. doi:10.5306/wjco.v2.i1.8

Zhu X, Guo J, He C, Geng H, Yu G, Li J, Zheng H, Ji X, Yan F (2016) Ultrasound triggered image-guided drug delivery to inhibit vascular reconstruction via paclitaxel-loaded microbubbles. Sci Rep 6:21683. doi:10.1038/srep21683

Zippel DB, Papa MZ (2005) The use of MR imaging guided focused ultrasound in breast cancer patients; a preliminary phase one study and review. Breast Cancer 12(1):32–38. doi:10.2325/jbcs.12.32

Intensity-Modulated Proton Beam Therapy of Prostate Cancer-History, Results, and Future Directions

Carl J. Rossi Jr.

Abstract

Proton beam radiation therapy is a form of external—beam radiation treatment which takes advantage of the superior physical properties of positively charged subatomic particles (i.e., low entrance dose and lack of exit dose) to deliver highly conformal radiation therapy with a lower integral dose (dose to normal tissue) than can be achieved with photon-based treatments. Proton beam radiation therapy first became available on an extremely limited basis in the late 1950s, and was initially used to treat prostate cancer in the late 1970s. More recently, intensity—modulated proton therapy (IMPT), in which all beam shaping and modulation is performed electromagnetically, has become available at a number of proton centers. This improvement in proton beam treatment delivery significantly expands the utility of proton therapy by allowing for treatment of complex target volumes such as the whole pelvis and by permitting the creation of highly individualized nonuniform dose distributions, including the use of simultaneous integrated boosting. This chapter will review the history of proton beam therapy of prostate cancer, beginning with the initial patient treatments at the Harvard Cyclotron Laboratory and continuing up to the present day, with particular emphasis being placed upon emerging trends in proton beam treatment technology and their potential impact on the future of proton beam therapy in prostate cancer.

Keywords

Protons · Prostate cancer · Intensity-modulated proton therapy

C.J. Rossi Jr. (✉)
Scripps Proton Therapy Center, 9730 Summers Ridge Road,
San Diego, CA 92121, USA
e-mail: Rossi.carl@scrippshealth.org

© Springer International Publishing AG 2017
J.Y.C. Wong et al. (eds.), *Advances in Radiation Oncology*,
Cancer Treatment and Research 172, DOI 10.1007/978-3-319-53235-6_5

1   Introduction

Prostate cancer presents a major oncological dilemma for the developed world. In the United States there will be an estimated 226,000 new cases diagnosed in 2015, with approximately 27,000 deaths from this disease (Society 2015). Prostate cancer is the second leading cause of cancer deaths among American men and accounts for approximately 10% of all cancer related deaths in men. A similar incidence and death rate is seen in Western Europe, with the lowest reported incidence being in Eastern/Southern Asia. Over the past twenty-five years the discovery and use of Prostate Specific Antigen (PSA) as a screening tool has led to both an increase in the number of cases being diagnosed and a decrease in the proportion of men being diagnosed with advanced disease. This trend towards diagnosis with organ-confined disease has prompted the development and refinement of treatment methods directed at the prostate in the entirely reasonable hope of providing long-term disease free survival and cure.

From the radiotherapy standpoint virtually all technical advances in prostate cancer treatment have been implemented to reduce normal tissue toxicity by limiting the volume of adjacent bladder and especially rectum that receive moderate to high doses of radiation. A direct consequence of this improvement in dose conformality has been dose escalation, a successful treatment strategy whose favorable impact on biochemical freedom from relapse which has been tested and confirmed in one proton beam-based prospective randomized trial, and in numerous prospective non-randomized series.

The unique physical properties inherent in proton beams makes them particularly attractive to the radiation oncologist, for they permit a reduction in "integral dose" (defined as the total radiation dose given to the patient) over and above anything which can be achieved with any photon-based external beam treatment systems (Suit et al. 1977, 2003; Suit 2002).

However, proton beam therapy of prostate cancer is not without its detractors. Critics often correctly point out that a multitude of effective treatment methods exist for prostate cancer and that modern X-ray therapy employing intensity-modulated techniques (IMRT) and image-guided treatment delivery (IGRT) yield similar outcomes at less monetary cost to society, while still others question the wisdom of aggressively treating prostate cancer at all (Zietman 2007, 2008, 2016; Trofimov et al. 2007). This chapter will discuss the technical aspects of proton therapy, review the published experience to date with passive—scattered proton therapy, and discuss the impact of the ongoing clinical implementation of intensity—modulated proton therapy in the treatment of prostate cancer.

2   Technical Aspects of Proton Therapy

Protons are subatomic particles which are found within the atomic nucleus, indeed, they are the most abundant subatomic particle in the Universe. The clinical appeal of protons lies in their physical properties-in contrast to X-rays, which are massless and changeless and are therefore only sparsely attenuated by passing through relatively low-density material such as the human body, protons are characterized by an energy deposition pattern in which the majority of their ionizing effect is found at the very distal end of the particle's path. Beyond that point, the particle comes to rest and no further ionizing radiation is deposited. As a result, an unmodulated proton beam will have an extremely low "entrance dose", a high dose spike at some energy and tissue density dependent depth, and no dose beyond that point. This is a description of the classic "Bragg Peak", discovered by physicist William Bragg in 1903, and the clinical utility of a particle with these properties is readily apparent. Indeed, the first published proposal to employ protons in radiation oncology appeared in Wilson's 1946 paper (Wilson 1946) with preliminary clinical efforts beginning in the late 1950s at the Harvard Cyclotron Laboratory, the Lawrence Berkeley Laboratory, and the Svedberg Laboratory in Sweden (Miller 1995; Olsen et al. 2007; Bonnett 1993).

The heart of all proton beam therapy centers is a particle accelerator, currently either a synchrotron or cyclotron, which is capable of accelerating protons to energies of 225–250 meV (=velocities of $\sim$100,000 miles/second), producing a maximal range in human tissue of $\sim$36 cm. After being extracted from the accelerator the protons are transported to the treatment room in a "beam line", a metal tube inside of which a high vacuum (akin to interplanetary space) is maintained. The beam line is surrounded by various focusing magnets which prevent the proton stream from striking the walls of the tube, while other "switching" magnets shunt the proton stream into whichever treatment room they are needed. Treatment rooms either utilize "fixed" beams, in which the treatment nozzle is fixed in position and all patient movement is by means of a robotic couch, or isocentric gantries in which the nozzle can rotate completely around the patient.

While a monoenergetic, unmodulated proton beam may be ideal for treating an extremely small tumor (such as a uveal melanoma) since the vast majority of clinical situations require radiation delivery to large, irregularly shaped targets, it is necessary to modulate the proton beam so that, the target volume can be irradiated in a homogeneous (or, as we shall see, a non-homogeneous) manner. This can be accomplished by one of two methods commonly referred to as passive-scatter proton therapy (PSPT) or intensity-modulated proton therapy (IMPT).

PSPT was the first method employed in clinical proton therapy, and it remains in widespread use to this day (Lomax 2009; Schippers and Lomax 2011). In fact, the majority of patients treated in the history of proton therapy have been irradiated with PSPT. As is illustrated below, this technique begins by taking a small (3–5 mm) proton beam and propagating this beam through a variety of physical devices whose ultimate purpose is to spread out the monoenergetic Bragg Peak so that, in effect, a uniform dose "plateau" is created which encompasses the desired target volume. Many of these devices such as the aperture and tissue compensator are patient—specific and beam—specific; for example, if a patient is to be treated with two fields there are two separate, unique sets of apertures and boluses required, each of which must be uniquely identified so as to assure that the proper aperture/bolus pair is being used in each beam.

One inevitable consequence of such a beam shaping is that while the radiation dose within the target is generally extremely uniform, it is not possible to significantly vary the radiation dose within that target if such is (as is often the case) clinically desirable. Another consequence is that the entrance and dose, or dose proximal to the target, is somewhat increased and in general is approximately 50–70% of the dose through the plateau. Of course, since there is no contribution to the entrance dose from any contralateral beam this still results in dose distributions which deliver a lower integral dose then is the case with intensity modulated X-ray therapy but, as we shall see, there exist more advanced proton therapy techniques which substantially decrease this proximal dose. A typical passive scatter treatment nozzle with associated hardware is illustrated in Fig. 1.

In contrast, intensity—modulated proton therapy obviates the need for physical beam—shaping devices. In IMPT a small (3–5 mm) beam of protons is electromagnetically scanned over the target volume, with dose being deposited in effect "layer by layer", with the typical layer thickness being on the order of 1 mm. Bragg Peak placement is achieved by dynamically varying the energy of the proton beam (Lomax 1999). Thus, treatment delivery is analogous to the operation of a 3-Dimensional printer that creates a complex, solid object by precisely depositing varying thicknesses of material. With IMPT, treatment dose can be optimized to the target itself and what is more, the delivery of differential radiation doses within the target becomes both feasible and easily achievable. In addition, since the beam manipulation is performed electromagnetically and not by patient-specific physical devices, IMPT plans can be rapidly altered (often within 24 h) to reflect changes in

Fig. 1 A typical passive scatter treatment nozzle with associated hardware

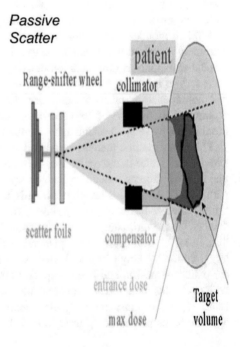

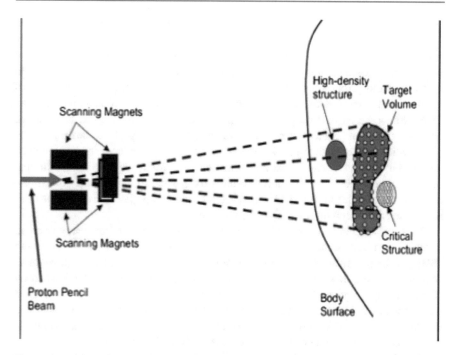

Fig. 2 A diagram of a typical IMPT treatment nozzle

patient anatomy and tumor configuration. The first IMPT treatment systems were developed in the early 2000s (Lomax et al. 2004), and this proton treatment method became available in the United States in 2008. Rapid advances in this technology have led to the construction of "IMPT-only" treatment facilities and indeed the vast majority of recently commissioned proton centers, and those under construction, are designed to employ this technology as their sole means of proton beam treatment delivery. A diagram of a typical IMPT treatment nozzle is shown in Fig. 2.

3 Treatment Planning

Whether employing PSPT or IMPT, all proton beam therapy planning, like modern X-ray therapy planning, is based upon creating a three-dimensional reconstruction of the target and adjacent normal tissues. In general, the patient positioning and immobilization techniques which are utilized in X-ray therapy are equally applicable to proton beam treatment. Similarly, the concepts of gross tumor volume (GTV) and clinical target volume (CTV) are also identical to those used in IMRT, however, the unique physical characteristics of a proton beam result in a modification of the X-ray therapy planning target volume (PTV) into either a beam— specific PTV (in the case of PSPT), or a "Scanning Target Volume" in IMPT

(Lomax et al. 2004). One of the primary differences between proton therapy and X-ray therapy dosimetry lies in the uncertainty as to exactly where a proton of any given energy will come to a stop. This "range uncertainty" is partly due to the need to convert tissue densities obtained from CT (which are quantified as Hounsfield Units) to proton stopping power; this process typically adds a range uncertainty of up to 3% to the precise location at which any given proton will come to rest (Lomax 2009). Since the protons range is also significantly affected by tissue density, it is a common planning practice to avoid to the greatest extent possible beam arrangements which traverse anatomic structures (such as small or large intestine) which vary widely in density and in anatomic location. This partly explains the reason that the vast majority of prostate cancer patients treated with protons have their treatment delivered through a left and right lateral field as this field arrangement minimizes density uncertainties within the beam path.

Another dosimetric issue which is unique to proton and other heavy charged particle beam treatment is the need to account for the Relative Biologic Effectiveness (RBE) of the proton so as to proscribe a radiation dose whose biologic equivalent is accurately linked to known doses and risks of normal tissue injury established by X-ray therapy. In general, a relative biologic effectiveness (RBE) of 1.1 is assumed for protons as compared to megavoltage X-rays and although this approximation is undoubtedly an oversimplification it has clinically proven to be an accurate value for predicting both disease response and the risk of normal tissue injury.

The clinical implementation of IMPT has, in a fashion analogous to what was seen with the implementation of IMRT, resulted in the introduction of additional complexity into the treatment planning process. For one thing, the ability to deliver differential radiation doses within any given target volume means that (again, in a fashion identical to IMRT) in effect a proton "fluence map" is created. Not only does this result in quality assurance needs which are identical to those utilized in IMRT, combining this fluence map with the confounding factors of proton range uncertainty as well as patient positional uncertainty has led to the introduction of a property known as "robustness" in IMPT planning (Lomax 1999, 2008; Lomax et al. 2004). Robustness is in effect a probability analysis which graphically displays (typically by means of dose—volume histograms) the likely range of dose distributions for any given beam arrangement and the probability that any one given treatment plan will accurately and reproducibly irradiate the target structure while simultaneously minimizing radiation dose to normal tissues. Robustness is influenced by a number of factors including the degree of patient immobilization, the depth of the target, the density of the tissues proximal to the target, and whether or not the patient is being treated with a single—field optimization (in which all proton beams "see" the entirety of the target) or a multi-field optimization (in which any one given beam may only "see" a portion of the target, with the summation of all beams resulting in the desired radiation dose to the target). Because of its favorable anatomic location IMPT prostate plans tend to be very robust although they are still sensitive to factors such as patient rotation (which may alter the density of bone between the skin surface and the prostate) and the presence of distensible organs such as the bladder or rectum within the beam path.

4 Early Proton Beam Treatment Results

The ability to use proton beam therapy to treat deep organs was and remains greatly dependent on the concurrent development of cross-sectional imaging technology (CT, MRI) and modern computers, hence it is not surprising that proton beam therapy of prostate cancer did not commence until the late 1970s. Beginning in 1977, Shipley and associates at the Massachusetts General Hospital (MGH) initiated a Phase I trial in which proton beam radiotherapy was used to deliver a boost dose to patients with locally advanced disease who were also receiving photon radiotherapy. At that time, this boost dose was felt to be over and above what could be safely given with existing 2-Dimensional photon technology. Seventeen patients with stage T2–T4 disease received a perineally-directed proton beam boost of 2000–2600 rads (given at a rate of 180–200 rads per day) which was proceeded by treatment of the prostate and pelvis to a dose of 5040 rads with 10 MV photons delivered as a four-field box. A perineal approach was mandated because this was the only anatomical pathway that allowed the 160 meV proton beam generated by the Harvard Cyclotron to reliably encompass the entire prostate gland. Acutely, the treatment was well tolerated and after a follow up period ranging from 12 to 27 months no severe late rectal reactions were noted (Shipley et al. 1979).

These favorable toxicity results led directly to the initiation of a prospective randomized trial designed to test the benefits of proton beam dose escalation in patients with locally advanced disease. Patients with stage T3–T4 tumors were chosen as it was felt that this group stood to benefit the most from dose escalation. All patients received 50.4 Gy to the prostate and pelvis with megavoltage photons. They were then randomized to receive either an additional 16.8 Gy of photons (for a total prostate dose of 67.2 Gy) or 25.2 GyE of protons for a total prostate dose of 75.6 Gy. Adjuvant hormonal therapy was not permitted. The limited availability of the Harvard Cyclotron significantly impacted patient accrual; nonetheless, two hundred and two patients were eventually enrolled, with one hundred and three being treated in the high dose proton boost arm and ninety-nine in the standard dose arm.

With a median follow up of 61 months there were no differences seen in overall survival, disease-specific survival, total relapse-free survival, or local control between the arms. Patients with high-grade tumors who were treated on the high dose arm did experience a trend improvement in local control at five and eight years (92 and 77% vs. 80 and 60%, p = 0.89). Patients whose digital rectal exams normalized following treatment and who underwent subsequent prostate biopsy revealed a lower positive biopsy rate in the high dose arm (28 vs. 45%) and, perhaps most surprisingly, the local control rates for patients with Gleason grade 4–5 tumors (57 patients total) were significantly better at five and eight years in the high dose patients (94 and 84% vs. 68 and 19%, p = 0.0014). High dose treatment was associated with an increase in late grade 1–2 rectal bleeding (32 vs. 12%, p = 0.02) (Shipley et al. 1995).

Some critics have repeatedly and in my opinion incorrectly cited these results as evidence that proton-beam dose escalation is of doubtful utility. It should be noted that the patients treated in this trial were at a high risk of not only local failure but also of distant failure and therefore one should not be surprised that overall survival was unaffected. In addition, patients with these adverse characteristics would not, if undergoing treatment today, receive radiotherapy as monotherapy and instead would be treated with a multi-modality approach. I believe that the two most important points learned from this study are (1) high dose radiotherapy did decrease local failure, and this decrease was most profound in those patients with the most aggressive tumors and (2) Dose-escalation by means of a perineal proton beam (an approach which has virtually universally been abandoned today as higher energy machines become available) could be performed safely with acceptable toxicity.

The improvement in local control seen with dose escalation prompted a very logical question: If patients with earlier stage disease who are less likely to have already experienced metastatic failure are treated with dose escalation will we see a positive effect on survival? This intriguing hypothesis has been tested in a prospective randomized multi-institution trial and its conclusions will be covered presently.

The completion in 1990 of the world's first hospital-based proton treatment center at Loma Linda University Medical Center (LLUMC) marked the beginning of a transition in proton beam therapy from the research laboratory setting to that of clinical radiation oncology (Slater et al. 1988, 1992). Beginning in late 1991 prostate patients at LLUMC was treated on a clinical trial that set out to confirm the efficacy and toxicity data generated at MGH. Between December 1991 and December 1995 643 patients were treated to total prostate radiation doses of 74–75 GyE. Patients who were deemed to be at a low risk for occult nodal metastasis were treated with lateral proton beams alone while those who were felt to benefit from elective nodal radiation received 45 Gy to the pelvis with 18–23 MV photons delivered via a multi-field 3-D conformal technique. Patient characteristics are shown in Table 1 (Slater et al. 1998).

Table 1 LLUMC Patient Characteristics

		# Patients
Stage	1A/1B	28
	1C	91
	2A	157
	2B	173
	2C	157
	3	37
Gleason	2–5	232
	6–7	324
	8–10	54
Initial PSA	≤ 4.0	53
	4.1–10.0	280
	10.0–20.0	175
	> 20.0	85

With a median follow up of 43 months, the overall biochemical disease-free survival (bNED) rate was 79% as per the original American Society for Therapeutic Radiology and Oncology (ASTRO) definition of three successively rising PSA values above a nadir equating to biochemical failure. The risk of biochemical failure was strongly dependent on the pre-treatment PSA with five-year bNED survival rates varying from 53% in patients with pre-treatment PSA's of 20–50 to 100% with PSA's of <4.1 (Fig. 3). bNED survival was also significantly influenced by post-treatment PSA nadir (Fig. 4). A multi-variant analysis of failure predictors

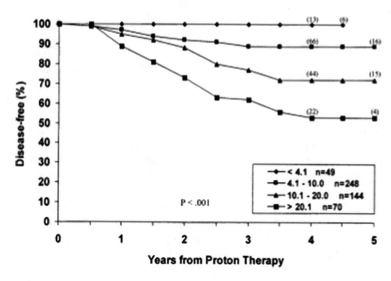

Fig. 3 bNED survival in relation to pre-treatment PSA

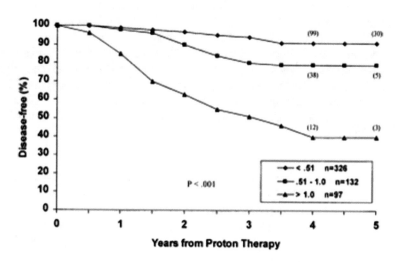

Fig. 4 bNED survival in relation to post-treatment PSA nadir

Table 2 Predictors of local/distant failure, initial LLUMC experience

		Local failure (%) 5 year	p	Distant metastasis (%) 5 year	p
Initial PSA	≤ 4.0	0		0	
	4.1–10.0	3	0.06	4	< 0.001
	10.0–20.0	4		12	
	> 20.0	16		17	
Gleason	2–5	2		6	
	6–7	6	0.01	6	0.11
	8–10	19		24	
T stage	1A/1B	4		0	
	1C	0		0	
	2A	2	0.009	5	< 0.001
	2B	5		7	
	2C	11		15	
	3	20		27	

demonstrated that initial stage, PSA, and Gleason Score were all strong predictors of biochemical failure at five years (Table 2). Similar to what was reported in the MGH trial, treatment was by and large well tolerated. Acute toxicity was minimal and all patients completed the prescribed course of radiotherapy. Proctitis remained the most common late toxicity with Grade 2 toxicity occurring in 21% of patients at three years; for the majority of patients this represented a single episode of rectal bleeding. No ≥ Grade 3 GI toxicity was seen. Grade 2 GU toxicity (primarily gross hematuria) was seen in 5.4% of patients at three years, with two patients developing Grade 3 bladder toxicity. Interestingly, no significant difference in late toxicity was seen between those patients treated with protons alone and those receiving pelvic X-ray therapy. The excellent biochemical control rates and acceptable toxicity seen in this trial confirmed the earlier MGH data and led to the implementation of a prospective randomized dose escalation study in organ confined prostate cancer.

A further update of the initial LLUMC experience was published in 2004. This study encompassed 1255 patients with stage T1–T3 disease who were treated with proton beam radiotherapy alone (i.e., no prior or concurrent hormonal therapy) to a dose of 74–75 GyE. As was seen in the earlier trial initial PSA, Gleason Grade, and PSA nadir were all strong predictors of bNED survival (Fig. 5a–c). Treatment continued to be well tolerated with rates of RTOG Grade ≥ 3 GI/GU late morbidity of <1% (Slater et al. 2004).

5   PROG 95-09 Trial

Beginning in 1996, LLUMC and MGH embarked on the Proton Radiation Oncology Group/American College of Radiology (PROG/ACR) 95-09 trial, a prospective, randomized dose-escalation study for patients with organ-confined

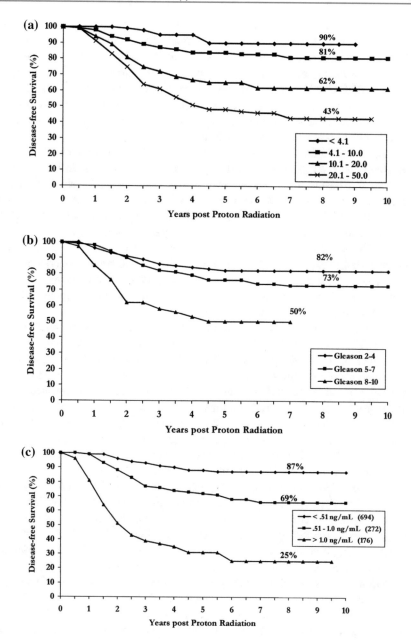

Fig. 5 Effect of pre-treatment PSA on bNED survival (a) Gleason score on bNED survival (b) PSA nadir on bNED survival (c)

prostate cancer. This study was designed to test the hypothesis that dose escalation from 70.2 to 79.2 GyE would result in a statistically significant decrease in local failure, biochemical failure, and overall survival. Eligibility criteria included stage T1b–T2b disease (as per the 1992 American Joint Committee on Cancer staging system), a PSA of ≤ 15 ng/ml, and no evidence of metastatic disease on imaging studies (bone scan, abdominal-pelvic CT scan). Gleason score was not an exclusion criterion, and no prior or concurrent androgen-depravation therapy was permitted. Pre-treatment patient characteristics are shown in Table 3.

Patients were randomly assigned to receive a total prostate dose of 70.2 or 79.2 GyE. Radiotherapy was administered sequentially in two phases. In Phase I, conformal proton beams were used to treat the prostate alone. Depending on randomization either 19.8 or 28.8 GyE in 11 or 16 fractions was delivered. The clinical target volume (CTV) was the prostate with a 5 mm margin. Beam arrangement was facility dependent with patients at LLUMC being treated with lateral proton beams of 225–250 meV energy, while at MGH a perineal 160 meV proton beam was employed. Before each proton beam treatment, a water balloon was inserted into the rectum and inflated with 100 ml of saline; this served the dual purpose of distending the rectum lumen to decrease the volume of rectum receiving any radiation and minimizing prostate motion.

In the second phase of treatment all patients received 50.4 Gy of photons given in 1.8 Gy fractions. The CTV was the prostate and seminal vesicles. No effort was made to include the pelvic lymphatics. Three-dimensional planning was used on all patients and photon energies of 10–23 MV were employed. The use of photons for this portion of the treatment was solely to allow both institutions to participate in this trial, for at the time the trial commenced MGH patients were still restricted to treatment at the Harvard Cyclotron Laboratory and the limited throughput of that facility meant that the most efficient use of protons was as a boost and not as monotherapy. The randomization schema is shown in Fig. 6. A total of 393 patients were randomized between January 1996 and December 1999.

The results of the trial were initially published in Zietman et al. (2005), with an update in Zietman et al. (2010). At a median follow-up of 8.9 years there is a persistent and statistically significant increase in biochemical freedom from relapse amongst patients randomized to the high dose arm (Fig. 7a, b). This difference was seen when using both the original ASTRO and the more recent Phoenix definition (in which biochemical failure = a PSA elevation of >2 ng/ml above a nadir). Subgroup analysis showed a particularly strong benefit in 10 year bNED survival amongst the "low risk" patients (defined as PSA < 10 ng/ml, and Gleason score < 7 and stage < t2b), with 92.2% of high dose patients being disease free versus 78.8% for standard dose (p = 0.0001). A strong trend towards unproved bNED similar was also seen in the intermediate risk patients but this has not reached statistical significance (Fig. 8). In addition, patients in the standard dose arm are twice as likely to have been started on androgen depravation therapy as high dose patients (22 vs. 11, p = 0.47) with such treatment usually being initiated due to a rising PSA. To date, there is no statistically significant difference in overall survival between the arms.

Table 3 Pre-treatment patient characteristics PROG 95-09 trial

| | Assigned Dose | | | |
| | 70.2 GyE (n = 196) | | 79.2 GyE (n = 195) | |
Characteristic	No.	%	No.	%
Age, years				
45-59	43	22	34	17
60-69	92	47	106	54
70-79	61	31	55	28
≥ 80	1	0.5	0	
Median	67		66	
Range	45-91		47-78	
Race				
White	175	89	178	91
Hispanic	4	2	7	3
Black	12	6	5	3
Other	5	3	5	3
PSA, ng/mL				
< 5	54	28	47	24
5 to < 10	114	58	119	61
10-15	28	14	29	15
Median	6.3		6.2	
Range	1.24-14.68		0.67-14.30	
Karnofsky performance status				
80	8	4	9	5
90	52	27	47	24
100	136	69	139	71
Combined Gleason				
2-6	148	75	147	75
7	29	15	30	15
8-10	18	9	15	8
Unknown	1	1	3	2
T stage				
T1b	1	1	0	
T1c	120	61	120	61
T2a	43	22	50	26
T2b	32	16	25	13
N stage				
N0	0		2	1
NX	196	100	193	99
Risk groups*				
Low	111	57	116	59
Intermediate	75	38	69	35
High	10	5	7	4
Not classified	0		3	2

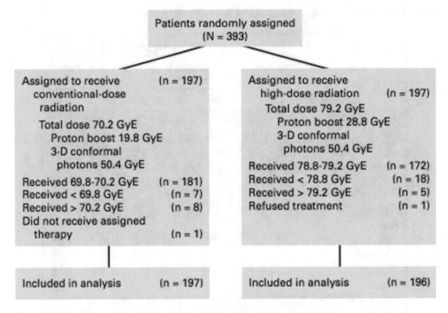

Fig. 6 PROG 95-09 randomization schemata

As was seen in the previously reported proton trials treatment was well tolerated. Only 2% of patients in both arms have experienced late GU toxicities of Grade ≥ 3 and 1% have experienced late GI toxicity of Grade ≥ 3. Interestingly, as opposed to what has been reported in some photon-based randomized dose escalation trials high dose radiotherapy delivered via a conformal proton beam boost did not result in an increase in late Grade ≥ 3 GI morbidity amongst the high dose patients (Table 4). This encouraging finding has been confirmed in a patient-reported sensitive quality of life instrument which did not report any greater morbidity than the physician-reported scores, and which revealed equal and high satisfaction with quality of life between both arms (Talcott et al. 2010).

Thus, the PROG/ACR 9509 trial provides "Level One" evidence verifying the importance of radiation dose-escalation in organ confined prostate cancer and while this study was not designed to directly compare the efficacy of conformal proton beam radiotherapy against other conformal techniques or modalities it does demonstrate that conformal proton beam radiotherapy is an effective treatment for this disease, with minimal risk of severe treatment-induced toxicity (Goitein and Cox 2008; Goitein 2010).

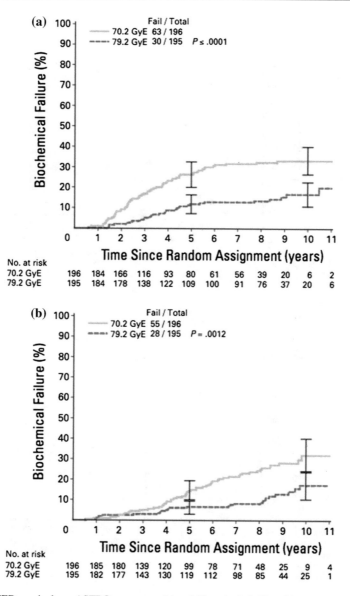

Fig. 7 bNED survival per ASTRO consensus (a) and Phoenix definition (b)

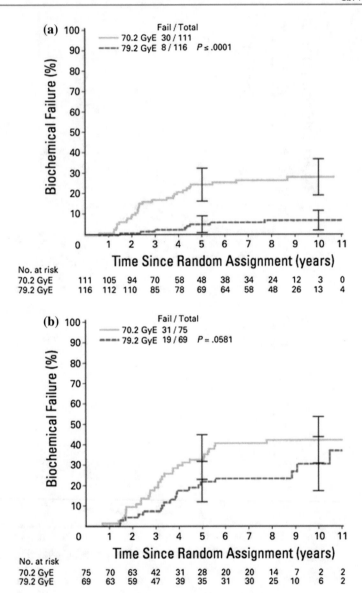

Fig. 8 bNED survival by low (a) and intermediate risk (b) group

6   University of Florida Experience

The University of Florida Proton Therapy Institute commenced prostate cancer treatment in the summer of 2006. From 2006 thru 2010 patients were treated on one of several prospective trials, all of which delivered 78–82 Gy (RBE) in 2 Gy

Table 4 Sequel of treatment PROG 95-09 trial

	Grade 2 (%)	Grade 3 (%)
GI	21	0
GU	5.4	0.3
Total	26	0.3

fractions. After excluding patients who also received concurrent chemotherapy, received IMRT for elective pelvic node radiation, GI/GU follow up data were unavailable, and patients with less than 2-year biochemical follow-up for reasons other than death 1214 patients remained eligible for analysis. Virtually all patients were treated with either lateral or posterior-oblique fields, IMRT treatment of pelvic nodes was performed in those with >15% risk of node involvement per nomogram, and androgen-depravation therapy was administered to 18% of the patients.

With a median follow up of 5.5 years, freedom biochemical failure was 99% in the low-risk patients, 94% in the intermediate risk patients, and 74% in the high-risk patients. Statistically significant predictors of biochemical included Gleason Score (4–7 vs. 8 vs. 9–10; p = 0.02), PSA (0 < 10 vs. 10–20 vs. >20; p = 0.02), perineural invasion (yes vs. no; P = 0.01), and percentage of positive zones on biopsy (<50% vs. ≥ 50%; P = 0.02).

Grade 3+ Acute/late GU toxicity was seen in 5.4% of patients (70/1289), with 58/70 being late events, 9 being acute events, and 3 patients who experienced both acute and late events. One patient experienced a Grade 4 toxicity, while no Grade 5 events have occurred. The primary reason for Grade 3 toxicity in both the acute and late patients was obstruction. Late Grade 3 GU toxicity was associated with use of androgen suppressive therapy (P = 0.0243), prescription anticoagulants (P = 0.0316), prostate volume < 40 cc vs. 40–60 cc vs. >60 cc (P < 0.0001), pretreatment alpha-blocker use (P < 0.0001), diabetes (P = 0.0210), pretreatment TURP (P < 0.0001), any pretreatment urologic symptom management (P < 0.0001) and numerous bladder and bladder wall dose-volume histogram parameters. The five-year actuarial incidence of late Grade 3 GI toxicity was 0.6%. The authors reported that both the rates of biochemical freedom from relapse and GU/GI toxicity compare favorably with large published IMRT series. The authors also note that while the incidence of bladder and rectal toxicity are similar to what is reported with IMRT, the primary benefit of proton beam therapy over IMRT is not in reducing the volume of bladder, rectum, or penile bulb receiving a high dose but in the volume of these structures receiving moderate doses (30–60 Gy), and this dose reduction may be expected to result in less erectile dysfunction, diarrhea, and bowel urgency as opposed to less rectal bleeding, urethritis, or urethral stricture (Mendenhall et al. 2012, 2014; Bryant et al. 2016).

7 Intensity-Modulated Proton Therapy

The recent development and deployment of Intensity-Modulated Proton Therapy (IMPT) now permits proton beam threat to be given in a fashion similar to IMRT, while using a beam that carries with it all of the physical advantages of protons over X-rays.

IMPT is being rapidly integrated into clinical proton beam therapy. It first became available in the United States in 2008 when the University of Texas MD Anderson Proton Treatment Center deployed this capability in one treatment room and it is now found in a number of existing centers, as well as being installed from inception at most new facilities being constructed worldwide. The Scripps Proton Therapy Center became the first "IMPT only" center in the United States when it opened in 2014.

To date, there exists only one published comparison of quality of life (QOL)/toxicity in men treated with proton beam therapy for localized prostate cancer between those who were treated with passively scattered proton therapy and intensity modulated proton therapy. Pugh and colleagues at M.D. Anderson performed a comparison between 226 men treated with PSPT and 65 men treated with IMPT. Quality-of-life was assessed by the expanded prostate cancer Index composite questionnaire (EPIC) which was administered at baseline and every 3–6 months after proton beam therapy. Clinically meaningful differences in quality of life were defined as $\geq 0.5 \times$ baseline standard deviation. In addition, the cumulative incidence of modified RTOG grade ≥ 2 GI or GU toxicity and the need for argon plasma coagulation (APC) were determined by the Kaplan–Meier method. Both groups of patients were treated with opposed right and left lateral beams with both fields being treated daily, and all patients received a total dose of 76 Gray (RBE) delivered in 38 fractions. The authors noted that both PSPT and IMPT conferred low rates of grade ≥ 2 GI and GU toxicity with preservation of meaningful sexual and urinary QOL at 24 months. A "modest yet clinically meaningful decrement in bowel QOL" was seen throughout the follow-up period, but there were no differences seen in toxicity or QOL between the two different delivery techniques. The authors did note that many of the patients treated with IMPT were some of the first patients treated with this technique both at their institution and within North America and hence postulated that the possible existence of a "learning curve effect" could have skewed the results somewhat (Pugh et al. 2013).

8 IMPT-Examples

The following treatment plans serve well to illustrate the flexibility and capability of IMPT in various clinical situations:

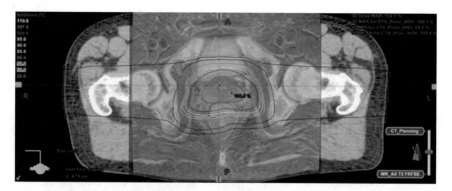

Fig. 9 The isodose image illustrates coverage of the prostate gland with simultaneousdose-escalation of the MRI-defined DIL

1. Conventional fractionation with simultaneous integrated boost (SIB) of a dominant intra-prostatic lesion (DIL). This 53-year-old gentleman had organ confined, intermediate risk prostate cancer. His IMPT planning included a thin-slice CT of the pelvis and multi-parametric MRI, both of which were performed with him in his treatment position. A SpaceOAR rectal spacer was also placed prior to imaging. The isodose image illustrates coverage of the prostate gland with simultaneous dose-escalation of the MRI-defined DIL (Fig. 9).

   Dose-volume histograms (DVH) for this patient are shown below. In this case, the patient underwent adaptive pelvic CT and MRI scans weekly during treatment to monitor the stability of his rectal spacer. The resulting composite DVH nicely illustrates both the high dose conformity achievable with IMPT and the low dose to the anterior rectal wall (pink contour) courtesy of the spacer (Fig. 10a).

   In order to monitor the status of his rectal spacer this patient underwent weekly adaptive pelvic CT and MRI scans. The dose-volume histogram demonstrates the reproducibility of his treatment plan while also illustrating the utility of the rectal spacer in reducing radiation dose to the anterior rectal wall (pink isodose lines) (Fig. 10b).
2. High-risk prostate cancer with treatment of the whole pelvis, plus prostate gland including SIB of DIL (Fig. 11).
3. Modestly Hypofractionated IMPT including SIB directed at DIL (Fig. 12).

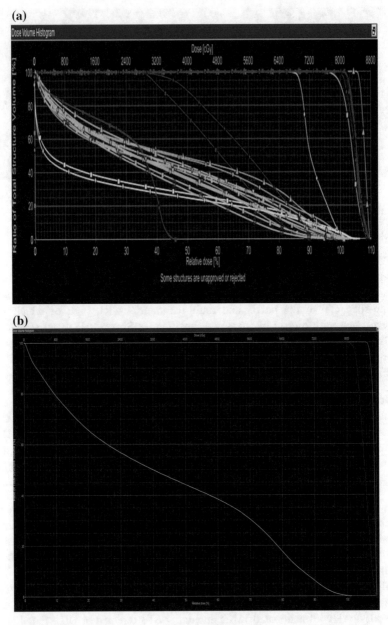

Fig. 10 **a** Composite DVH for patient with SpaceOAR Rectal Spacer. Prostate is in Red, DIL is Blue, Anterior Rectal Wall Pink, Whole Rectum Green, Bladder yellow. **b** Magnified View of static DVH, DIL in Orange, Prostate in Red, Anterior Rectal Wall Pink

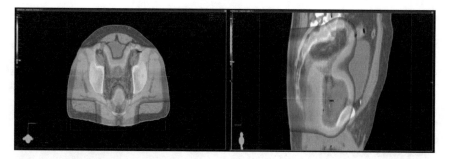

Fig. 11 High-risk prostate cancer with treatment of the whole pelvis, plus prostate gland includingSIB of DIL

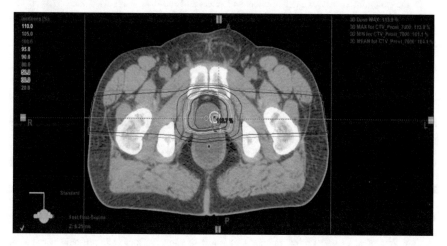

Fig. 12 Modestly hypofractionated IMPT including SIB directed at DIL

9 Conclusion

The implementation of IMPT has brought about a substantial leap in clinical capabilities including the ability to efficiently treat large, complex shapes while simultaneously producing both uniform and non-uniform dose distributions. In prostate cancer treatment these improved capabilities are at last bringing to proton therapy the same clinical utility which has existed with IMRT for the past decade and carries with it the promise of further improving the clinical utility of this treatment modality. Although to date the limited data on direct comparisons between IMPT and PSPT has shown little if any difference in efficacy or morbidity it is reasonable to anticipate that as the availability of IMPT becomes more widespread the further reduction in normal tissue doses associated with this modality will begin to manifest themselves as clinically meaningful differences in toxicity as compare to PSPT and IMRT-based treatment systems.

References

Bonnett DE (1993) Current developments in proton therapy: a review. Phys Med Biol 38 (10):1371–1392

Bryant C et al (2016) Five-year biochemical results, toxicity, and patient-reported quality of life after delivery of dose-escalated image guided proton therapy for prostate cancer. Int J Radiat Oncol Biol Phys 95(1):422–434

Goitein M (2010) Trials and tribulations in charged particle radiotherapy. Radiother Oncol 95 (1):23–31

Goitein M, Cox JD (2008) Should randomized clinical trials be required for proton radiotherapy? J Clin Oncol 26(2):175–176

Lomax A (1999) Intensity modulation methods for proton radiotherapy. Phys Med Biol 44 (1):185–205

Lomax AJ (2008) Intensity modulated proton therapy and its sensitivity to treatment uncertainties 2: the potential effects of inter-fraction and inter-field motions. Phys Med Biol 53(4):1043–1056

Lomax AJ (2009) Charged particle therapy: the physics of interaction. Cancer J 15(4):285–291

Lomax AJ et al (2004a) The clinical potential of intensity modulated proton therapy. Z Med Phys 14(3):147–152

Lomax AJ et al (2004b) Treatment planning and verification of proton therapy using spot scanning: initial experiences. Med Phys 31(11):3150–3157

Mendenhall NP et al (2012) Early outcomes from three prospective trials of image-guided proton therapy for prostate cancer. Int J Radiat Oncol Biol Phys 82(1):213–221

Mendenhall NP et al (2014) Five-year outcomes from 3 prospective trials of image-guided proton therapy for prostate cancer. Int J Radiat Oncol Biol Phys 88(3):596–602

Miller DW (1995) A review of proton beam radiation therapy. Med Phys 22(11 Pt 2):1943–1954

Olsen DR et al (2007) Proton therapy—a systematic review of clinical effectiveness. Radiother Oncol 83(2):123–132

Pugh TJ et al (2013) Quality of life and toxicity from passively scattered and spot-scanning proton beam therapy for localized prostate cancer. Int J Radiat Oncol Biol Phys 87(5):946–953

Schippers JM, Lomax AJ (2011) Emerging technologies in proton therapy. Acta Oncol 50(6):838–850

Shipley WU et al (1979) Proton radiation as boost therapy for localized prostatic carcinoma. JAMA 241(18):1912–1915

Shipley WU et al (1995) Advanced prostate cancer: the results of a randomized comparative trial of high dose irradiation boosting with conformal protons compared with conventional dose irradiation using photons alone. Int J Radiat Oncol Biol Phys 32(1):3–12

Slater JM, Miller DW, Archambeau JO (1988) Development of a hospital-based proton beam treatment center. Int J Radiat Oncol Biol Phys 14(4):761–775

Slater JM et al (1992) The proton treatment center at Loma Linda University Medical Center: rationale for and description of its development. Int J Radiat Oncol Biol Phys 22(2):383–389

Slater JD et al (1998) Conformal proton therapy for prostate carcinoma. Int J Radiat Oncol Biol Phys 42(2):299–304

Slater JD et al (2004) Proton therapy for prostate cancer: the initial Loma Linda University experience. Int J Radiat Oncol Biol Phys 59(2):348–352

Society AC (2015) Cancer facts and figures 2015

Suit H (2002) The Gray Lecture 2001: coming technical advances in radiation oncology. Int J Radiat Oncol Biol Phys 53(4):798–809

Suit HD et al (1977) Clinical experience and expectation with protons and heavy ions. Int J Radiat Oncol Biol Phys 3:115–125

Suit H et al (2003) Proton beams to replace photon beams in radical dose treatments. Acta Oncol 42(8):800–808

Talcott JA et al (2010) Patient-reported long-term outcomes after conventional and high-dose combined proton and photon radiation for early prostate cancer. JAMA 303(11):1046–1053

Trofimov A et al (2007) Radiotherapy treatment of early-stage prostate cancer with IMRT and protons: a treatment planning comparison. Int J Radiat Oncol Biol Phys 69(2):444–453

Wilson RR (1946) Radiological use of fast protons. Radiology 47(5):487–491

Zietman AL (2007) The Titanic and the Iceberg: prostate proton therapy and health care economics. J Clin Oncol 25(24):3565–3566

Zietman A (2008) Active surveillance: a safe, low-cost prognostic test for prostate cancer. BJU Int 101(9):1059–1060

Zietman AL (2016) Making radiation therapy for prostate cancer more economical and more convenient. J Clin Oncol 34(20):2323–2324

Zietman AL et al (2005) Comparison of conventional-dose vs high-dose conformal radiation therapy in clinically localized adenocarcinoma of the prostate: a randomized controlled trial. JAMA 294(10):1233–1239

Zietman AL et al (2010) Randomized trial comparing conventional-dose with high-dose conformal radiation therapy in early-stage adenocarcinoma of the prostate: long-term results from proton radiation oncology group/american college of radiology 95-09. J Clin Oncol 28(7):1106–1111

IGRT and Hypofractionation for Primary Tumors

Sagus Sampath

Abstract

Advancements in radiation planning and delivery have resulted in the ability to safely deliver higher doses per fraction to the tumor while also sparing normal tissue. Known as hypofractionated radiation therapy (HRT), or stereotactic ablative radiation therapy (SABR), this technique has been developed in multiple sites outside the brain, including lung, prostate, and pancreas. Accompanying such treatment is some form of image guided radiation therapy (IGRT). Localization of these tumors requires high quality soft tissue imaging, in addition to the ability to ascertain tumor location *during* radiation delivery. This chapter will outline the role of IGRT as it pertains to HRT treatment schemes for various malignancies.

Keywords

Hypofractionation · Image guided · Radiotherapy · Stereotactic

List of Abbreviations

HRT	Hypofractionated radiation therapy
SABR	Stereotactic ablative radiation therapy
IGRT	Image guided radiation therapy
NSCLC	Non-small cell lung cancer
CT	Computed tomography
PTV	Planning target volume
CBCT	Cone beam computed tomography
4DCT	Four-dimensional computed tomography

S. Sampath (✉)
Department of Radiation Oncology, City of Hope,
1500 E. Duarte Rd, Duarte, CA 91010, USA
e-mail: ssampath@coh.org

© Springer International Publishing AG 2017
J.Y.C. Wong et al. (eds.), *Advances in Radiation Oncology*,
Cancer Treatment and Research 172, DOI 10.1007/978-3-319-53235-6_6

AVB   Audio-visual feedback
kV   Kilovoltage
IMRT   Intensity modulated radiation therapy
RTOG   Radiation therapy oncology group
KIM   Kilovoltage intrafraction monitoring
MV   Megavoltage
ERB   Endo-rectal balloon
Gy   Gray
XRT   External beam radiotherapy
SBRT   Stereotactic body radiation therapy
LED   Light emitting diode
ITV   Internal target volume

1   Introduction

Hypofractionated radiation therapy (HRT) when given with definitive intent is defined as delivering doses per fraction that are higher than conventional radiation, typically greater than 4 Gy. These higher doses have clinically demonstrated superior benefit to conventional 2 Gy/day treatment in specific disease sites, such as stage I NSCLC. In order to safely administer such higher doses, understanding the position of the tumor during simulation and treatment is essential. Advances in linear-accelerator-based imaging, placement of fiducial markers, and patient-assisted devices, have enabled the clinician to deliver HRT with higher levels of certainty, facilitating narrower treatment margins around the tumor. This chapter will describe examples of these advances, as it pertains to specific solid tumor types, including lung, prostate, and pancreatic cancers.

2   Non-small Cell Lung Cancer (NSCLC)

Treatment planning. Stereotactic ablative radiation therapy (SABR) is considered a standard-of-care treatment option for patients with medically inoperable stage 1 NSCLC. One major challenge with treatment delivery is the ability to account and manage motion of the lung tumor. During the treatment planning, one option is to obtain a computed tomography (CT) scan at 3 timepoints: end-expiration, end-inspiration, and free breathing. A more sophisticated approach is to use a four-dimensional CT scan, which provides additional detail regarding the tumor trajectory between the peak and nadir. This approach can facilitate the use of narrow planning target volume (PTV) margins, thereby reducing normal tissue dose (Wang et al. 2009).

Image guidance. Cone-beam CT (CBCT) is now a standard imaging modality available on most linear accelerators, and is critical for verification of tumor position prior to treatment. Studies have shown that aligning to bony anatomy is not a substitute for aligning to the tumor soft tissue, as the first method can still result in significant shifts to match the tumor position (Corradetti et al. 2013). However, intra-fraction motion, or tumor motion that occurs during radiation delivery, is another important issue that can impact the accuracy of treatment. With 4D CT planning, recommended PTV margins around the gross tumor and motion are 5 mm (Corradetti et al. 2013). The purpose of this margin is to encompass tumor motion or migration during each treatment, in addition to daily setup differences between each treatment fraction. Corradetti et al. examined CBCT scans in 87 patients that were taken before and after each fraction (Corradetti et al. 2013). The mean shifts ranged from 1.1 to 1.6 mm, with 27 and 10% of shifts exceeding 3 and 5 mm, respectively.

Intra-fraction motion. Multiple strategies have been used to address the quandary of lung tumor motion during the time of the radiation delivery. These approaches include limiting the tumor motion itself, with external compression devices, or employing bio-feedback so that patient restricts their breathing on their own within a pre-specified window. Tumors are generally treated throughout the entire trajectory, under the presumption that the trajectory itself is being restricted. An alternative approach, known as *gating*, is to turn on the beam only during a specific range of the tumor's trajectory. More complex are tumor-tracking techniques. These various options are outlined below.

External compression was one of the first techniques used to address tumor motion in lung SBRT. The compression paddle is applied below the xiphoid in order to restrict tumor motion (Fig. 1: http://qfix.com/qfix-products/sbrt.asp). The goal was to limit the motion to less than 1 cm, using fluoroscopic guidance. Another option is to use a vacuum chamber around the patient, which restricts the amplitude of respiratory excursion (Fig. 2: http://ecatalog.elekta.com/oncology/oncology/breast-_-thorax-positioning-and-immobilization/products/0/22325/22341/20231/breast-_-thorax-positioning-and-immobilization.aspx). Li et al. examined positioning data from over 2000 CBCT scans from patients receiving lung SBRT (Li et al. 2011). There were no significant differences in the intra-fraction motion between an evacuated cushion with, or without abdominal compression. Image guidance with CBCT prior to delivery was sufficient to provide treatment that allowed for a 5 mm PTV margin. They concluded that performance status (ECOG 2 vs. 0-1) was a significant factor for cranial-caudal drift.

Audiovisual biofeedback (AVB) allows for patients to be an active participant in managing their tumor motion. Specialized eyewear can display a particular breathing pattern that is customized to the patient, which the patient can then follow during simulation, pre-treatment image guidance, and therapy. Lee et al. compared the consistency of displacement (or amplitude), and periodicity of breathing patterns as seen on MRI, in patients receiving AVB versus free breathing (Lee et al. 2016). They showed a significantly higher level of consistency in the AVB cohort,

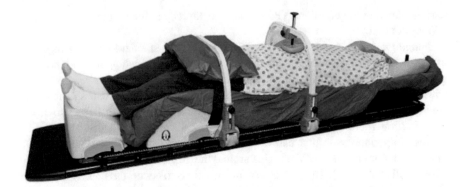

Fig. 1 External compression was one of the first techniques used to address tumor motion in lung SBRT

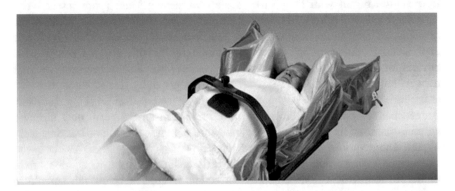

Fig. 2 Image guidance with CBCT prior to delivery was sufficient to provide treatment that allowed for a 5 mm PTV margin

for both inter-fraction and intra-fraction breathing. AVB had the strongest benefit with periodicity (70% improvement compared to free-breathing) compared to displacement. These results have spawned the development of a phase II multi-institutional randomized trial in Australia comparing AVB versus the free-breathing approach (Pollock et al. 2015).

Even when controlling or restricting the motion trajectory, it is still quite common for tumors to have displacements of more than 1 cm, especially those located in the lower lobes. In these cases, delivering dose during a limited range in the trajectory, or *gating*, can facilitate using narrower PTV margins and also expose less normal lung tissue (Jang et al. 2014). In addition, the process of gating itself has not been shown to impact tumor motion variability, highlighting the reproducibility of this approach (Saito et al. 2014). Advances have been made to use fiducial marker motion data generated from on-board kilo-voltage (kV) imaging (Ali et al. 2011; Wan et al. 2016). This has led to development of emerging technologies such as gated-CBCT and tumor-tracking treatment delivery.

The implantation of small inert metal markers near or within a tumor target to guide setup accuracy is not a novel concept. Before the advent of CBCT, this was the main approach for localizing the prostate gland and helped foster the coupling of dose-escalation with narrower PTV margins. Techniques of Implanting such markers in the lung have dramatically improved over the past 10 years, with advances in electromagnetic navigational bronchoscopy. A recent report by Minnich et al. indicated marker retention rates exceeding 90% (Minnich et al. 2015). Others have shown similar outcomes, with very low rates of complications and minimal intra-fraction migration (Nabavizadeh et al. 2014; Rong et al. 2015). These markers can be used for localization on the CBCT, and are also seen on intra-fraction kV images during arc-IMRT delivery. This allows for opportunity to correct for shifts that can occur during longer treatment delivery sessions.

One limitation of inert markers is the reliance of obtaining serial imaging repeatedly during the delivery fraction, and the inevitable inherent time lag in receiving the marker positional data and the ability for the therapist to intervene if necessary. With this mind, the feasibility of placing electro-magnetic transponder fiducials (Calypso Inc, Seattle, WA) in the lung were first reported in a pilot study of 7 patients (Shah et al. 2013). Two markers were placed per patient using bronchoscopic guidance. Placement into the lung itself was difficult, and therefore markers were placed into the most distal bronchus that was closest to the tumor. Thirteen of the 14 markers remained stable and were able to be tracked by the system. Based on this data, the Calypso system is now approved for intra-fraction motion monitoring and gating in lung cancer patients.

Active tumor tracking is the ability of the linear accelerator to shape the radiation beam to match the contour of the lung tumor, but treating it during the entire trajectory. The benefit to this approach is a shorter treatment time compared to gating, which can minimize risk for intra-fraction positional changes in the tumor and/or patient. One phantom study has demonstrated feasibility to reconstruct motion of the fiducial marker data to improve imaging artifact of CBCT due to patient breathing (Ali et al. 2011). This is an important development that can provide real-time motion data to the linear accelerator to assist with tracking. A new linear accelerator platform has been developed with a gimble-pivoting mechanism to permit simultaneous tracking and treatment of the lung tumor throughout the respiratory cycle (Vero Inc) The commissioning and quality assurance report is presented by Solberg et al. (2014). Clinical outcome data in the United States are still pending.

3 Prostate Cancer—Intact Gland

There have been remarkable advances in the technology of radiation treatment delivery for prostate cancer over the past 20 years. The advent of intensity modulated radiation therapy (IMRT), with more conformal dose distributions and steeper dose gradients next to normal tissue, enabled clinicians to employ narrower

PTV margins. This also enabled the ability to increase the potency of treatment by increasing the prescription dose. Doses as high as 86 Gy are now used in the definitive setting with conventional fractionation, with excellent outcomes and acceptable toxicity (Spratt et al. 2013). Hypofractionated dosing schedules have also been studied to increase patient convenience. The Radiation Therapy Oncology Group (RTOG) protocol 0415 was recently published by Lee et al., indicating that 70 Gy in 28 fractions is not inferior to conventionally fractionated treatment (73.8 Gy in 41 fractions) (Lee et al. 2016). SBRT has also been studied for low-risk and intermediate-risk prostate cancer, with greater than five year follow-up (Hannan et al. 2016; Katz et al. 2013). With dose escalation to 50 Gy in 5 fractions, Hannan et al. report biochemical control rates of 100% at five years (Hannan et al. 2016). As clinical outcomes from more potent dose schedules continue to emerge, there have also been a parallel of advancements in image-guidance to monitor and limit intra-fraction motion.

The only commercially available wireless radiotransponder fiducial system (Calypso Inc, Seattle, WA) was originally pioneered in patients with prostate cancer (Willoughby et al. 2006). Kupelian et al. reported multi-insitutional intra-fraction motion data on 35 patients (Kupelian et al. 2007). They found that displacement of the beacons exceeded 3 mm in more than 40% of treatment sessions. Motion trajectory was unpredictable in majority of cases. Radiotransponder beacons were used in the SBRT trial by Hannan et al., although intra-fraction motion data have not been reported. The majority of the clinical experience comes from patients treated using the Cyberknife platform, which uses orthogonal kV images to assess implanted marker motion at multiple time-points during delivery. A report of pooled outcomes using the Cyberknife system has been recently published by King et al. (2013).

Alternatives to wireless transponders are also being explored, given several limitations with this system, most notably imaging artifact on MRI. Keal et al. report on a novel approach known as kilovoltage intrafraction monitoring (KIM), using inert metal fiducial markers (Keall et al. 2016). A major advantage with KIM is it uses the standard kV-imager already built into the standard modern linear accelerator without necessity to purchase any additional hardware. In a preliminary study of 6 patients, they assessed the impact of KIM as a method for reducing gating events using a 3 mm/5 s action threshold, compared to patients without KIM. Out of 200 delivered fractions, 15% had a gating event. Percentage of beam-on time with the prostate being >3 mm away from isocenter was reduced in patients who had KIM (24% vs. 73%). The accuracy of KIM was also measured as <0.3 mm in all 3 dimensions by comparing it to simultaneously acquired kv/MV triangulation data. Given that the majority of published prostate SBRT studies did not use Calypso, this approach to intra-fraction motion management may have far-reaching clinical impact.

The use of an endo-rectal balloon (ERB) may overcome daily variation in rectal distention and peristalsis. This physiologic motion is the dominating contributor to intra-fraction motion of the prostate gland. Langen et al. demonstrated that the magnitude of intra-fraction motion using Calypso was largest in the

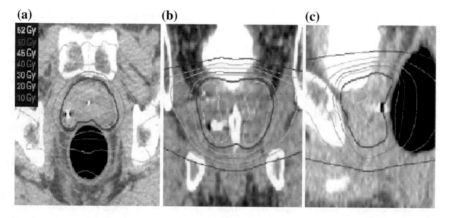

Fig. 3 Rectal balloon placement for prostate SBRT (Boike et al., Journal of Clinical Oncology © 2011). Reprinted with permission

anterior-posterior direction, with both positional drift and transient pulsatile motion (Langen et al. 2008). The total elapsed treatment time also had a significant impact on the motion, with larger movements seen with longer treatment times. In the setting of SBRT, such displacement of the target organ can result in under-dosing the PTV. To assess the potential benefit of ERB, Wang et al. compared the motion between 30 patients who were treated with and without ERB (Wang et al. 2012). They report that the ERB group had significant decreases in the motion in all dimensions, especially the anterior-posterior direction. In the University of Texas phase I prostate SBRT trial, daily endorectal balloon was used for simulation and treatment (Hannan et al. 2016). The rectal catheter was filled a pre-determined quantity of air, thereby fixing the interface between the anterior rectal wall and the prostate itself (Fig. 3). Another purpose of the ERB is to also *displace* the lateral and posterior rectal wall away from the PTV, facilitating lower doses received to these areas. The lack of any grade 2 or higher late gastro-intestinal toxicities in the 45 Gy arm, with a median follow-up of 74 months, illustrates the benefit with this technique (Hannan et al. 2016). The 45 Gy starting dose was the highest 5-fraction dose reported in the literature to date. Intra-fraction motion data has not been reported for this trial.

4   Prostate Cancer Following Prostatectomy

Salvage XRT is a standard treatment recommendation to treat biochemical recurrence of prostate cancer following radical prostatectomy. IMRT is now considered the preferred technique to optimize sparing of adjacent rectal tissues. Given the lack of a solid tumor target, radiation delivery in this setting presents multiple challenges. As IMRT inherently results in sharper dose gradients away from the target volume, intra-fraction data on the location of the tumor bed is critical. The definition of the CTV itself is fundamentally based on the relationship between the bladder and rectum. After multiple reports of successful implantation of fiducial markers in the intact-gland, a similar approach was started in the prostate bed.

Inter- and Intra-fraction motion data from 20 patients who received Calypso implantation was presented by Klayton et al. (2012). Prostate bed displacement was measured after aligning to bony landmarks. The shift in the superior-inferior direction exceeded 5 mm in more than 21% of delivered fractions. During delivery, motion was predominant in the posterior direction toward the rectum. Approximately 15% of all treatments were interrupted due to motion threshold being exceeded. It is possible that ERB may be useful to minimize motion of the prostate bed. In the absence of markers, soft tissue imaging with CBCT is essential to visualize the rectal wall. Besides traditional x, y, and z translation movements, yaw, pitch, and roll changes have also been shown to be contributors to intra-fractional target changes using Calypso (Zhu et al. 2013). Real-time adaptive planning strategies may be important in order maximize target coverage. It is proposed by Zhu et al. that intra-fraction data obtained early in the treatment course can be helpful in the decision making process to modify the existing treatment plan (Zhu et al. 2013).

To date, there are no published 5-fraction SBRT studies in the treatment of the prostate bed, analogous to the approach in the intact-gland setting. Hypofractionation schedules over 4-5 weeks have been explored. There is a clinical trial studying a 5-fraction technique which is actively accruing patients (clinicaltrials. gov), employing fiducial marker placement, CBCT, and ERB. Both intra- and inter-fraction motion will need to be considered for the successful implementation of this technique.

5 Pancreatic Cancer

Given that local failure was observed in 30-50% of patients with unresectable pancreatic cancer with conventional fractionation, the intention of SBRT in this setting was to develop a more potent local therapy (Willett et al. 2005). Colleagues from Stanford recently published their long-term experience, including patients receiving single-fraction and multi-fraction SBRT. They reported a 12-month crude local failure rate of approximately 10%, and 12-month survival of 30–35% (Pollom et al. 2014). Herman et al. reported a median survival of 13 months in 49 patients using a 5-fraction scheme (Herman et al. 2015).

In an earlier publication, Chang et al. outlined their treatment planning and simulation techniques (Chang et al. 2009). Patients were treated using a robotic radiosurgery system (Cyberknife, Accuray Inc, Sunnyvale, CA). Placement of fiducial markers into or around the pancreas has been shown to be safe using an endoscopic ultrasound (EUS) technique, although a traditional CT-guided percutaneous approach is the most common (Park et al. 2010). Approximately 1–2 weeks later, patients received a 4D-CT simulation with contrast (after 2004) and a PET/CT scan. GTV was delineated on the various phases of the 4D-CT and constituted a combined internal target volume. A 2–3 mm margin was then added to create the PTV.

6 Image-Guided Therapy

Chang et al. describe their approach to image guidance and respiratory management using the Cyberknife platform (Chang et al. 2009). The Cyberknife imaging system consists of 2 diagnostic orthogonal X-ray sources in the ceiling paired with detectors on the ground, enabling real-time images to verify bony anatomy and fiducial marker location during treatment. Outlining the fiducial markers on the 4D-CT is thus crucial to creating an internal motion trajectory, which is then paired with external motion trajectory data. The Synchrony respiratory tracking system uses motion data from LEDs placed on the chest wall of the patient. A model is generated from the LED and fiducial marker data to enable the linear accelerator to monitor the tumor motion during beam-on delivery, and make adjustments to the beam based on change changes in motion.

Such real-time tracking of tumor motion is critical, since it has been demonstrated that range of tumor trajectory at the time of 4D-CT simulation may not replicable at time of treatment (Minn et al. 2009). Minn et al. indicate that in the superior-inferior direction, the range of the centroid motion during simulation was 0.9–28.8 mm, compared to 0.5–12.7 mm during treatment. This suggests that the amplitude of the tumor motion can sometimes *decrease* compared to simulation, and therefore careful intra-fraction monitoring of tumor fiducials is essential to avoid missing the target. In patients receiving a 3–5 week fractionation regimen Len et al. describe differences in cranial-caudal motion magnitude between 4DCT and tumor motion seen on CBCT (Lens et al. 2014). Differences exceed 5 mm in 17% of the fractions delivered. The authors suggested employing breath-hold treatment techniques to address this issue.

Relying on external motion data alone during treatment may also be inadequate, as highlighted by Li et al. They performed the first clinical study assessing the geometric accuracy of gated Rapidarc treatment. Patients had fiducial marker placement in or near the tumor, and location of these markers were identified on the kV image portal prior to each beam-on delivery during the gating process. The distance between the ITV and the markers on the kV images were very small. The largest difference was in the cranial caudal direction, where a 1.5 mm margin was calculated. However, there were cases where the difference exceeded 2 mm, which approaches the uncertainty margin used in SBRT planning.

The Calypso marker system has also been used to monitor inter- and intra-fraction motion in pancreatic cancer. In their initial experience, Shinohara et al. demonstrated feasibility of marker implantation (Shinohara et al. 2012). They also report novel intra-fraction motion that was higher than anticipated, with a mean shift of 7 and 12 mm in the superior and inferior dimensions, respectively. They also suggested that implementing a breath-hold gating technique may be prudent.

7 Conclusions

With the advent of SBRT and shorter radiation treatment schedules, it is now of paramount importance that accurate and reproducible localization of the target be achieved. Both inter- and intra-fraction verification of target localization are necessary in order to ensure optimal outcomes, given the sharper dose gradients seen in SBRT planning. This is accomplished with highly complex imaging technology, that is becoming increasingly integrated with the treatment delivery platform. Each solid tumor type presents a unique set of treatment delivery challenges which require an individualized approach. Several strategies to account for intra-fraction tumor motion and deformation based on tumor type have been presented in this chapter. Future advancements are anticipated in the area of adaptive radiation planning and delivery based on real-time inter- and intra-fraction imaging data.

References

Ali I et al (2011) An algorithm to extract three-dimensional motion by marker tracking in the kV projections from an on-board imager: four-dimensional cone-beam CT and tumor tracking implications. J Appl Clin Med Phys 12(2):3407

Chang DT et al (2009) Stereotactic radiotherapy for unresectable adenocarcinoma of the pancreas. Cancer 115(3):665–672

Corradetti MN et al (2013) A moving target: Image guidance for stereotactic body radiation therapy for early-stage non-small cell lung cancer. Pract Radiat Oncol 3(4):307–315

Hannan R et al (2016) Stereotactic body radiation therapy for low and intermediate risk prostate cancer—results from a multi-institutional clinical trial. Eur J Cancer 59:142–151

Herman JM et al (2015) Phase 2 multi-institutional trial evaluating gemcitabine and stereotactic body radiotherapy for patients with locally advanced unresectable pancreatic adenocarcinoma. Cancer 121(7):1128–1137

Jang SS et al (2014) The impact of respiratory gating on lung dosimetry in stereotactic body radiotherapy for lung cancer. Phys Med 30(6):682–689

Katz AJ et al (2013) Stereotactic body radiotherapy for localized prostate cancer: disease control and quality of life at 6 years. Radiat Oncol 8:118

Keall PJ et al (2016) Real-time 3D image guidance using a standard LINAC: measured motion, accuracy, and precision of the first prospective clinical trial of kilovoltage intrafraction monitoring-guided gating for prostate cancer radiation therapy. Int J Radiat Oncol Biol Phys 94 (5):1015–1021

King CR et al (2013) Stereotactic body radiotherapy for localized prostate cancer: pooled analysis from a multi-institutional consortium of prospective phase II trials. Radiother Oncol 109 (2):217–221

Klayton T et al (2012) Prostate bed motion during intensity-modulated radiotherapy treatment. Int J Radiat Oncol Biol Phys 84(1):130–136

Kupelian P et al (2007) Multi-institutional clinical experience with the Calypso system in localization and continuous, real-time monitoring of the prostate gland during external radiotherapy. Int J Radiat Oncol Biol Phys 67(4):1088–1098

Langen KM et al (2008) Observations on real-time prostate gland motion using electromagnetic tracking. Int J Radiat Oncol Biol Phys 71(4):1084–1090

Lee D et al (2016a) Audiovisual biofeedback improves cine-magnetic resonance imaging measured lung tumor motion consistency. Int J Radiat Oncol Biol Phys 94(3):628–636

Lee WR et al (2016b) Randomized phase III noninferiority study comparing two radiotherapy fractionation schedules in patients with low-risk prostate cancer. J Clin Oncol 34(20):2325–2332

Lens E et al (2014) Differences in respiratory-induced pancreatic tumor motion between 4D treatment planning CT and daily cone beam CT, measured using intratumoral fiducials. Acta Oncol 53(9):1257–1264

Li W et al (2011) Effect of immobilization and performance status on intrafraction motion for stereotactic lung radiotherapy: analysis of 133 patients. Int J Radiat Oncol Biol Phys 81 (5):1568–1575

Minn AY et al (2009) Pancreatic tumor motion on a single planning 4D-CT does not correlate with intrafraction tumor motion during treatment. Am J Clin Oncol 32(4):364–368

Minnich DJ et al (2015) Retention rate of electromagnetic navigation bronchoscopic placed fiducial markers for lung radiosurgery. Ann Thorac Surg 100(4):1163–1165 Discussion 1165–1166

Nabavizadeh N et al (2014) Electromagnetic navigational bronchoscopy-guided fiducial markers for lung stereotactic body radiation therapy: analysis of safety, feasibility, and interfraction stability. J Bronchology Interv Pulmonol 21(2):123–130

Park WG et al (2010) EUS-guided gold fiducial insertion for image-guided radiation therapy of pancreatic cancer: 50 successful cases without fluoroscopy. Gastrointest Endosc 71(3):513–518

Pollock S et al (2015) Audiovisual biofeedback breathing guidance for lung cancer patients receiving radiotherapy: a multi-institutional phase II randomised clinical trial. BMC Cancer 15:526

Pollom EL et al (2014) Single-versus multifraction stereotactic body radiation therapy for pancreatic adenocarcinoma: outcomes and toxicity. Int J Radiat Oncol Biol Phys 90(4):918–925

Rong Y et al (2015) Minimal inter-fractional fiducial migration during image-guided lung stereotactic body radiotherapy using superlock nitinol coil fiducial markers. PLoS ONE 10(7): e0131945

Saito T et al (2014) Respiratory gating during stereotactic body radiotherapy for lung cancer reduces tumor position variability. PLoS ONE 9(11):e112824

Shah AP et al (2013) Real-time tumor tracking in the lung using an electromagnetic tracking system. Int J Radiat Oncol Biol Phys 86(3):477–483

Shinohara ET et al (2012) Feasibility of electromagnetic transponder use to monitor inter- and intrafractional motion in locally advanced pancreatic cancer patients. Int J Radiat Oncol Biol Phys 83(2):566–573

Solberg TD et al (2014) Commissioning and initial stereotactic ablative radiotherapy experience with Vero. J Appl Clin Med Phys 15(2):4685

Spratt DE et al (2013) Long-term survival and toxicity in patients treated with high-dose intensity modulated radiation therapy for localized prostate cancer. Int J Radiat Oncol Biol Phys 85 (3):686–692

Wan H et al (2016) Automated patient setup and gating using cone beam computed tomography projections. Phys Med Biol 61(6):2552–2561

Wang L et al (2009) Dosimetric comparison of stereotactic body radiotherapy using 4D CT and multiphase CT images for treatment planning of lung cancer: evaluation of the impact on daily dose coverage. Radiother Oncol 91(3):314–324

Wang KK et al (2012) A study to quantify the effectiveness of daily endorectal balloon for prostate intrafraction motion management. Int J Radiat Oncol Biol Phys 83(3):1055–1063

Willett CG et al (2005) Locally advanced pancreatic cancer. J Clin Oncol 23(20):4538–4544
Willoughby TR et al (2006) Target localization and real-time tracking using the Calypso 4D
    localization system in patients with localized prostate cancer. Int J Radiat Oncol Biol Phys 65
    (2):528–534
Zhu M et al (2013) Adaptive radiation therapy for postprostatectomy patients using real-time
    electromagnetic target motion tracking during external beam radiation therapy. Int J Radiat
    Oncol Biol Phys 85(4):1038–1044

The Impact of IGRT on Normal Tissue Toxicity

Timothy E. Schultheiss

Abstract

Image Guided Radiation Therapy (IGRT) deploys advanced imaging techniques prior to each treatment to ensure the highest possible agreement between the planned treatment geometry and the daily set-up. This agreement includes both the patient position and the localization of the internal target and normal structures. This process reduces non-tumor tissues within the target volume to a minimum. IGRT is now commonly accompanied by altered fractionation schemes, usually hypofractionation. With the small-volume, high-dose-per-fraction treatments, the profile of treatment morbidities may change, compared to conventional 3D treatment. This chapter explores how these morbidities may change with the use of IGRT.

Keywords

Image guided radiation therapy · Normal tissue toxicity

1 Introduction

Technological advances in radiation oncology have largely focused on delivering as much dose as possible to the target volume while minimizing normal tissue (NT) morbidity.[1] This has been accomplished by deploying increasingly complex

---

[1]Only recently has de-escalation of target dose become a serious line of investigation in radiation oncology.

T.E. Schultheiss (✉)
Department of Radiation Oncology, City of hope, 1500 East Durate Road,
Durate, CA 91010, USA
e-mail: Schultheiss@coh.org

© Springer International Publishing AG 2017
J.Y.C. Wong et al. (eds.), *Advances in Radiation Oncology*,
Cancer Treatment and Research 172, DOI 10.1007/978-3-319-53235-6_7

field arrangements of increasingly smaller beamlets and arcs and by using immobilization and imaging to ensure proper patient positioning and targeting of the
planning target volume.[2] The result has been sharper dose gradients at the margin of
the high dose region and lower doses to normal tissues. If no change is made in the
dose per fraction or in the total tumor dose, then normal tissue toxicity will necessarily be reduced because normal tissue doses are reduced. However, as technology has improved, tumor doses have been escalated, generally (or at least
initially) by increasing the number of fractions rather than the dose per fraction.
Under the assumption that as tumor doses increase, the same dose limits on normal
tissue are respected, then the NT dose per fraction will decrease, again decreasing
the morbidity. Thus it is self-evident that deploying IGRT either while keeping
target doses the same, or while increasing them but keeping NT tissue doses the
same will decrease NT morbidity if the target dose per fraction is held constant or
will hold NT morbidity constant if the target dose per fraction is increased. The
exception to this statement is the morbidity to normal tissues within the target
volume itself.

We will explore three scenarios where a tradeoff occurs between local control
and NT morbidity when IGRT replaces conventional treatments. We investigate
these scenarios primarily with respect to the changes in NT morbidity. Some
increase in local control will be assumed so that dose escalation may be justified,
but it is the potential increase in NT morbidity that will be explored in order to
determine how much the target dose may be safely increased.

The first scenario is the use of IGRT to escalate target dose with conventional
fractionation where the NT doses are also increased but the NT dose per fraction
decreases. To explore this scenario requires knowledge of the fractionation effects
on normal tissues. The volume effects will not greatly impact the morbidity in this
case since the relative dose distribution would not be expected to change
dramatically.

The second scenario is the use of IGRT to escalate the effective target dose by
deploying hypofractionation in addition to IGRT. This technique is often limited to
small volume treatments, with a concomitant small volume of irradiated NT. In this
situation, the volume effect can be paramount and may even result in the nature of
the NT morbidity being different from what would typically be observed when large
NT organ volumes are irradiated.

Finally, the third scenario is the use of single fraction IGRT, which can be
considered as the limit of hypofractionated IGRT. The tissue at risk in this scenario
is very commonly nervous tissue.

The radiobiological considerations in these three scenarios may be different and
will be discussed separately.

---

[2]In this chapter, IGRT will be assumed to include daily volumetric imaging prior to treatment.
Early definitions of IGRT included multimodality imaging to define better the target volume. In
this chapter, we will consider only the impact of daily imaging on NT responses. In IGRT like in
quantum mechanics, we assume you know where something is only when you look for it.

2   Radiobiological Foundations

2.1   A Brief History

IGRT highlights the longstanding discussion regarding the relative importance of dose versus volume in radiation induced normal tissue toxicity. The specific issue is whether toxicity is more sensitive to changes in irradiated volume at a constant dose or changes in dose at a constant volume. Historically, most technical improvements in radiation dose delivery (custom blocking, CT simulation, conformal therapy, IMRT, IGRT, adaptive treatment) have been claimed to have the potential to increase the tumor dose (local control) and/or decrease normal tissue doses/volumes (morbidity) by improving the targeting of the radiation treatment. In the 1970s and 1980s, the same objective was attempted by manipulating the fractionation schedule using split course treatments and searching for the best dose per fraction whether deployed in conventional, hypofractionation, or hyperfractionation schedules. These efforts met with limited success, but the emphasis on "tighter" dose distributions and better definition of treatment objectives as exemplified by the publication ICRU 50 ultimately led to greater success (IRCU 50, 1993). The proof-of-principle study in controlling dose distributions was RTOG 94-06, A Phase I/II Dose Escalation Study Using Three Dimensional Conformal Radiation Therapy for Adenocarcinoma of the Prostate(Michalski et al. 2000). The genesis of this RTOG study was an NCI-sponsored cooperative study "National Collaborative Radiation Therapy Trials: 3-D Dose Escalation Study for Prostate Cancer." Rapid advances in delivery technology and 3D dose calculations made it possible to transition from the introduction of conformal radiation therapy in the mid 1990s to IGRT with helical tomotherapy in less than 10 years. IGRT using arc therapy on C-arm linacs followed rapidly thereafter.

2.2   Some Biological Considerations

How NT morbidity changes with changes in dose and volume depends upon how the tissue is organized morphologically and the pathogenesis of the injury. A useful concept used in discussing NT morbidity is the functional subunit, FSU, first introduced in radiation oncology by Withers et al. (1988). The FSU is a construct to model how the organ or tissue is organized, but in some cases the idea has been carried beyond its connection to reality. Withers et al. argued that FSUs could be organized either in parallel, when the loss of some FSU's would not necessary result in a radiation injury, or in series where the loss of a single FSU would yield an injury. In the former case, FSU's organized in parallel is a tautology. If an organ has FSU's, logic demands that they are organized in parallel. Those organs that have functional reserve can be said to have FSU's. In those organs, part of the organ can be lost and the remainder of the organ can fulfill its function. The lung, kidneys, and liver are some obvious examples. However, if an organ fails when a single component fails, then the entire organ functions as a single unit and there are no *sub*units. If there is no functional reserve, that is, if no part of the organ accomplishes a portion of the task of the organ as a whole, then there is a single functional unit.

In radiation response, not just the tissue organization, but the pathogenesis is relevant to the determination of FSU's. Veno-oclusive disease is a potential radiation injury, but it is fundamentally a complication of the whole liver (Klaus Trott, personal communication). Radiation induced liver disease, formerly known as radiation hepatitis, is a complication that manifests at higher doses to a fractional portion of the liver(Dawson et al. 2002; Lawrence et al. 1995). Thus a single organ may have different FSU's depending on the injury type.

The spinal cord is generally held to be the paradigm of an organ made of serial functional subunits. However, the fundamental function of the spinal cord is to transmit reliably a signal from the brain to a remote tissue or vice versa. If part of the spinal cord is damaged, the signal is not reduced, it is interrupted. The spinal cord acts as one, single electrical cable.

The confusion that led to the erroneous concept that organs without subunits have serial architecture probably had its genesis in the fact that the original version of the critical element model (a volume effects model) assumed a complication was the result of a lesion of sufficient size occurring anywhere in the organ it risk, as in the spinal cord (Schultheiss et al. 1983). The probability of a lesion occurring in a fractional volume, v, of uniformly irradiated tissue was estimated by

$$P(D, v) = 1 - (1 - P(D, 1))^v$$

.

where P(D, 1) is the probability of a lesion occurring if the entire organ is irradiated to dose D. This formula was derived using the simple notion that the probability of a lesion *not* occurring in the organ was the product of the probabilities of its not occurring in all subvolumes of the organ. This model is easily generalized to an inhomogeneous dose distribution, and it has the advantage that the probability of complication is based on the dose response function of a uniformly irradiated whole organ, the most likely form that clinical data of that era would take. However, the mathematical "trick" of using subvolumes does not imply the existence of FSU's.

Jackson and colleagues developed a similar model for organs with actual FSU's (Jackson and Kutcher 1993; Jackson et al. 1995). Rather than the production of a single lesion, they modeled a volume *element* as having suffered a binary level of damage. The endpoint was reached if a sufficient number of volume elements, presumed to be FSU's, suffered damage. Unfortunately, this formalism requires the dose response function for the FSU in order to determine the organ response. It is not possible to determine the dose response function of a partially irradiated organ based on the dose response of the whole organ. One can see how the division of a so-called serial organ encouraged the mistaken association of these volume elements with FSU's, as they truly are in an organ with functional reserve.

Both the critical element model and the parallel architecture model are examples of what is known in reliability systems as a k-out-of-N system; the system fails if k of the N elements of the system fail, and is denoted as a k-out-of-N:F. The critical element model is a 1-out-of-N:F system and the parallel model is a k-out-of-N system. A k-out-of-N:G system is good (G) if k of the component remain functional. There are consecutive k-out-of-N systems where a linear system fails if k *consecutive* components fail. The critical element or serial model is a k-out-of-N system with *k = 1*. The parallel architecture model of Jackson et al. is a nonconsecutive k-out-of-N system, where N is the number of FSU's and k is the number that must fail to elicit a radiation complication. Tumors are typically modeled as k-out-of-N:G systems with *k = 1*. That is, as long as a single clonogen is good, the tumor is viable. More complex models can be made by adding higher dimensions, i.e. two and three dimensional k-out-of-N systems. However, consecutive k-out-of-N systems are mathematically very complex (or at least tedious), and higher dimensional systems have the disadvantage of being simultaneously nearly intractable while having too many independent variates in the model to be statistically useful for modeling normal tissue responses.

3 Fractionation Scenarios

3.1 Conventionally Fractionated Treatments

Image guidance today is primarily achieved with commercially available on-board systems used for daily volumetric imaging in radiation therapy setups such as cone beam CT and megavoltage CT. Open MRI coupled with rotational Co-60 beams has been developed recently and ultrasound imaging is still commercially available. Early versions of daily CT scanning involved scanning on a CT simulator prior to treatment and transferring the patient to a treatment table using a transfer board (Lattanzi et al. 1998). The authors concluded, "With daily isocenter correction of setup and organ motion errors by CT imaging, PTV margins can be significantly reduced or eliminated. We believe this will facilitate further dose escalation in high-risk patients with minimal risk of increased morbidity." This technique was compared to the use of transabdominal ultrasound in the treatment position for prostate cancer (Lattanzi et al. 1999). The two were found to be "functionally equivalent."

Thus even as conformal therapy was transitioning to IMRT in the 1990s, efforts to deploy IGRT were already being made. Outside of SRS treatments, these initial efforts were primarily focused on reducing the CTV-PTV margin by reducing set-up variations and imaging the target volume every day. The objective was to increase tumor dose without increasing morbidity. Megavoltage CT was being deployed with a prototype helical tomotherapy for the same purpose (Mackie et al. 1995; Yang et al. 1997). In-room CT was also deployed later with varying success (Owen et al. 2009).

In an extensive study of set-up variations versus the frequency of imaging in IGRT, Han et al. determined the likelihood of a decrease in coverage of the target volume and an increase in NT irradiated volumes when imaging occurred at frequencies of 0, 20, 40, and 60% versus daily (100%) imaging (Han et al. 2012). Even at an imaging frequency of 60%, the lung volume receiving 0.8 Gy per day and the heart volume receiving 1.2 Gy per day increased by more than 20% in 10% of the fractions. The CTV receiving 95% of the daily dose (1.8 Gy) decreased by more than 20% in 5% of the fractions. This is primary evidence that by deploying daily image guidance, the NT doses can be decreased and target doses increased. Complications rates and the types of side effects would not change. Conversely, if the target dose did not change, complication rates could decrease without affecting the types of complications. This was observed by Chung et al. in prostate cancer (Chung et al. 2009).

It is important not to overstate the effect of image guidance. Clearly, an advantage is seen since the NT DVH is shifted to lower doses (and the PTV DVH becomes steeper). However, it is important to acknowledge that part of this shift is a result of reduced margins afforded by daily imaging (IGRT) and part results from improved dose fall-off away from the target due to improved dose *delivery* technology (IMRT). It is difficult to find in the literature clinical studies that compare similar IMRT techniques with dissimilar imaging protocols. It is the imaging that distinguishes IGRT from IMRT.

3.2 Hypofractionated Treatment

The failure of early hypofractionation resulted from a lack of understanding of radiobiology and the response of normal tissues to radiation. It was believed, or more accurately hoped that morbidity from increases in daily doses could be offset by lengthening the interfraction interval. Furthermore, the biological consequence of increasing the dose per fraction was underestimated. Unfortunately these early attempts were undertaken when field shaping was unsophisticated, volume effects were underestimated, and treatments were frequently delivered using one field per day. By the late 1980s, hypofractionation, often combined with split course treatments, was largely abandoned in the definitive setting (Overgaard et al. 1988; Parsons et al. 1980). Late complications, which are more sensitive to changes in dose per fraction than tumors, increased without a compensating increase in tumor control because the relative dose distributions were not altered.

By sparing normal tissues, IGRT reduces both the dose per fraction and the volume of NT irradiated without reducing the tumor dose. Increasing the dose per fraction to the tumor so that the NT dose per fraction remains approximately constant would still leave a smaller volume of NT irradiated. Using hypofractionation, investigators have tested the hypothesis the NT morbidity will not increase because reduced irradiated volumes will compensate for any increase in dose per fraction. The truth to this hypothesis largely rests on the nature of the volume effect and the pathogenesis of the NT morbidity.

As discussed above, prostate cancer was among the sites where IGRT was deployed early in its history, initially with conventional fractionation. Because doses were being escalated to 80 Gy and higher, overall treatment times were extending beyond 8 weeks. In part to shorten the overall duration of treatment, hypofractionation trials were initiated. In general, the GI late toxicities are similar into those seen with the best conformal or IMRT results. However, there is a strong tendency to report slightly greater GU toxicity in IGRT than in conformal treatments, although severe late GU toxicity is rare.

Rectal toxicity generally includes symptoms of radiation proctitis (urgency, frequency, mucus discharge, pain) or rectal bleeding. Rectal bleeding would not be expected to be very volume dependent, but to depend rather more on dose; however, Wu et al. reported no rectal bleeding in 72 patients treated with a schedule of 16×3.4 Gy (Wu et al. 2012). In this report, as in several others (King et al. 2009; Madsen et al. 2007; Pollack et al. 2013), GU toxicity was a greater problem than GI toxicity.

The relatively greater incidence of GU toxicity in IGRT for the prostate can be reasonably explained by the fact that the urethra is in the high dose volume whereas the rectum can largely be excluded from the target volume. Obviously as the target dose is escalated, so are the doses to most GU tissues that are at risk for radiation injury.

A somewhat similar effect occurs in the lung. The relative frequency of toxicity changes in two ways when conformal fields shrink to SBRT fields with the concomitant increase in dose per fraction (Kollar and Rengan 2014). As seen in animal models (Van Der Veen et al. 2016), there is a shift from early to late effects as the volume is reduced. Furthermore, at the higher doses per fraction, the central normal structures become more likely to express morbidity than peripheral lung parenchyma. These effects are independent of yet a third possibility–spatial variation in lung sensitivity as seen in mouse models and attributed to the spatial variation in target structure for radiation pneumonitis (Tucker et al. 1997).

In the CNS, both brain and spinal cord, there appear to be no changes in the types of normal tissue morbidity that result from reducing volumes and number of fractions while increasing the dose per fraction. The obvious exception is that neurocognitive deficits result from large volume treatment of CNS. However, one must still be cognizant of differing sensitivity of different regions. For example, there is some evidence that thoracic spinal cord is less sensitive than the cervical cord. The lumbar cord is also less sensitive, possibly owing to its being myelinated with Schwann cells rather than oligodendrocytes.

In addition to dose and volume factors associated with normal tissue responses in changing from conventional fractionation and target volumes to hypofractionation and image guided target volumes, different biological factors and responses may come into play at larger doses per fraction. With higher biological doses that result from higher doses per fraction, not only are direct effects observed, but the microenvironment in the target region is altered by release of inflammatory mediators and molecular factors that may alter vascular permeability, induce changes in fibroblasts, and impact the endothelial cell compartment (Song et al. 2014; Zeng et al. 2014). Research has concentrated on the impact of these effects on tumor response and tumor growth, but the impact on normal structures inside the IGRT target volume has received relatively little attention.

3.3 Single Fraction Treatments

Reoxygenation, redistribution or reassortment, repair, and repopulation comprise the 4 R's of radiotherapy. Reoxygenation is probably irrelevant to normal tissue and repopulation is not very important in late injury. Clearly reassortment and repair are not factors if single fraction treatments are used. Thus single fraction treatments cannot benefit from the traditional advantages of fractionation, which generally reduce normal tissue injury while simultaneously enhancing tumor sensitivity. Of course there are many examples of failed single-fraction efforts in the history of radiation oncology. The success of single fraction IGRT can be largely attributed to the significant geometrical advances of IGRT and the fact that we have learned the cost of treating large volumes using single fractions.

There may some biological advantages to single fractions as described elsewhere in this volume. See *Optimizing radiation dose and fractionation* in the Chapter "Advances in Immunotherapy." However, it seems any putative advantages would not outweigh the advantages of fractionation. High-dose radiation treatments may impact tumor control through stromal effects not predicted by classical radiobiological considerations (Brown et al. 2014; Hellevik and Martinez-Zubiaurre 2014). However, these stromal effects are not dependent on the radiation being given in a single fraction.

One might be tempted to believe that the probability of a geographic miss would increase with fractionation. However, the probability of a miss is the same if equal care is given to N fractions in a single patient or in single fractions to N patients.

Thus from biological and physical arguments, fractionated treatment still appears to be advantageous. The advantage of single fraction treatments comes primarily in patient convenience and especially for palliative cases (Greco et al. 2011).

4 Conclusions

The emphasis of this chapter is not to list the normal tissue complications observed in IGRT. It is to describe how morbidity profile and pathogenesis might change in going from conventional treatments to image guided treatments. In deploying image guided treatments, effective doses are generally escalated, dose per fraction increases, and volumes are decreased. If the tumor dose is increased solely by increasing the number of fractions as was done in the early days of IGRT for prostate cancer, then the character of the morbidities is unlikely to change although the relative frequency might as a result of increased morbidity to the normal tissues in the target volumes and decreases elsewhere.

Hypofractionation and single fraction IGRT are almost always associated with small-target-volume treatment. The small target volumes can result in significant changes in the normal tissues at risk, the types of morbidities elicited, and a shift from early to late effects. When using high doses per fraction, the likelihood increases that the morbidity will be associated with local necrosis and late fibrosis. Combining high doses per fraction and small volumes can result in morbidities rarely seen in conventional treatments, such as those seen in central lung structures after SBRT.

There seems to be little to recommend single fraction treatments over hypofractionation. In nearly all cases, the biology for normal tissue recovery and tumor cell kill seems to favor some fractionation. The statistics of treatment set up do not favor single fraction treatments. Patient convenience is the only measure in which single fraction treatments have an advantage. This may be important in palliative cases, if a cogent argument for image guided treatment can be made in the palliative setting.

References

Brown JM, Carlson DJ, Brenner DJ (2014) The tumor radiobiology of SRS and SBRT: are more than the 5 Rs involved? Int J Radiat Oncol Biol Phys 88:254–262

Chung HT, Xia P, Chan LW et al (2009) Does image-guided radiotherapy improve toxicity profile in whole pelvic-treated high-risk prostate cancer? Comparison between IG-IMRT and IMRT. Int J Radiat Oncol Biol Phys 73:53–60

Dawson LA, Normolle D, Balter JM et al (2002) Analysis of radiation-induced liver disease using the Lyman NTCP model. Int J Radiat Oncol Biol Phys 53:810–821

Greco C, Zelefsky MJ, Lovelock M et al (2011) Predictors of local control after single-dose stereotactic image-guided. Intensity-modulated radiotherapy for extracranial metastases. Int J Radiat Oncol Biol Phys 79:1151–1157

Han C, Schiffner DC, Schultheiss TE et al (2012) Residual setup errors and dose variations with less-than-daily image guided patient setup in external beam radiotherapy for esophageal cancer. Radioth Oncol 102:309–314

Hellevik T, Martinez-Zubiaurre I (2014) Radiotherapy and the tumor stroma: the importance of dose and fractionation. Front Oncol 4:1–12

International Commission on Radiation Units and Measurements: ICRU Report 50 (1993) Prescribing, recording and reporting photon beam therapy Prescribing, Recording and Reporting Photon Beam Therapy, Bethesda

Jackson A, Kutcher GJ (1993) Probability of radiation-induced complications for normal tissues with parallel architecture subject to non-uniform irradiation. Med Phys 20:613–625

Jackson A, Ten Haken RK, Robertson JM et al (1995) Analysis of clinical complication data for radiation hepatitis using a parallel architecture model. Int J Radiat Oncol Biol Phys 31:883–891

King CR, Brooks JD, Gill H et al (2009) Stereotactic body radiotherapy for localized prostate cancer: interim results of a prospective phase ii clinical trial. Int J Radiat Oncol Biol Phys 73:1043–1048

Kollar L, Rengan R (2014) Stereotactic body radiotherapy. Semin Oncol 41:776–789

Lattanzi J, Mcneeley S, Pinover W et al (1999) A comparison of daily CT localization to a daily ultrasound-based system in prostate cancer. Int J Radiat Oncol Biol Phys 43:719–725

Lattanzi J, Mcneely S, Hanlon A et al (1998) Daily CT localization for correcting portal errors in the treatment of prostate cancer. Int J Radiat Oncol Biol Phys 41:1079–1086

Lawrence TS, Robertson JM, Anscher MS et al (1995) Hepatic toxicity resulting from cancer treatment. Int J Radiat Oncol Biol Phys 31:1237–1248

Mackie TR, Holmes TW, Reckwerdt PJ et al (1995) Tomotherapy: optimized planning and delivery of radiation therapy. Int J Imaging Syst Technol 6:43–55

Madsen BL, Hsi RA, Pham HT et al (2007) Stereotactic hypofractionated accurate radiotherapy of the prostate (SHARP) 335 Gy in five fractions for localized disease: first clinical trial results. Int J Radiat Oncol Biol Phys 67:1099–1105

Michalski JM, Purdy JA, Winter K et al (2000) Preliminary report of toxicity following 3D radiation therapy for prostate cancer on 3DOG/RTOG 9406. Int J Radiat Oncol Biol Phys 46:391–402

Overgaard J, Hjelm-Hansen M, Johansen LV et al (1988) Comparison of conventional and Split-course radiotherapy as primary treatment in carcinoma of the larynx. Acta Oncol 27:147–152

Owen R, Kron T, Foroudi F et al (2009) Comparison of CT on rails with electronic portal imaging for positioning of prostate cancer patients with implanted fiducial markers. Int J Radiat Oncol Biol Phys 74:906–912

Parsons JT, Bova FJ, Million RR (1980) A re-evaluation of split-course technique for squamous cell carcinoma of the head and neck. Int J Radiat Oncol Biol Phys 6:1645–1652

Pollack A, Walker G, Horwitz EM et al (2013) Randomized trial of hypofractionated external-beam radiotherapy for prostate cancer. J Clini Oncol 31:3860–3868

Schultheiss TE, Orton CG, Peck RA (1983) Models in radiotherapy: volume effects. Med Phys 10:410–415

Song CW, Kim MS, Cho LC et al (2014) Radiobiological basis of SBRT and SRS. Int J Clin Oncol 19:570–578

Tucker SL, Liao ZX, Travis EL (1997) Estimation of the spatial distribution of target cells for radiation pneumonitis in mouse lung. Int J Radiat Oncol Biol Phys 38:1055–1066

van der Veen SJ, Faber H, Ghobadi G et al (2016) Decreasing irradiated rat lung volume changes dose-limiting toxicity from early to late effects. Int J Radiat Oncol Biol Phys 94:163–171

Withers HR, Taylor JMG, Maciejewski B (1988) Treatment volume and tissue tolerance. Int J Radiat Oncol Biol Phys 14:751–759

Wu JSY, Brasher PMA, El-Gayed A et al (2012) Phase II study of hypofractionated image-guided radiotherapy for localized prostate cancer: outcomes of 55 Gy in 16 fractions at 34 Gy per fraction. Radioth Oncol 103:210–216

Yang JN, Mackie TR, Reckwerdt P et al (1997) An investigation of tomotherapy beam delivery. Med Phys 24:425–436

Zeng J, Baik C, Bhatia S et al (2014) Combination of stereotactic ablative body radiation with targeted therapies. Lancet Oncol 15:e426–e434

Biologic and Image Guided Systemic Radiotherapy

Jeffrey Y.C. Wong, Susanta Hui, Savita V. Dandapani and An Liu

Abstract

Radiotherapy has traditionally been used as a therapy directed to the primary site of disease to achieve local and regional control. This role is rapidly changing with radiotherapy now playing an integral part of systemic therapy in patients with metastatic disease. Stereotactic body radiotherapy to each oligometastatic site is now actively being evaluated as a means to more definitively control disease and contribute to a longer progression free interval. Irradiation of a tumor site can result in clinically important immuno-modulatory systemic effects which when combined with certain immunotherapy agents can result in abscopal responses at unirradiated sites harboring macroscopic and microscopic disease. Technological advances have now made the delivery of targeted systemic radiotherapy a reality. Systemic radiotherapy can be biologically guided as in the case of radiolabeled peptide analogs or immunologically guided as in the case of radiolabeled antibodies directed against tumor associated antigens. Recent advances in intensity modulated radiation therapy allow for radiation dose sculpting to the entire body resulting in a more targeted form of total body irradiation, also referred to as total marrow irradiation. This targeting is CT image guided to a specific anatomic region, but in the future is expected to incorporate PET and MRI based functional imaging allowing for systemic

J.Y.C. Wong (✉) · S. Hui · S.V. Dandapani · A. Liu
Department of Radiation Oncology, City of Hope, Duarte, CA 91010, USA
e-mail: jwong@coh.org

S. Hui
e-mail: shui@coh.org

S.V. Dandapani
e-mail: sdandapani@coh.org

A. Liu
e-mail: aliu@coh.org

© Springer International Publishing AG 2017
J.Y.C. Wong et al. (eds.), *Advances in Radiation Oncology*,
Cancer Treatment and Research 172, DOI 10.1007/978-3-319-53235-6_8

radiotherapy which is biologically guided based on the unique physiologic, phenotypic and genotypic properties of the tumor. This chapter will summarize the progress, current state and future directions of targeted systemic radiotherapy. The treatment of hematopoietic malignancies is used to illustrate important principles which are applicable to other malignant conditions.

Keywords
Total marrow irradiation · Radioimmunotherapy · Total body irradiation · Bone marrow transplantation

1   Introduction

Radiation therapy has traditionally been utilized as a local regional therapy to optimize local control at the primary site or at a symptomatic site of metastatic disease. This treatment paradigm is rapidly changing with radiotherapy now playing a critical role as an integral part of systemic therapy in patients with metastatic disease. For example, a distinct subset of patients with oligometastatic disease is now recognized, with disease characterized by lower tumor burden, limited metastatic sites, and a longer timeline towards progression (Weichselbaum and Hellman 2011). Stereotactic body radiotherapy (SBRT) to each tumor site is now actively being evaluated as a means to more definitively control macroscopic disease and contribute to a longer progression free interval in this population (Salama et al. 2008). Irradiation of a tumor site in patients with metastatic disease can result in clinically important immuno-modulatory systemic effects which when combined with certain immunotherapy agents can result in abscopal immune responses at unirradiated sites harboring macroscopic and microscopic disease (Formenti and Demaria 2012, 2005).

Technological advances have now made the delivery of targeted systemic radiotherapy a reality. Systemic radiotherapy can be targeted to cancer cells at the cellular level. These can be biologically guided as in the case of radiolabeled peptide analogs to somatostatin in the treatment of neuroendocrine tumors, or immunologically guided as in the case of radiolabeled antibodies directed against tumor associated antigens expressed by solid tumors and hematopoietic malignancies, also known as radioimmunotherapy (RIT) (Jurcic et al. 2016).

Recent advances in intensity modulated radiation therapy (IMRT) delivery systems allow for radiation dose targeting and sculpting to the entire body resulting in a more targeted form of total body irradiation (TBI), also referred to as total marrow irradiation (TMI) (Wong et al. 2006, 2009; Schultheiss et al. 2007). This targeted form of systemic radiotherapy is image guided and to specific anatomic regions identified on CT, but in the future is expected to incorporate PET and MRI based functional imaging allowing for image guided targeted systemic radiotherapy to also be biologically guided based on the unique physiologic, phenotypic and genotypic properties of the tumor. This chapter will summarize the progress, current state and future directions of targeted systemic radiotherapy. Although the treatment of hematopoietic malignancies is used as an example, the principles outlined are applicable to other malignancies.

2 Total Body Irradiation: The Earliest Form of Systemic Radiotherapy

Total body irradiation (TBI) is one of the earliest forms of systemic radiotherapy and understanding its potential benefits and limitations provides the basis for developing new more targeted systemic radiotherapy approaches. TBI is a non-conformal, non-targeted form of systemic radiotherapy and was initially evaluated as a single modality therapy in patients with advanced leukemias, lymphomas and solid tumors. The first leukemia patient was treated with TBI in 1927 (Teschendorf 1927). In 1932 a specially designed room for TBI was developed at Memorial Sloan Kettering (Heublein 1932). In the 1950s units specifically designed to deliver TBI were developed at the Naval Medical Research Unit in Bethesda (Draeger et al. 1953), Oak Ridge National Laboratories (Hayes et al. 1964; Andrews et al. 1962) and City of Hope (Jacobs and Pape 1960, 1961). Jacobs and Marasso at City of Hope reported their four year experience treating 52 patients with advanced acute and chronic leukemia, Hodgkin's and non-Hodgkin's lymphoma, multiple myeloma and a variety of solid tumors (Jacobs and Marasso 1965). Doses as low as 40 cGy resulted in palliation of symptoms in patients with leukemia. Pancytopenia was dose limiting and five patients received autologous or allogeneic marrow reinfusion.

The first use of TBI as part of the conditioning regimen for hematopoietic cell transplant (HCT) delivered the dose in a single fraction and was reported by Thomas et al. (1959). Although engraftment was successful, relapse occurred within 12 weeks suggesting that TBI alone was insufficient to prevent relapse. Since then chemotherapy, usually cyclophosphamide (Cy) has been combined with TBI. Since these initial pioneering efforts, TBI continues to be an important part of conditioning regimens in patients undergoing HCT. In a recent survey of the Center for International Blood and Transplant Research (CIBMTR) Database which surveyed 596 centers in 52 countries and included 219341 patients, TBI was utilized in 46% of patients undergoing allogeneic and 10% of autologous HCT (Hong et al. 2012). The primary indications for HCT in acute myelogenous leukemia (AML) and acute lymphoblastic leukemia (ALL) are patients in first remission with intermediate to high risk features, induction failure, relapse, or in second remission or beyond. Patients with myelodysplastic syndrome (MDS) with high risk features or evolving to an acute state are also candidates for HCT. Patients with chronic myelogenous leukemia (CML) and chronic lymphocytic leukemia (CLL) undergo HCT much less frequently given the efficacy of current systemic therapies.

A primary role of TBI as part of the conditioning regimen just prior to HCT is the eradication of malignant cells. In patients undergoing allogeneic HCT, TBI also provides a powerful means of immunosuppression to prevent rejection of donor hematopoietic cells. TBI offers distinct advantages compared to chemotherapy. Unlike chemotherapy, delivery of radiation therapy to the tumor site is not dependent on blood supply or influenced by inter-patient variability of drug absorption, metabolism, biodistribution, or clearance kinetics. Radiation therapy can reach potential sanctuary sites, such as testes and brain. Chemotherapy resistant clones that develop may still be sensitive to irradiation.

The available data demonstrate that application of the same radiobiologic principles successfully employed for conventional field radiotherapy, such as fractionation, hyperfractionation, and organ shielding, have also helped to improve the therapeutic ratio of TBI with reduced toxicities and improved outcomes (Deeg et al. 1986; Girinsky et al. 2000; Labar et al. 1992; Shank et al. 1990). The effect of dose-rate appears to be modest above 5 centigray (cGy)/minute and diminishes if TBI is fractionated as opposed to a single fraction (Travis et al. 1985; Tarbell et al. 1987; Sampath et al. 2005; Weiner et al. 1986; Ozsahin et al. 1992). Typical TBI schedules today deliver a total dose of 10–16 (Gray) Gy at 1.2–1.35 Gy per fraction three times per day, 1.5–2 Gy per fraction twice a day or 3–4 Gy per fraction once a day with a minimum of 4–6 h between fractions. Patients are usually treated at extended SSD (source to skin distance) to encompass the entire body in a single field. As a result dose-rates are in the range of 5–30 cGy/minute. Many centers utilize lung shielding to reduce median lung doses to 8–10 Gy and reduce the incidence of pneumonitis. Others have utilized renal shielding to reduce long term nephrotoxicity (Rhoades et al. 1997). Hepatic shielding has been attempted by some groups to reduce hepatotoxicity especially when TBI is combined with busulfan (Bu) (Einsele et al. 2003) although one group in a small series of patients concluded that this may increase relapse rates due to under treatment of disease (Anderson et al. 2001).

Non-TBI chemotherapy only conditioning regimens offer no obvious advantage in reducing toxicities or improving control rates compared to TBI containing regimens, and in some randomized trials have been shown to be inferior (Blaise et al. 1992; Dusenbery et al. 1995; Ringden et al. 1996; Bunin et al. 2003). Most studies have compared TBI-Cy to the BuCy regimens. Hartman et al. (1998) performed a meta-analysis of 5 published randomized trials. Survival and disease free survival were better with TBI-based regimens compared to BuCy although the differences were not statistically significant. A significantly greater incidence of sinusoidal obstructive syndrome (SOS) (also known as veno-occlusive disease) was observed with the BuCy regimens. Recently, Gupta et al. (2011) performed a meta-analysis of seven randomized HCT trials involving 730 patients with leukemia randomized between BuCy and TBI-Cy. TBI-Cy was associated with a modest but non-significant reduction in all cause mortality and relapse rates. Since the early randomized trials utilized suboptimal dosing of busulfan, more recent comparison studies have been done. In a prospective cohort comparison study of 1483 patients, patients undergoing intravenous BU regimens experienced a statistically significant increase in 2 year overall survival (OS) compared to those undergoing a TBI containing conditioning regimen. The survival difference was only seen for early stage AML and not seen for intermediate or advanced AML, CML or MDS, and hepatotoxicity was greater with IV-Bu (Bredeson et al. 2013).

TBI containing and chemotherapy only conditioning regimens have traditionally been myeloablative. Myeloablative regimens are associated with a treatment related mortality (TRM) or no-relapse mortality (NRM) rate of about 20–30%. In a recent summary report of the CIBMTR of patients undergoing a myeloablative regimens prior to HLA matched allogeneic HCT, the main cause of death was relapse of primary disease (48%) but treatment related causes including graft versus host disease (GVHD), infection, and organ failure accounted for 17, 14 and 5% of deaths, respectively. As a result older patients (greater than age 55–60) or patients with co-morbidities are often not able to tolerate standard myeloablative TBI containing regimens.

As a result non-myeloablative (NMA) and reduced intensity conditioning (RIC) regimens have been developed which utilize lower chemotherapy or TBI doses (Deeg and Sandmaier 2010). These regimens are usually associated with fewer acute toxicities, are primarily used as a method of immunosuppression to allow engraftment of donor cells and rely more on graft versus tumor (GVT) effects to eradicate disease. RIC and NMA regimens offer a larger spectrum of patients a HCT option, but being less myeloablative can be associated with increased relapse rates. For example, in a recent multi-center phase III randomized trial, 272 patients, age 18–65 years old with AML in first remission or with MDS, were randomized to either a myeloablative or RIC regimen (Scott et al. 2015). With the RIC group the relapse rate was significantly higher (48.3% vs. 13.5%, $p < 0.01$) and the relapse free survival (RFS) rate was significantly lower (47.3% vs. 67.7%, $p < 0.01$), resulting in an 18 month overall survival difference of 67.7% versus 77.4% ($p = 0.07$).

3 Rationale for Targeted Systemic Radiotherapy and TBI

Targeted forms of TBI and systemic radiotherapy have the potential to significantly reduce organ dose and associated acute and late toxicities. With regards to TBI and HCT, several groups have demonstrated a reduction in radiation related complications with reduction in dose to critical normal organs including pneumonitis, nephrotoxicity and cataract formation (Fig. 1) (Sampath et al. 2005; Cheng et al. 2008; Hall et al. 2015). This could also potentially reduce TRM rates of radiation condition regimens allowing for a broader spectrum of patients to undergo radiation containing conditioning regimens, including patients who are older or those with co-morbidities who would otherwise not tolerate standard TBI.

RIC regimens can be associated with increased relapsed rates as noted earlier. Attempts to add TBI to RIC chemotherapy regimens to improve relapse rates have been challenging because of additional toxicities. For example Petropolous et al.

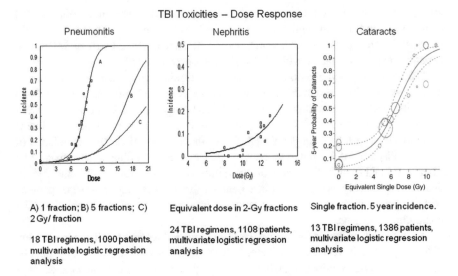

Fig. 1 Select examples of radiation dose-toxicity curves demonstrating that a reduction in dose to normal organs is associated with a decrease in late organ toxicities such as pneumonitis, nephritis and cataract formation (Sampath et al. 2005; Cheng et al. 2008; Hall et al. 2015)

(2006) reported that combining 9 Gy (3 Gy/day) TBI with the RIC regimen fludarabine (Flu) and melphalan (Mel) was not possible in adults because of increased mucositis. More targeted forms of TBI combined with RIC may be better tolerated and may potentially improve relapse rates compared to RIC chemotherapy regimens alone.

The primary reason for a more targeted form of TBI is to improve the therapeutic ratio by reducing normal organ dose and toxicities allowing for the potential to increase dose to tumor and improve long term outcomes. The available clinical data indicate that there is a dose response for most cancers including acute leukemia. Chloromas (also known as granulocytic or myeloid sarcomas) are extramedullary tumors of myeloid leukemia cells. Although relatively radiosensitive, Chak et al. (1983) demonstrated local control rates at 2 Gy per day of approximately 20% at doses less than 10 Gy, 40% at doses of 10–20 Gy and over 80% at doses of >20 Gy. They recommended a dose of 30 Gy at 2 Gy per day for optimal local control. More recently, Bakst et al. observed only one local failure at 6 Gy and recommended at least 20–24 Gy at 2 Gy/day (Bakst and Wolden 2012).

A dose response relationship has also been observed with the TBI experience. Two randomized phase II single institution trials have compared Cy combined with 12 Gy at 2 Gy/day or 15.75 Gy at 2.25 Gy/day. In a trial of 116 patients with CML in chronic phase, the higher dose resulted in a significantly lower relapse rate (0% vs. 25% $p = 0.008$), but higher treatment related mortality rate (24% 12 Gy and 34% 15.75 Gy, $p = 0.13$), and as a result no significant change in overall survival (Clift et al. 1991). In a separate report of 71 patients with AML in first remission, relapse rate was also decreased with the higher dose (14% vs. 39% $p = 0.06$), but these gains were offset by an increase in TRM rate (38% vs. 19%, $p = 0.05$), resulting in no difference in overall survival between the two arms (Clift et al. 1998). The increase in TRM rate was due to an increase in lung, liver and mucous membrane toxicities (Appelbaum et al. 1992). In several retrospective reports from the group in Genoa (Scarpati et al. 1989), relapse rate and survival was significantly decreased if TBI dose was >9.9 Gy (3.3 Gy/day). In an analysis of the CIBMTR and City of Hope Cancer Center databases, Marks et al. (2006) reported that patients with ALL beyond first remission receiving TBI-CY conditioning regimens had a lower relapse rate and increased disease free survival if the TBI dose was $\geq$13 Gy. Finally, Kal et al. (2006), compared results of different TBI regimens published in three randomized trials, four studies comparing results of two to three TBI regimens, and nine studies reporting on one TBI regimen. Using linear-quadratic principles, a biologically effective dose (BED) was calculated for each TBI regimen to normalize for differences in dose per fraction, number of fractions and dose-rates of the different regimens. Higher BED values were associated with a lower relapse rate and higher disease-free survival and overall survival rates.

In summary, despite use of fractionated schedules and organ shielding, escalation of TBI dose has been difficult due to dose-limiting normal tissue toxicities. This has limited total doses of most TBI conditioning regimens to approximately 16 Gy or less. Gains in disease control with TBI dose escalation are associated with an increase in regimen related toxicities and non-relapse mortality in some studies, resulting in no improvement in overall survival. New more targeted strategies are clearly needed to allow further dose escalation without associated increase in side effects. With regards to HCT, two targeted systemic radiotherapy strategies have been evaluated in the clinic and are discussed below, biologically targeted radioimmunotherapy (RIT) and image guided-IMRT based total marrow irradiation (TMI).

4 Radioimmunotherapy: Biologically Targeted Systemic Radiotherapy

Radioimmunotherapy (RIT) is a form of targeted systemic radiotherapy that utilizes monoclonal antibodies or related immunoconstructs linked to radionuclides. Radiolabeled antibodies have been evaluated as a form of therapy in solid tumors and hematopoietic malignancies. A number of detailed reviews on this topic have been published (Jurcic et al. 2016; Speer 2013). This section will focus on the use of RIT as a form of targeted TBI for leukemia.

The majority of the experience has been with antibodies targeting CD20 on B cells in patients with non-Hodgkin's lymphoma. RIT has also been applied to other hematopoietic malignancies including leukemia. Table 1 lists the antigens that

Table 1 Radioimmunotherapy target antigens in acute leukemia

Target	Disease	Expressed by
CD33	Myeloid leukemia	Promyelocytes to mature myeloid cells AML blasts (not ALL blasts) Not hematopoietic stem cells or ALL blasts
CD45	AML, ALL	Virtually all hematopoietic stem cells except plasma cells 90% of AML and ALL
CD66	AML, ALL	Mature myeloid and monocytic cells Not on AML blasts (relies on cross-fire effect)
CD22	ALL	B-cell acute lymphoblastic leukemia

Table 2 Radionuclides used in RIT of acute leukemia

Radionuclide	Particles emitted	Half life	Energy (MeV)	Path length	Comments
Iodine-131 (^{131}I)	β, γ	8.1 days	0.6	0.8 mm	Dehalogenation
Yttrium-90 (^{90}Y)	β	2.7 days	2.3	2.7 mm	Goes to bone, liver
Rhenium-188 (^{188}Re)	β, γ	17 h	2.1	2.4 mm	Goes to kidney
Bismuth-213 (^{213}Bi)	α, γ	46 min	6.0	84 μm	Requires fast targeting
Actinium-225 (^{225}Ac)	α, γ	10 days	8	50–80 μm	Difficult to generate

radiolabeled antibodies have been developed against to target AML and ALL. Table 2 lists the radionuclides that have been linked to these antibodies and evaluated in clinical trials.

Selection of the appropriate radionuclide for RIT is based on availability, half-life, energy path length, and ease of labeling to the antibody. ^{131}I is both a β and γ emitter. The γ emission allows for imaging and assessing biodistribution of the RIT. The β energy emission provides the therapeutic RIT effect. The disadvantage is that γ radiation travels far and increases exposures to normal tissues as well as to surrounding medical personnel. ^{131}I will also disassociate from the antibody, a process called dehalogenation, especially if the antibody is internalized into the cell after antigen binding, which reduces radiation dose to the target cell.

^{90}Y is a radiometal commonly used in RIT and is a pure β emitter. The mean β emission range is approximately 2.7 mm compared to 0.8 mm for ^{131}I ^{90}Y β emissions travel only a few mm and thus mainly affect the cells which are targeted or adjacent malignant cells through what is termed a cross-fire effect. To monitor biodistribution of ^{90}Y RIT requires the co-administration of the same antibody radiolabeled with the γ-emitting radiometal ^{111}In which allows for visualization biodistribution by planar and SPECT imaging. Some have hypothesized that the path length of ^{90}Y β emissions are too long for the treatment of microscopic disease although there are no clinical data to date to support this.

α emitters are the most recent radioisotope to be exploited. α emitters have higher linear energy transfer (LET) than either γ or β emitters. In addition, the effective range of α emitter's effect is shorter (range of 40–80 μM) thus potentially further reducing the normal toxicity and potentially making it more suitable for the treatment of microscopic disease. The utilization of α-emitters has been limited by their availability and short half-life.

RIT directed against CD33 has been evaluated as single modality therapy in pilot and phase I trials in acute myeloid leukemia. The CD33 antigen is a 67-kD glycoprotein expressed on most myeloid leukemias and leukemia progenitors but not on normal stem cells. Anti-CD33 RIT has been developed and evaluated using the murine M195 and the HuM195 (linituzumab) humanized antibodies by the group at Memorial Sloan-Kettering Cancer Center (MSKCC). A phase I trial at MSKCC reported on the feasibility of administering ^{131}I-CD33 antibodies (M195 and HuM195) in 31 patients and demonstrated that dose escalation to 135 mCi/m^2 achieved myelosuppression and allowed 8 patients to proceed to bone marrow transplant, with three patients remaining in complete remission at 59, 87, and 90 months (Burke et al. 2003). Rosenblat et al. (2010) evaluated HuM195 anti-CD33 radiolabeled with the α-emitter [213]Bi administered after cytarabine in a Phase I/II trial in patients with newly diagnosed, refractory or relapsed AML. The RIT agent was shown to be tolerable at all dose levels. Although 77% of patients had >20% decrease in marrow blasts with the addition of RIT compared to only 40% with cytarabine alone, the response rate was only 19% at the maximum tolerated dose (MTD) of 37 MBq/kg with a median duration of response of 6 months. Due to the short half life of [213]Bi, HuM195 has recently been evaluated in a phase I trial labeled with the α-emitter [225]Ac by the same group with an overall response rate of 29% reported (Jurcic et al. 2015).

RIT has also been evaluated as part of conditioning regimens in patients with leukemia undergoing allogeneic HCT. RIT has been combined with established myeloablative or reduced intensity regimens. Table 3 lists select trials that have combined RIT with non-TBI conditioning regimens. Marrow doses have ranged from 3 to 47 Gy with mean marrow doses depending on the agent ranging from 11–36 Gy at the MTD. Almost all trials have demonstrated the feasibility of combining RIT with established conditioning regimens and acceptable TRM rates. Results have been are encouraging, although the experience to date has been limited to phase I and II trials, at a limited number of centers, and in a relatively small number of patients.

Combining RIT with TBI containing regimens has also been evaluated and has demonstrated the limits of dose escalation (Table 4). Matthews et al. (1999) combined ^{131}I-BC8 anti-CD45 RIT with the myeloablative conditioning regimen of 12 Gy TBI and Cy is a phase I trial. RIT was escalated based on estimated dose to the bone marrow. One case of non-engraftment occurred with the combination of 12 Gy TBI and 31 Gy RIT. A RIT marrow dose of 24 Gy in combination with 12 Gy TBI was determined to be the MTD. Bunjes et al. (2002) combined [188]Re labeled anti-CD66 RIT with myeloablative conditioning regimen which included TBI to 12 Gy. This agent has greater biodistribution and dose to kidney than other

Table 3 Select hct trials combining RIT with myeloablative or reduced intensity conditioning regimens

First Author year	Antibody (target)	No.	Disease	HCT	Marrow dose (Gy)	Response	Toxicities
Burke et al. (2003) Phase I	131I-M195 or Hu195 (CD33)	31	AML relapsed AML refractory CML-AP MDS advanced	Bu/Cy	2.72–14.7	3 CR 59 +, 87 +, and 90 + months	TRM 65%
Pagel et al. (2006) Phase I/II	131I-BC8 (CD45)	46	AML CR1	Bu/Cy	5.3–19 Mean 11.3	3 yr DFS 61%	3 yr TRM 21%
Pagel et al. (2009) Phase I	131I-BC8 (CD45)	58	AML advanced MDS high risk Age >50	RIC: Flu + TBI (2 Gy)	6.3–46.9 At MTD 36	1 yr OS 41%	1 yr TRM 22%
Mawad et al. (2014) Phase I	131I-BC8 (CD45)	58	AML advanced MDS high risk Age <50	RIC: Flu + TBI (2 Gy)	12–43.3 Mean 27	1 yr OS 73% 1 yr RFS 67%	1 yr TRM 0%
Koenecke et al. (2008) Phase I/II	188Re-BW 250/183 (CD66)	21	AML high risk MDS advanced	Bu/Cy or RIC	4.95–21.3 Mean 10.9	DFS 43% median follow-up 42 months	1 yr TRM 28.6%
Ringhoffer et al. (2005) Phase I/II	188Re- or 90Y-BW 250/183 (CD66)	20	AML, MDS Age 55–65	Flu + ATG or Mel	21.9 ± 8.4	1 yr OS 70% 2 yr OS 52%	Cumulative TRM 25%
Lauter et al. (2009) Phase II	188Re-BW 250/183 (CD66)	22	AML advanced Age >54	RIC: Flu/Bu/campath		2 yr OS 40% 2 yr DFS 41%	2 yr TRM 23%

HCT hematopoietic cell transplantation; *RIT* radioimmunotherapy; *AML* acute myelogenous leukemia; *CML-AP* chronic myelogenous leukemia in acute phase; *MDS* myelodysplastic syndrome; *CR* complete remission; *CR1* first complete remission; *Bu* busulfan; *Cy* cyclophosphamide; *RIC* reduced intensity conditioning regimen; *Flu* fludarabine; *TBI* total body irradiation; *Gy* Gray; *ATG* anti-thymocyte globulin; *Mel* melphalan; *DFS* disease free survival; *RFS* relapse free survival; *OS* overall survival; *TRM* treatment related mortality

Table 4 Select HCT Trials Combining RIT and TBI (12 Gy)

First Author year	Antibody (target)	No.	Disease	HCT	RIT marrow dose (Gy)	Response	Toxicities
Appelbaum et al. (1992) Phase I	^{131}I-p67 (CD33)	4	AML Relapse, second CR	Cy/TBI (12 Gy)	1.7–5.56	3 of 4 CR 195–477 days	Low marrow doses
Matthews et al. (1999) Phase I	^{131}I-BC8 (CD45)	44	AML, ALL beyond first remission	Cy/TBI (12 Gy)	4–31 24 at MTD	AML: 7/25 (28%) NED 15-89 months ALL: 3/9 NED at 23, 58, 70 months	One engraftment failure at 31 Gy RIT + 12 Gy TBI
Bunjes (2002) Phase I/II	^{188}Re-BW 250/183 (CD66)	57	High risk AML and MDS $\leq$25% marrow blasts	Cy/TBI (12 Gy) TBI/Cy/TT Bu/Cy	15.5 ± 5.1	DFS 54% DFS 64% (n = 44) if $\leq$15% blasts DFS 8% (n = 13) if >15% blasts	14% late renal toxicity Radiation nephropathy in 6 patients (4/6 if > 12 Gy) 26 month TRM 30%
Zenz et al. (2006) Phase I	^{188}Re-BW 250/183 (CD66)	20	Ph + ALL advanced CML	Bu/Cy or Cy/TBI (12 Gy) kidney shielded to 6 Gy	13.3 ± 1.1	4 yr OS 29% relapse rate cumulative 40%	1 yr TRM 20%

HCT hematopoietic cell transplantation; *RIT* radioimmunotherapy; *AML* = acute myelogenous leukemia; *ALL* = acute lymphoblastic leukemia; *CML* = chronic myelogenous leukemia; *MDS* = myelodysplastic syndrome; *CR* = complete remission; *CR1* = first complete remission; *NED* = no evidence of disease; *Bu* = busulfan; *Cy* = cyclophosphamide; *TT* = thiotepa; *TBI* = total body irradiation; *Gy* = Gray; *DFS* = disease free survival; *OS* = overall survival; *TRM* = treatment related mortality agents. Late renal toxicity was seen in 14% and in 4 of 6 patients if the total renal dose exceeded 12 Gy. Renal toxicity was reduced in a subsequent study of the same agent when renal shielding was utilized with TBI (Zenz et al. 2006).

RIT as a form of targeted systemic radiotherapy and a form of targeted TBI for acute leukemia patients undergoing HCT is theoretically attractive with encouraging results and acceptable toxicities, yet challenges still remain. The availability of these agents, expertise and resources needed to perform myeloablative RIT is limited to only a few centers. The technology is therefore currently not easily exportable for wide use making further clinical evaluation of these agents beyond the phase I and II trial setting difficult. There is inter-patient variability in the biodistribution and pharmacokinetics for these agents. In many trials, a small subset of patients does not receive the therapy infusion after demonstrating suboptimal biodistribution of the pre-therapy infusion. Although the amount of administered radioactivity and agent is determined by the treating physician, the actual radiation doses to the intended target sites and organs is not and can vary from patient to patient adding a degree of uncertainty to the anticipated toxicities and efficacy.

5   Total Marrow Irradiation: Image Guided Systemic Targeted Radiotherapy

5.1   Background and Rationale

Recent technological advances in radiotherapy systems now allow for the delivery of a image guided IMRT to large regions of the body allowing for more targeted forms of TBI and therefore targeted whole body or systemic radiotherapy. These new forms of image guided targeted TBI are often referred to as total marrow irradiation (TMI). The Tomotherapy HiArt System® was the first system used to deliver targeted TMI. Tomotherapy integrates CT image-guided radiotherapy and helical delivery of IMRT in a single device. Specifically, a 6 MV linear accelerator is mounted on a CT ring gantry and rotates around the patient as the patient translates through the ring. The maximum target size possible is approximately 60 cm in width by approximately 160 cm in length (Beavis 2004). More recently, other groups have successfully used linear accelerators with volumetric arc-based image guided IMRT (also referred to as VMAT) capabilities to deliver TMI (Han et al. 2011; Aydogan et al. 2011; Fogliata et al. 2011; Patel et al. 2014).

The first delivery of TMI as part of the conditioning regimen in patients undergoing autologous or allogeneic HCT began in 2005 (Wong et al. 2006, 2009; Schultheiss et al. 2007; Wong et al. 2013; Somlo et al. 2011; Rosenthal et al. 2011; Stein et al. 2012). Figure 2 shows the typical conformal dose distribution pattern that is achieved to the designated target structure, with simultaneous reduction of dose to critical organs. Table 5 compares the median doses for various normal organs at risk (OAR) delivered through standard TBI to 12 Gy with 50% transmission block lung shielding and electron boost to the underlying chest wall versus TMI to 12 Gy to the

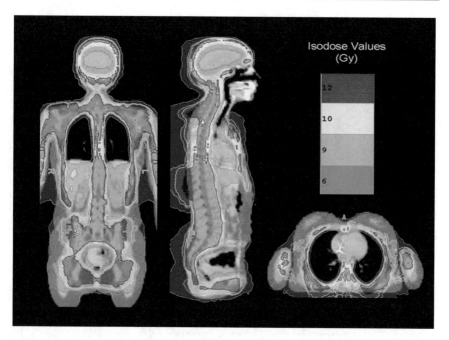

Fig. 2 Radiotherapy dose color wash demonstrating typical dose distribution of a patient treated with TMI. The target structure is skeletal bone

skeletal bone. Significant reduction in dose and volume of organ receiving full dose is observed compared to standard TBI for all critical organs.

This approach offers the treatment team more control of radiation dose delivery to target regions and organs compared to targeted radiopharmaceutical approaches. The physician can simultaneously reduce dose to organs or any other user-defined avoidance structure, while simultaneously increasing dose to particular target regions depending on the tumor burden and clinical situation. Figure 3 shows median organ doses and Fig. 4 lung dose-volume histogram (DVH) plots for standard TBI to 12 Gy versus TMI at 12 and 20 Gy in the same patient. At TMI doses to 20 Gy, median doses to all organs are still below that of TBI to 12 Gy. The lung DVH plots demonstrate that at 20 Gy TMI median lung doses remain below that of TBI 12 Gy with lung shielding but the D_{80} (minimum dose to at least 80% of the lung volume) is comparable, which predicts for similar pneumonitis risks for TMI 20 Gy and TBI 12 Gy. Table 6 compares median organ doses between TMI plans to 12 Gy (target structure is bone) compared to TBI plans to 12 Gy using 50% transmission blocks to shield lung.

5.2 Methodology Used at City of Hope

5.2.1 CT Simulation and Immobilization

All patients undergo CT simulation for treatment planning purposes. The patient is scanned supine with arms at side on a CT simulator. Two planning CT scans are

Table 5 Completed TMI Trials at City of Hope

Type of trial (NCT no.)	Type of HCT	Disease type	No.	Targets (dose)	TMI Dose levels (Gy)	Fraction and Schedule	Chemo-therapy
Phase I (Somlo et al. 2011) (00112827)	Autologous (tandem)	MM stage I-III responding or stable	25	bone	10,12,14,16,18	2 Gy QD-BID x 5 days	Mel
Phase II (Somlo et al.2015) (00112827)	Autologous (tandem)	MM stage I-III responding or stable	54	bone	16	2 Gy BID x 5 days	Mel
Pilot (Rosenthal et al. 2011) (00800150)	Allogeneic	Advanced disease ineligible for myeloablative regimens >50 yrs old, co-morbidities,	33	bone, nodes, spleen, testes, brain	12	1.5 Gy BID x 4 days	Flu/ Mel
Phase I (Wong et al. 2013) (00540995)	Allogeneic	AML, ALL relapsed or refractory with active disease not eligible for standard HCT	20	bone, nodes, testes, spleen, liver, brain	12, 13.5	1.5 BID x 4-5 days	BU/ VP16
Phase I (Stein et al. 2015) (02446964)	Allogeneic	AML, ALL relapsed or refractory with active disease not eligible for standard HCT	51	bone, nodes, testes, spleen, liver, brain	12, 13.5, 15, 16, 17, 18, 19, 20	1.5 BID x 4-5 days	Cy/ VP16

HCT hematopoietic cell transplantation; *AML* acute myelogenous leukemia; *ALL* acute lymphoblastic leukemia; *MM* multiple myeloma; *QD* once per day; *BID* twice per day; *Bu* busulfan; *Cy* cyclophosphamide; *Flu* fludarabine; *Mel* melphalan; *VP-16* etoposide; *TMI* total marrow irradiation; *Gy* Gray

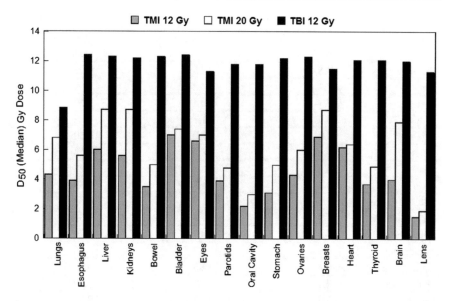

Fig. 3 Median organ doses from treatment plans for TBI 12 Gy, TMI 12 Gy and TMI 20 Gy planned on the same patient. Median organ doses are *lower* with TMI at 20 Gy compared to TBI 12 Gy, predicting that dose escalation of TMI to 20 Gy in patients should result in *lower* organ doses and reduced side effects compared to standard TBI 12 Gy

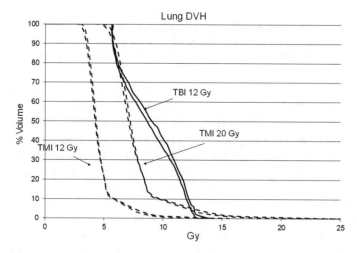

Fig. 4 Comparison of dose-volume histogram (DVH) plots for lung with TMI 12 Gy, TMI 20 Gy versus standard TBI to 12 Gy in the same patient. Standard TBI utilized 10 MV photons to deliver 12 Gy. Fifty percent attenuation blocks were used to shield the lungs. Electrons were used to deliver 6 Gy to the rib cage underlying the lung blocks. The lung DVH plots demonstrate that at 20 Gy TMI median lung doses remain *below* that of TBI 12 Gy with lung shielding but the D_{80} (minimum dose to at least 80% of the lung volume) is comparable, suggesting that pneumonitis risks for TMI 20 Gy may be similar to TBI 12 Gy

Table 6 Median dose to normal organs with TMI compared to standard TBI to deliver 12 Gy

Organ at risk	Median dose (Gy) TMI	Median dose (Gy) TBI	TMI/TBI median dose
Bladder	7.5	12.3	0.61
Brain	7.1	12.2	0.58
Breast	7.7	12.4	0.62
Esophagus	4.9	11.7	0.42
Orbits	6.0	12.0	0.50
Heart	6.1	11.5	0.53
Lens	2.3	10.5	0.22
Liver	6.9	11.7	0.59
Left Kidney	7.4	11.9	0.62
Right Kidney	6.9	11.9	0.58
Left Lung	6.3	9.0	0.70
Right Lung	6.4	9.7	0.66
Optic Nerve	6.4	12.3	0.52
Oral Cavity	2.5	12.5	0.20
Ovary	7.0	12.5	0.56
Parotids	4.6	13.1	0.35
Rectum	4.8	12.6	0.38
Small intestine	5.0	12.5	0.40
Stomach	4.6	11.5	0.40
Thyroid	4.4	12.6	0.35

Data is an average of comparison plans from 6 patients at City of Hope (unpublished data)
Standard TBI utilized 10 MV photons to deliver 12 Gy. Fifty percent attenuation blocks were used
to shield the lungs. Electrons were used to deliver 6 Gy to the rib cage underlying the lung blocks

performed, one to plan body regions from head to pelvis and the other to plan for lower extremities. The body CT scan is obtained with normal shallow breathing. 4D CT scan data are acquired for chest and abdomen. If 4D CT is not available, shallow inspiration and expiration breath hold CT scans can be acquired instead. The normal shallow breathing CT data set is used for dose calculation and planning. The 4D CT datasets are registered to the planning CT to account for any organ motion during respiration. AccuForm™ (CIVCO Medical Systems, Kalona, IA) cushion is used in combination with Silverman headrest to support and stabilize the head and neck. A body vac-lok™ bag (CIVCO Medical Systems, Kalona, IA) and a thermoplastic head and shoulder mask are used as additional immobilization devices. The patient's arms, legs and feet are positioned using a vac-lok bag to enhance comfort and repositioning accuracy. Oral contrast is used to help visualize the esophagus. Couch height is approximately 10 cm below the isocenter of the gantry and patient is positioned on the couch so that the top of the head is approximately 5 cm from the end of the couch. Those settings are used to maximize the available length for the CT scanning and treatment delivery.

Target delineation: Target and avoidance structures and normal organs are contoured on an Eclipse™ treatment planning system (Varian Medical Systems, Palo Alto, CA) or similar planning system. Avoidance structures contoured are user defined and usually include lungs, heart, kidneys, liver, esophagus, oral cavity, parotid glands, thyroid gland, eyes, lens, optic chiasm and nerves, brain, stomach, small and large intestine, breasts, rectum, testes, ovary and bladder. Depending on the clinical circumstances, clinical trial or center, potential target structures can include skeletal bone, spleen, testes and major lymph node chains. In some clinical trials brain and liver are target structures. The 4D CT datasets are registered to the planning CT so that the contours of ribs, esophagus, kidneys, spleen and liver are enlarged to account for the organ movements during respiration. An additional 3 to 5 cm margin is usually added to the CTV to define the PTV target. Our center has added up to 10 cm margins in areas where larger setup uncertainty is observed, such as in the regions of the shoulder, arms, thighs, and posterior spinous processes. Spinal cord (part of the target) is outlined separately so to avoid hot spots in the spinal canal during planning. At some centers such as City of Hope, the mandible and maxillary bones are excluded from the target in an effort to minimize oral cavity dose and mucositis.

5.2.2 Treatment Planning with a Helical Tomographic Delivery System (Tomotherapy)

DICOM-RT images are transferred to the Hi-Art™ Tomotherapy treatment planning system (Accuray Inc. Palo Alto, CA). Helical Tomotherapy plan is designed such that a minimum of 85% of the target received the prescribed dose. For the body treatment plan, jaw size of 5 cm, pitch of 0.287 and modulation factor of 2.5 are used for most patients as a balance of treatment time and plan quality. Plan quality index is comprised of target dose uniformity and critical organ doses. Since the first TMI patient treated in 2005, TMI treatment planning efforts at City of Hope have continued to evolve. Median organ doses with current planning methods are now lower than previously published (Wong et al. 2006). Our current approach is to perform plan optimization in two stages. Critical organ sparing is optimized before target dose uniformity optimization is done resulting in being able to escalate target doses without a proportionate increase in normal organ dose (Stein et al. 2015). Legs and feet are planned in Tomo-Direct mode. A 5 cm jaw size is used. Gantry angles of 0 and 180° are selected. Composite dose of body plan and leg plan is generated to double check there is no dose gap or overlap at the junction.

5.2.3 Treatment Planning with a VMAT Conventional Linear Accelerator System

TMI can be planned and treated using a conventional linear accelerators with VMAT capability as well. Multiple dynamic IMRT arcs with usually 3–4 isocenters are used to cover target regions. Collimator angles are varied for each arc to increase the planning degree of freedom and plan quality. After the plan of the body is finalized, the lower extremities are planned with two or three additional AP-PA fields given the lack of sensitive organs in this area. AP-PA fields are opened at 40 cm × 40cm and gapped at 50% isodose line at midplane (Han et al. 2011; Aydogan et al. 2011).

5.2.4 Treatment Delivery

Our current procedure involves initial laser alignment of the patient in the vac-lok bag and thermoplastic mask. Verification CT positioning scans are performed prior to each treatment session using multiple cone beam CT scans (CBCTs) or one megavoltage CT (MVCT) scan from orbit to ischial tuberosities and is fused to the planning CT. Registration and couch shifts are reviewed and approved by attending physician before treatment is delivered. The Tomotherapy has a maximum treatment length of approximately 150 cm. A jaw size of 5 cm and pitch of 0.287 usually result a beam-on of time of approximately 25 min to treat the upper body. On the Tomotherapy system, the patient translates through the unit head first to treat from the head to proximal thighs and is then re-setup and translates through the unit feet first to treat the lower extremities. Treatment of legs has a beam-on of time of approximately 10 min. With a conventional linear accelerator with VMAT capability, it is recommended the verification CBCT to be performed for each isocenter before treatment delivery. The total treatment time is similar to TMI delivery using a helical topographic approach.

5.2.5 Comparison to TBI Planning and Delivery

Table 7 compares the steps needed to plan and deliver TBI versus TMI. The TBI technique currently used at City of Hope is similar to that developed at Memorial Sloan Kettering Cancer Center (Shank et al. 1990). Briefly, patients are treated using a C-arm linac in the standing position at extended SSD of approximately 400 cm. The most common fractionation schedule is 1.2 Gy three times a day for 10–11 fractions using alternating AP and PA fields. A compensator is made for each patient to achieve a uniform dose. Fifty percent transmission blocks are used to shield the lung for each fraction. Electrons are used to treat the rib cage underlying the lung blocks. The time and resources needed for planning and delivery of TMI is

Table 7 Comparison of TBI versus TMI planning and preparation

	TBI	TMI
Day 1	• TBI measurement: thickness, SSD, positioning, gantry angle, hand position • CT Simulation for chest wall e boost treatment planning	• Immobilization • Whole body CT simulation
Day 2–4	• TBI calculation • Fabricate compensator and lung blocks • Set up—lung block placement and port films • Generate e boost plan • 2nd calculation QA verification	• Contour • Plan optimization • Phantom QA
Day 5	• Position standing—harness and lung blocks • Treatment: 20 min beam-on time for 2 Gy fraction	• Position in mask and vac-lock • Treatment: 35 min beam-on time for 2 Gy fraction

comparable to TBI. Centers actively involved in HCT and already treating patients with TBI should also be able to adopt TMI as part of their HCT program.

5.3 Results of TMI Clinical Trials

Initial preclinical dosimetric studies comparing TMI and TBI demonstrated that TMI could result in median organ doses that were approximately 15–65% of the prescribed dose to the target structure (bone) depending on organ site. These preclinical studies were hypothesis generating and predicted that TMI could result in a reduction of acute toxicities and the potential to dose escalate to marrow without an increase TRM rates compared to TBI containing regimens. Clinical trials would need to validate this hypothesis.

5.3.1 Tandem Autologous Mel-TMI HCT in Multiple Myeloma

The TMI trials at City of Hope have evolved through several phases. Patients undergoing HCT were first treated with TMI containing conditioning regimens in 2005. The initial trial evaluated TMI as part of a conditioning regimen in patients with multiple myeloma undergoing autologous tandem HCT. Since this was the first in human trial evaluating TMI, the trial was designed in part to address initial concerns of possible increased toxicities with TMI due to higher dose-rates compared to TBI. TMI would be evaluated without concurrent chemotherapy using a fractionation schedule and a fraction size comparable to TBI. This would allow us to evaluate the acute toxicities and determine the MTD of TMI alone in this population (Wong et al. 2006; Somlo et al. 2011).

Patients with Salmon-Durie stage I-III multiple myeloma and with stable or responding disease after first line therapy, underwent tandem autologous HCT. The first autologous HCT used the standard conditioning regimen of Mel at 200 mg/m^2. This was followed a minimum of 6 weeks later by a second autologous HCT using TMI as the conditioning regimen. TMI dose was escalated from 10 Gy to 18 Gy at 2 Gy fractions delivered twice a day with a minimum interval between fractions of 6 h. The TMI target structure was bone (Fig. 2). The trial design was a modification of a standard tandem autologous HCT regimen which utilized Mel at 200 mg/m^2 as a conditioning regimen for both tandem HCT.

Of 22 patients, reversible NCI grade 3 non-hematologic toxicities were as follows: nausea/emesis in 3 patients, enteritis in 2 patients and mucositis in no patients. Dose limiting toxicities were not observed until a TMI dose of 18 Gy (1 patient with reversible grade 3 pneumonitis, congestive heart failure and enteritis, and 1 patient with grade 3 hypotension), establishing the MTD at 16 Gy. With dose escalation to 18 Gy, median organ doses still remained below that for standard TBI to 12 Gy (Somlo et al. 2011), ranging from 11 to 81% of the prescribed bone dose.

The observation of radiation pneumonitis in one of three patients at 18 Gy TMI is consistent with predications made by initial preclinical planning studies. Table 8 displays the D_{80}, D_{50} (median) and D_{20} doses points for lung averaged for all

Table 8 Total Lung D_{80}, D_{50} and D_{20} DVH Doses for Patients with Multiple Myeloma Undergoing TMI

	N	D_{80}	D_{50}	D_{10}
TBI 12 Gy[a]	3	7.0	9.4	12.3
TMI 10 Gy	3	4.5	4.9	6.8
TMI 12 Gy	4	5.6	6.2	8.4
TMI 14 Gy	3	6.4	6.9	9.4
TMI 16 Gy	3	6.4	7.1	10.7
TMI 18 Gy	3	6.9	7.6	11.2

[a]Based on TBI plans from first 3 TMI patients (dose level 1) with 50% transmission lung blocks and 6 Gy electron boost to underlying chest wall
D_{80} minimum dose to that 80% of the organ receives; D_{50} minimum dose that 50% of the organ receives; D_{20} minimum dose that 20% of the organ receives

patients at each dose level. This shows the D_{80} point of 6.9 Gy which is similar to the D_{80} of 7 Gy which is observed with standard TBI to 12 Gy with 50% transmission lung blocks.

A phase II tandem autologous HCT trial of Mel followed by 16 Gy TMI has been completed (Somlo et al. 2015). A total of 54 patients were entered on the Phase I and II trials. No grade 4 toxicities, treatment related mortality, or non-engraftment was observed in either the Phase I or II trials. The median age was 54 years (31–67). Four patients were stage I, 18 stage II and 32 stage III. Forty-four of the 54 pts received TMI (28 at the MTD of 16 Gy). Best responses included complete response in 22, very good partial response in 8 and partial response or stable disease in 14. Median follow-up of alive pts was 73 months (27–117). In an intent-to-treat analysis median progression free survival (PFS) for the 54 pts was 52 months (95% CI 34.4-not reached), and median overall survival (OS) was not reached. PFS and OS at 5 years was 43% (95% CI 31–59) and 66% (95% CI 54–81), respectively. For pts enrolled at 16 Gy, the PFS and OS at 5 years were 48% (34–69) and 73% (59–90). The authors concluded that TMI of 16 Gy was feasible following Mel and the long-term safety and PFS/OS were encouraging.

5.3.2 TMLI (Total Marrow and Lymphoid Irradiation) Added to an Established RIC Regimen (Flu-Mel) as a Conditioning Regimen for Allogeneic HCT in Older Patients with Acute Leukemia

As noted earlier RIC regimen can be associated with an increase in relapse rates (Scott et al. 2015), yet adding standard TBI to RIC regimen has resulted in unacceptable toxicities in adults (Petropoulos et al. 2006). At City of Hope a pilot trial evaluated the feasibility of combining TMLI with the established RIC regimen of fludarabine and melphalan. The hypothesis was that given the targeted nature of the radiotherapy it would be better tolerated than standard TBI in combination with Flu-Mel. The target structures for TMLI included bone, as well as major lymph node regions (TLI) and spleen to optimize the immunosuppression needed for allogeneic HCT and since these regions potentially harbored disease. Brain and testes were included as target regions in patients with ALL.

TMLI at 12 Gy (1.5 Gy BID) was combined with Flu (25 mg/m^2/d × 5 days) and Mel (140 mg/m^2) followed by allogeneic HCT in patients with advanced hematologic malignancies and who were older than age 50 or with co-morbidities and were ineligible for standard TBI myeloablative regimens. At study entry marrow blasts had to be <10% or reduced by over 50% after induction chemotherapy. The initial results of the first 33 patients have been reported (Rosenthal et al. 2011). Nineteen patients had AML and 3 ALL. Twenty-two were felt to be at very high risk having disease in induction failure, relapse, second or third remission or with a history of prior HCT. The TRM rate at 1 and 2 years was 19% and 25% respectively, which compared favorably to the 30-40% rates reported for Flu and Mel alone in a similar patient population (Giralt et al. 2001, 2002; Ritchie et al. 2003; de Lima et al. 2004). With a median follow-up for living patients of 14.7 months, 1-year overall survival, event free survival, and non–relapse-related mortality were 75, 65, and 19%, respectively. The authors concluded that the addition of TMLI to RIC is feasible and safe and could be offered to patients with advanced hematologic malignancies who might not otherwise be candidates for RIC. A recent updated analysis of 60 patients on this trial with a median follow-up of 5 years demonstrates similar TRM, relapse, event-free survival and overall survival rates (unpublished data). Further studies are needed to determine whether the addition of TMLI to an RIC regimen provides additional benefit compared to RIC regimens alone.

5.3.3 TMLI as an Alternative to TBI as Part of a Radiation Containing Myeloablative Conditioning Regimen in Allogeneic HCT

A previous trial at City of Hope demonstrated the feasibility of combining 12 Gy TBI, Bu and VP-16 as a conditioning regimen for poor risk acute leukemia patients undergoing allogeneic HCT (Stein et al. 2011). This led to two successor phase I trials evaluating the feasibility and defining the MTD of dose escalated TMLI with either Bu/VP-16 or Cy/VP-16 in poor risk acute leukemia. In both trials dose to the target structures bone, major lymph node chains, and spleen were escalated per standard phase I trial design. Target structures also included liver and brain which were kept at 12 Gy for all dose levels. Fraction schedule was 1.5–2 Gy BID over 4–5 days.

For the TMLI/Bu/VP-16 phase I trial the conditioning regimen was Bu days −12 to −8 (800 uM min), TMLI days −8 to −4, and VP-16 day −3 (30 mg/kg). TMI dose (Gy) was 12 (n = 18) and 13.5 (n = 2) at 1.5 Gy BID. Twenty patients with advanced acute leukemia were treated; 13 with induction failure, 5 in first relapse and 2 in second relapse. Nineteen patients still had detectable blasts in marrow prior to HCT with involvement ranging for 3 to 100% and 13 had circulating blasts prior to HCT ranging from 6–63%. Grade 4 dose limiting toxicities of stomatitis and sinusoidal obstructive syndrome (SOS) were seen at 13.5 Gy (Wong et al. 2013).

Hepatotoxicity was likely due the combination of Bu and a liver dose of 12 Gy, each of which has been associated with a risk of SOS.

TMLI dose escalation was also evaluated in combination with Cy and VP-16 (Stein et al. 2015). A phase I trial in 51 patients (age: median 34, range 16–57 years) with relapsed or refractory AML and ALL undergoing HCT with active disease and therefore conventionally ineligible for transplant, underwent a conditioning regimen of escalating doses of TMLI (range 12–20 Gy, days −10 to −6) with Cy (100 mg/kg day −3) and VP-16 (60 mg/kg day −5). Thirty-four were in induction failure, 14 in first relapse and 3 in second relapse. Fifty patients still had detectable blasts in marrow with involvement ranging form 5 to 98% and 27 had circulating blasts ranging from 6–85% prior to HCT. One patient at the 15 Gy level experienced Bearman scale (Bearman et al. 1988) grade 3 mucositis, but no other grade 3 dose limiting toxicities were observed up to 20 Gy. The maximum tolerated dose was declared at 20 Gy since as noted earlier TMLI planning indicated that prescribed target doses >20 Gy might deliver D_{80} doses to lung comparable to 12 TBI resulting in pneumonitis risks comparable to standard TBI. The post-transplant non-relapse mortality rate was 3.9% (95% CI: 0.7–12.0) at day 100 and 8.1% (95% CI: 2.5–18.0) at one year. The day +30 complete remission rate for all patients was 88 and 100% at 20 Gy. With a median follow-up if 24.6 months (3.3–72.0) of surviving patients, the overall one-year survival was 55.5% (95% CI: 40.7–68.1) and progression free survival 40.0% (95% CI: 26.4–53.2). Eleven patients are alive and in continuous complete remission at 1.6 to 6 + years. The authors concluded that TMLI/CY/VP16 conditioning regimen was feasible with acceptable toxicity at TMLI doses up to 20 Gy and with encouraging results for disease control for a very poor risk population not eligible for standard-of-care HCT regimens. A phase II trial is currently ongoing with the primary endpoint of 2 year progression free survival.

Figure 5 shows median (D_{50}) organ doses averaged for each dose level in the 51 patients undergoing TMLI combined with Cy and VP-16 and allogeneic HCT. Table 9 shows organ doses as a percentage of the prescribed target dose. Dose escalation to target structures up to 20 Gy was not associated with a proportionate increase in median organ doses for most critical organs. Median organ doses ranged from approximately 16–60% of the prescribed marrow dose with lung 44%, esophagus 33%, and oral cavity 28%. Lung D_{80} doses have been below 7.0 Gy even at the 20 Gy dose level. Figure 6 shows the level of dose uniformity within the target structure bone.

5.3.4 TMI Clinical Trials Performed at Other Institutions

Recently, other groups have evaluated TMI and TMLI containing conditioning regimens although the published experience to date is limited. Hui and colleagues at the University of Minnesota (Hui et al. 2007) reported on the first patient treated as part of a phase I autologous HCT trial in Ewing's sarcoma using TMI to 6 Gy (2 Gy per day), followed by Bu (targeted, 4 mg/kg days −8 to −6), Mel (50 mg/m^2 days −5 and −4) and thiotepa (250 mg/m^2 days −3 and −2). The regimen was well tolerated with only nausea and vomiting observed. Sheung et al. (2009) reported on

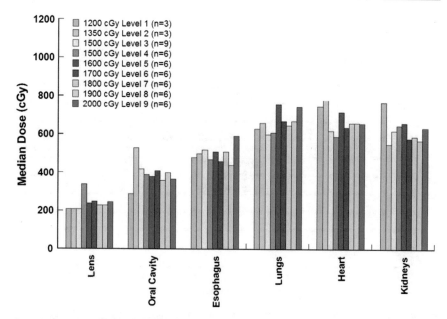

51 patients – median (D₅₀) dose at each level averaged

Fig. 5 Median (D_{50}) organ doses averaged for each dose level in 51 patients undergoing TMLI combined with Cy and VP-16 and allogeneic HCT. Dose escalation to target structures up to 20 Gy was not associated with a proportionate increase in median organ doses for most critical organs. Median organ doses ranged from approximately 16 to 60% of the prescribed marrow dose with lung 44%, esophagus 33%, and oral cavity 28%

Table 9 Median (D_{50}) organ dose as a percent of the prescribed target dose (n = 51)

Organs	Mean ± 1 SD	Range
Lens	15.0 ± 4.3	10.0–34.0
Oral cavity	24.3 ± 8.4	14.0–51.3
Rectum	33.1 ± 8.2	17.9–54.1
Esophagus	30.8 ± 5.8	16.3–44.2
Eyes	28.4 ± 13.0	13.1–71.9
Stomach	39.7 ± 7.4	27.1–58.3
Thyroid	44.6 ± 12.7	15.3–88.9
Parotids	39.6 ± 7.5	26.0–60.0
Lungs	41.5 ± 6.3	32.0–55.0
Heart	42.2 ± 10.3	28.8–69.2
Kidneys	37.9 ± 9.2	21.8–67.5
Small intestine	45.4 ± 6.9	26.8–61.1
Bladder	54.5 ± 12.5	25.3–89.2

SD standard deviation

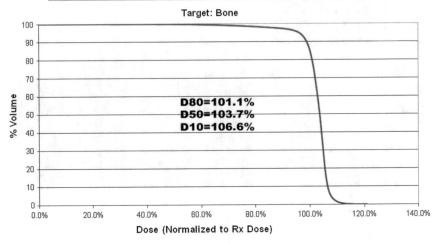

Target Organs	D80	D50	D10
Bone (n = 51)	101 % (97-106)	105 % (102-115)	109 % (104-119)

Fig. 6 Average D_{80}, D_{50} D_{10} Target Doses (as a percent of prescribed dose) in 51 Patients. DVH plot is a representative plot from one patient. This demonstrates the level of uniformity of dose to the bone compartment

3 patients conditioned with 8 Gy TMI at 2 Gy per day (days −6 to −3) combined with Mel at 140 mg/m² (day −2) prior to autologous HCT and observed only a single event of grade 3 toxicity (mucositis). Corvo et al. (2011) demonstrated the feasibility of adding a 2 Gy TMI boost to bone marrow and spleen after standard TBI 12 Gy (2 Gy BID) and Cy in 15 patients with AML and ALL undergoing allogeneic HCT and, with a median follow-up of 310 days, reported a cumulative TRM rate of 20%, relapse rate of 13% and disease free survival rate of 67%. Patel et al. (2014) were the first the deliver TMI using a VMAT approach with Flu and Bu. They reported on 14 patients most with advanced acute leukemia and established an MTD of 9 Gy (1.5 Gy BID). With a median follow-up of 1126 days TRM was 29%, RFS 43% and OS 50%.

Other centers in Europe, North America and Asia have also initiated similar trials but the early experience to date remains unpublished. Tables 10 and 11 list select TMI trials in multiple myeloma and leukemia that are ongoing. Most are pilot or phase I TMI dose escalation trials in patients with advanced, poor risk disease and are combined with RIC or myeloablative conditioning regimens. Most TMI schedules use 1.5 to 2 Gy fractions twice a day although some plan on using 3 to 4 Gy daily fractions.

5.3.5 High Dose-Rate and Organ Sparing

Clinical results have addressed initial concerns of TMI approaches. One concern was that the higher dose-rate with TMI (approximately ≥400 cGy/minute)

Table 10 Select TMI and TMLI trials currently open for accrual of patients with leukemia[a]

Institution	Type of trial	Type of HCT	Disease type	Age	Targets	TMI dose (Gy)	Fraction and schedule	Chemo therapy
City of Hope NCT02446964	Phase I	Allogeneic Haplo-identical	AML, ALL CR1 high risk, CR2, CR3, refractory	12–60	bone, spleen nodes	12, 14, 16, 18 20	1.5-2 Gy BID	Flu, Cy and post transplant Cy
City of Hope NCT02094794	Phase II	Allogeneic	AML or ALL, IF, relapsed or > CR2	18–60	bone, spleen, node, liver, brain	20 (12 to liver, brain)	2 Gy BID	Cy, VP16
U. Chicago NCT02333162	Phase I	Allogeneic	recurrent AML, ALL, MDS undergoing second HCT	18–75	Not Stated	NS	BID over 2-5 days	Flu, Mel
Case Comprehensive Cancer Center NCT02129582	Phase I	Allogeneic	ineligible for full myeloablative regimen AML, ALL, NHL, HL, MM, MDS, CLL, CML.	18–75	Not Stated	NS	BID over 4 days	Flu, Bu
U. Minnesota NCT00068556	Phase I	Allogeneic	ALL, AML CR2, CR3, Relapse, IF	pediatrics and adults	bone	15, 18, 21, 24	3 Gy QD	Flu, Cy
Ohio State NCT02122081	Pilot	Allogeneic	AML, ALL, MDS > 50 or comorbidities unable to undergo TBI based regimens;	18–75	bone, brain, testes	12	2 Gy BID	Cy

[a]Listed at www.cliniclatrials.gov

HCT hematopoietic cell transplantation; *AML* acute myelogenous leukemia; *ALL* acute lymphoblastic leukemia; *MM* multiple myeloma; *NHL* non-Hodgkin's lymphoma; *HL* Hodgkin's lymphoma; *MDS* myelodysplastic syndrome; *TBI* total body irradiation; *TMI* total marrow irradiation; *TMLI* total marrow and lymphoid irradiation; *CR1* first complete remission; *CR2* second complete remission; *CR3* third complete remission; *IF* induction failure; *QD* once per day; *BID* twice per day; *Bu* busulfan; *Flu* fludarabine; *Mel* melphalan; *Cy* cyclophosphamide; *VP-16* etoposide; *Gy* Gray

Table 11 Current TMI trials for patients with multiple myeloma[a]

Institution NCT trial no.	Type of trial	Type of HCT	Disease type	Age	Target	TMI dose levels (Gy)	Fraction and Schedule	Chemotherapy
City of Hope 01163357	Phase I	Allogeneic	MM refractory, relapsed prior auto HCT allowed	18–70	bone	12, then de-escalated to 9	1.5 Gy BID	Flu Mel Bortezomib
France multi-center 01794572	Phase I/II	Autologous	MM first relapse	18–65	bone	8, 10, 12, 14, 16	1–2 Gy BID over 4 d	Mel 140
Ottawa Regional 00800059	Phase I/II	Autologous	MM relapsed	18–60	bone	14, 16, 18 completed plan to go to 28	2 Gy BID	none
Marie Sklodowska- Curie Cancer Center, Poland 01665014	Pilot	Autologous tandem	MM in CR, VGPR, or PR	18–65	bone	12 Gy	4 Gy QD	Mel 200 second auto HCT
U. Illinois at Chicago 0202243860	Phase I	autologous	MM with high or intermediate risk of progression	18–75	bone	3, 6, 9, and 12	3 Gy QD	Mel 200
U. Illinois at Chicago 02043847	Phase I	Autologous	MM relapsed or refractory	18–75	bone	3, 6, and 9	3 Gy QD	Mel 200
U Rochester 01182233	Phase I	Autologous	MM	≤70	bone	10–20	2–4 Gy QD	Mel 200

[a]Listed at www.cliniclatrials.gov

HCT hematopoietic cell transplantation; *MM* multiple myeloma; *TMI* total marrow irradiation; *CR* complete remission; *VGPR* very good partial response; *PR* partial response; *QD* once per day; *BID* twice per day; *Mel* melphalan; *Gy* Gray compared to the low dose-rate with TBI (5–30 cGy/minute) would result in greater toxicity. The available toxicity data summarized earlier show that this is not the case. In addition, to the authors' knowledge there has not been a single reported case of non-engraftment. Finally, pre-clinical studies have demonstrated that dose-rate effects are not seen at dose-rates higher than approximately 25 cGy/minute and are significantly mitigated the more the TBI dose is fractionated (Travis et al. 1985; Tarbell et al. 1987). This may explain the lack of any dose-rate effect seen in the clinical trials to date.

Organ sparing has raised concerns of sparing of cancer cells. For example, in a study of 14 patients with refractory anemia undergoing allogeneic HCT and treated with Cy and TBI utilizing 95% attenuation lung and right hepatic lobe blocks, there was an increase in relapse rate (34% vs. 2%, $p = 0.0004$) and decrease in disease free survival (38% vs. 61%, $p = 0.16$) when compared to historical controls (Anderson et al. 2001). The authors hypothesized that 95% shielding of lung and liver may have shielded malignant cells or reduced immunosuppression and graft versus leukemia effect.

We have continued to monitor the rate and sites of extramedullary recurrences in patients treated with TMI regimens undergoing allogeneic HCT. Of 101 patients with a median follow-up of 12.8 months, 13 developed extramedullary relapses at 19 sites. The site of relapse was not dose-dependent, with 9 relapses occurring in the target region ($\geq$12 Gy), 5 relapses in regions receiving 10.1 to 11.4 Gy and 5 relapses in regions receiving 3.6 to 9.1 Gy (Kim et al. 2014). The risk of extramedullary relapse was comparable to that of standard TBI. In multivariate analysis extramedullary disease prior to HCT was the only predictor of extramedullary relapse. The use of TMI does not appear to increase the risk of relapse in non-target regions.

5.4 Future Directions

Ways to optimize dose delivery continue to be explored. Optimum dose schedules, fraction sizes, and chemotherapy regimens need to be defined. Larger fraction sizes of 3–4 Gy are being evaluated. Although this may be more time efficient, it diminishes the organ sparing effects of fractionation and hyperfractionation. Reduced fractionation combined with higher dose rates of TMI may increase the potential for organ toxicity particularly to the lungs, liver and kidneys.

The most appropriate target regions and target doses for a given patient population needs to be defined. The feasibility and benefit of dose escalation needs to be demonstrated in more trials. Other areas that need to be addressed are what patient population are TMI strategies most appropriate for and are TMI based regimens best used in patients who are poor risk and would do poorly with current regimens or in standard risk patients as a replacement for current TBI or on-TBI based regimens.

5.4.1 Multimodal and Functional Imaging for TMI Dose Painting and Response Assessment

An established principle in radiation oncology is that increased dose is needed to regions of higher tumor burden. Currently with TMI and other forms of image guided systemic radiotherapy dose escalation is to a CT based anatomic region such as bone and bone marrow. The assumption that the greater tumor burden is in the marrow and uniformly distributed throughout the bone and body for leukemia, multiple myeloma and other hematopoietic malignancies may not be the case. Future trials will explore the use of multi-modality and functional imaging to refine targeting and response assessment. [18]FDG- PET imaging and MRI including multi-parametric MRI are being actively being investigated to define areas of greater tumor burden, to define extramedullary disease and to assess response (Valls et al. 2016; Rubini et al. 2016). [^{18}F]-fluorothymidine, a DNA precursor which targets areas of greater DNA synthesis and cell proliferation, has demonstrated promise in detecting intramedullary distribution of acute leukemia and early recurrence (Vanderhoek et al. 2011).

Hematologic disease (especially leukemia) is assumed to be systemic, distributed homogeneously in the skeletal system and thus the iliac crest biopsy is the standard way to assess disease and to determine treatment management. In addition, the skeletal system micorenvironment and its compositional, structural, physiological, and functional units are assumed to be invariant. However, a small percentage of cells can become resistant and proliferate. As a result there have been new treatment strategies focusing in several areas: (1) the evolution of intrinsic cellular changes including stem cell clonogens, genetic mutations and various other ways to develop resistance to treatment and (2) the bone marrow (BM) "environment" which is beginning to be recognized as key contributing biological factor in hematological malignancies. The skeletal system is perhaps the largest and most complex physiological system. Pre-clinical studies indicate the important role the local BM environment plays in survival of leukemia cells or leukemia resistance after treatment (Kode et al. 2014; Konopleva and Jordan 2011; Raaijmakers 2011; Schepers et al. 2013). Recent pre-clinical studies with advanced imaging suggest structural and functional heterogeneity of BM (Lassailly et al. 2013; Naveiras et al. 2009).

The term functional total marrow irradiation or "fTMI" is coined to develop targeted radiation that incorporate functional information of the cancer, bone and marrow system, and interaction of cancer cells with BM macro- and the microenvironment. The path to develop and implement fTMI is complex and will develop over the next decades as the complex relation of hematologic cancers and its interaction with the BM environment and bone marrow hematopoiesis is better understood.

Hui and colleagues presented the concept of differential radiation targeting based on differences in bone marrow composition, namely active red marrow (RM), and yellow marrow (YM) or bone marrow adipose tissue or BMAT) as their functions are distinct. 3D mapping of marrow composition was developed using newly developed whole body DECT. In this framework, differential radiation to RM or YM was proposed (Fig. 7) (Magome et al. 2016). The radiation exposure was

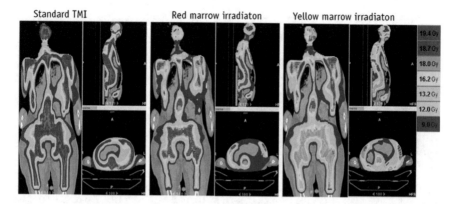

Fig. 7 Comparison of standard total marrow irradiation (TMI), *red marrow irradiation* (RMI), and *yellow marrow irradiation* (YMI). (A) Dose distributions of standard TMI, RMI, and YMI

significantly reduced to organs at risk (OARs) in RM and YM irradiation compared with standard total marrow irradiation (TMI). Although leukemia is prevalent in the vascularized marrow niche, regions of lower vascularity and higher hypoxia such as YM may function to enhance cancer resistance to systemic chemotherapy and radiation (Conklin 2004). Because cancer treatment changes marrow fat composition (Hui et al. 2015) individual factors including age and prior treatment may influence the distribution of marrow composition in different sites and possibly the distribution of viable tumor burden within the skeletal system.

A hybrid whole-body PET/DECT (3'-deoxy-3'[^{18}F]-fluorothymidine) imaging system, which is functional-anatomical-physiologic based imaging, offers the possibility of identifying spatial distribution of leukemia. Hui et al. observed highly heterogeneous distribution (systemic and focal lesions) of leukemia throughout the skeletal system. The majority of cells were systemic and uniformly distributed, but with additional regions of localized leukemia, that was associated with cortical bone in spine, proximal and distal femur, and pre-dominantly in RM regions. These data are hypothesis generating and raise the interesting possibility that heterogeneous distribution of leukemia could be associated with differences in the local marrow environment and possibly associated with different response characteristics to therapy.

Hui and colleagues simulated different TMI dose painting scenarios utilizing standard CT based imaging, FLT-PET based imaging and DCET based imaging (unpublished data). The full dose target region or planning tumor volume (PTV) for FLT or DECT based planning was dramatically reduced compared to the PTV of conventional TMI plan. Figure 8 shows color wash dose distributions of conventional, FLT, and DECT based TMI plans. With reduction in the volume of the target region, doses to critical organs could be reduced in FLT and DECT based TMI plans compared with the conventional TMI. In summary, multimodality image guided "fTMI" would allow for differential irradiation of regions with higher burden of chemo-resistant leukemia cells and the potential to more selectively increase dose and improve outcomes.

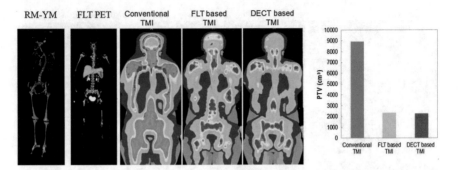

Fig. 8 Functional total marrow irradiation development (from *left* to *right*): 3D mapping BM composition using DECT (verified using water-fat MRI), FLT PET with DECT (not shown), dose painting comparison between conventional (CT based) total marrow irradiation (TMI), FLT imaging-based TMI, and DECT imaging-based TMI, and dose volume histograms of conventional (*blue*), FLT-based (*green*), DECT-based (*red*) TMI plans

6 Conclusions

In summary, strategies to deliver a more targeted form of TBI continue to be actively investigated in this emerging area through the use of newer image guided IMRT radiotherapy delivery systems. Although the follow-up has been short and the number of patients treated has been limited, initial results with TMI have been encouraging and demonstrate feasibility, acceptable toxicities, TRM rates that compare favorably to standard conditioning regimens, and encouraging response and survival rates in advanced disease. Dose escalation is possible when combined with certain drug combinations such as Cy/VP-16. TMI can now be delivered on more than one technology platform, through helical tomographic or VMAT based image guided IMRT delivery. The number of centers and trials continue to increase. Today TMI and TMLI trials are being performed or planned in centers in North America, Central America, Europe, Asia and Australia which demonstrates that this approach is exportable and reproducible at other centers. This emerging area will soon be positioned to carry out multicenter trials to answer important clinical questions that remain.

A potential advantage of TMI and TMLI is the ability to reduce doses to normal organs, thereby reducing toxicities and broadening the spectrum of patients able to tolerate radiation conditioning regimens, such as older patients or those with co-morbidities. As a result TMI and TMLI can be combined with established RIC regimens in an effort to improve outcomes. Another potential advantage is the ability to escalate target dose with acceptable toxicities. Although, TMI is represents a paradigm shift from standard TBI, its full clinical benefit needs to be validated through well-designed clinical trials. Ultimately trials need to demonstrate that TMI based conditioning regimens offer advantages over already established TBI and non-TBI containing conditioning regimens.

References

Anderson JE, Appelbaum FR, Schoch G et al (2001) Relapse after allogeneic bone marrow transplantation for refractory anemia is increased by shielding lungs and liver during total body irradiation. Biology Blood Marrow Transplan 7(3):163–170

Andrews GA, Sitterson BW, White DA et al (1962) Summary of clinical total-body irradiation program. Oak Ridge Institute of Nuclear Studies, Medical Division, Research Report, USA

Appelbaum FR, Matthews DC, Eary JF et al (1992) Use of radiolabeled anti-CD33 antibody to augment marrow irradiation prior to marrow transplantation for acute myelogenous leukemia. Transplantation 54:829–833

Aydogan B, Yeginer M, Kavak GO et al (2011) Total marrow irradiation with rapidarc volumetric arc therapy. Int J Radiat Oncol Biol Phys 81:592–599

Bakst R, Wolden S, Yahalom J (2012) Radiation therapy for chloroma (granulocytic sarcoma). Int J Radiat Onco Biol Phys 82(5):1816–1822

Bearman S, Appelbaum FR, Buckner CD et al (1988) Regimen-related toxicity in patients undergoing bone marrow transplantation. J Clin Oncol 6:1562–1568

Beavis AW (2004) Is tomotherapy the future of IMRT? British J Radio 77:285–295

Blaise D, Maraninchi D, Archimbaud E et al (1992) Allogeneic bone marrow transplantation for acute myeloid leukemia in first remission: A randomized trial of busulfan-cytoxan versus cytoxan-total body irradiation as a preparative regimen: A report from the Groupe d'Etudes de la Greffe de Moelle Osseuse. Blood 79:2578–2582

Bredeson C, LeRademacher J, Kato K et al (2013) Prospective cohort study comparing intravenous busulfan to total body irradiation in hematopoietic cell transplantation. Blood 122:3871–3878

Bunin N, Aplenc R, Kamani N et al (2003) Randomized trial of busulfan vs total body irradiation containing conditioning regimens for children with acute lymphoblastic leukemia: a pediatric blood and marrow transplant consortium study. Bone Marrow Transplant 32:543–548

Bunjes D (2002) 188Re-labeled anti-CD66 monoclonal antibody in stem cell transplantation for patients with high-risk acute myeloid leukemia. Leukemia Lymphoma 43:2125–2131

Burke JM, Caron PC, Papadopoulos EB et al (2003) Cytoreduction with iodine-131-anti-CD33 antibodies before bone marrow transplantation for advanced myeloid leukemias. Bone Marrow Transplant 32:549–556

Chak LY, Sapozink MD, Cox RS (1983) Extramedullary lesions in non-lymphocytic leukemia: results of radiation therapy. Int J Radiation Oncology Biol Phys 9:1173–1176

Cheng JC, Schultheiss TE, Nguyen KH, Wong JYC (2008) Acute toxicity in definitive versus postprostatectomy image-guided radiotherapy for prostate cancer. Int J Radiat Oncol Biol, Phys

Clift RA, Buckner CD, Appelbaum FR et al (1991) Allogeneic marrow transplantation in patients with chronic myeloid leukemia in the chronic phase: a randomized trial of two irradiation regimens. Blood 77:1660–1665

Clift RA, Buckner CD, Appelbaum FR et al (1998) Long-term follow-up of a randomized trial of two irradiation regimens for patients receiving allogeneic marrow transplants during first remission of acute myeloid leukemia. Blood 92:1455–1456

Conklin K (2004) Cancer chemotherapy and antioxidants. The Journal of Nutrition 134:3201S–3204S

Corvo R, Zeverino M, Vagge S et al (2011) Helical tomotherapy targeting total bone marrow after total body irradiation for patients with relapsed acute leukemia undergoing an allogeneic stem cell transplant. Radiother Oncol 98:382–386

de Lima M, Couriel D, Thall PF et al (2004) Once-daily intravenous busulfan and fludarabine: clinical and pharmacokinetic results of a myeloablative, reduced-toxicity conditioning regimen for allogeneic stem cell transplantation in AML and MDS. Blood 104:857–864

Deeg HJ, Sandmaier BM (2010) Who is fit for allogeneic transplantation? Blood 116:4762–4770

Deeg HJ, Sullivan KM, Buckner CD et al (1986) Marrow transplantation for acute nonlymphoblastic leukemia in first remission: toxicity and long-term follow-up of patients conditioned with single dose or fractionated total body irradiation. Bone Marrow Transplant 1:151–157

Draeger RH, Lee RH, Shea TE Jr et al (1953) Design of a radiocobalt large animal irradiator. Naval Medical Res Unit

Dusenbery KE, Daniels KA, McClure JS et al (1995) Randomized comparison of cyclophosphamide-total body irradiation versus busulfan-cyclophosphamide conditioning in autologous bone marrow transplantation for acute myeloid leukemia.[see comment]. Int J Radiat Oncol Biol Phys 31:119–128

Einsele H, Bamberg M, Budach W et al (2003) A new conditioning regimen involving total marrow irradiation, busulfan and cyclophosphamide followed by autologous PBSCT in patients with advanced multiple myeloma. Bone Marrow Transplant 32:593–599

Fogliata A, Cozzi L, Clivio A et al (2011) Preclinical assessment of volumetric modulated arc therapy for total marrow irradiation. Int J Radiat Oncol Biol Phys 80:628–636

Formenti SC, Demaria S (2005) Systemic effects of local radiotherapy. Lancet Oncol 10:718–726

Formenti SC, Demaria S (2012) Radiation therapy to convert the tumor into an insitu vaccine. Int J Radiat Oncol Biol Phys 84:879–880

Giralt S, Thall PF, Khouri I et al (2001) Melphalan and purine analog-containing preparative regimens: reduced intensity conditioning for patients with hematologic malignancies undergoing allogeneic progenitor cell transplantation. Blood 97:631–637

Giralt S, Aleman A, Anagnostopoulos A et al (2002) Fludarabine/melphalan conditioning for allogeneic transplantation in patients with multiple myeloma. Bone Marrow Transplant 30:367–373

Girinsky T, Benhamou E, Bourhis JH et al (2000) Prospective randomized comparison of single-dose versus hyperfractionated total-body irradiation in patients with hematologic malignancies. J Clin Oncol 18:981–986

Gupta T, Kannan S, Dantkale V et al (2011) Cyclophosphamide plus total body irradiation compared with busulfan plus cyclophosphamide as a conditioning regimen prior to hematopoietic stem cell transplantation in patients with leukemia: a systematic review and meta-analysis. Hematol Oncol Stem Cell Ther 4:17–29

Hall MD, Schultheiss TE, Smith DD et al (2015) Dose response for radiation cataractogeneisis: a meta-regression of hematopoietic stem cell transplantation regimens. Int J Radiat Oncol Biol Phys 91:22–29

Han C, Schultheisss TE, Wong JY (2011) Dosimetric study of volumetric modulated arc therapy fields for total marrow irradiation. Radiotherapy and Oncology 102(2):315–320

Hartman AR, Williams SF, Dillon JJ (1998) Survival, disease-free survival and adverse effects of conditioning for allogeneic bone marrow transplantation with busulfan/cyclophosphamide vs total body irradiation: a meta-analysis. Bone Marrow Transplant 22:439–443

Hayes RL, Oddie TH, Brucer M (1964) Dose comparison of two total-body irradiation facilities. Internat J Appl Radiation Isotopes 15:313–318

Heublein AC (1932) A preliminary report on continuous irradiation of the entire body. Radiology 18:1051–1060

Hong S, Barker C, Klein JP et al (2012) Trends in utilization of total body irradiation (TBI) Prior to hematopoietic cell transplantation (HCT) worldwide. Biology Blood Marrow Trans 18(2): S336–S337 [Abstract]

Hui SK, Verneris MR, Higgins P et al (2007) Helical tomotherapy targeting total bone marrow— first clinical experience at the University of Minnesota. Acta Oncol 46:250–255

Hui SK, Arentsen L, Sueblinvong T et al (2015) A phase I feasibility study of mylti-modality imaging assessing rapid expansion of marrow fat and decreased bone mineral density in cancer patients. Bone 73:90–97

Jacobs ML, Marasso FJ (1965) A four-year experience with total-body irradiation. Radiology 84:452–456

Jacobs ML, Pape L (1960) A total body irradiation chamber and its uses. Internat J Appl Radiation Isotopes 8:141–143

Jacobs ML, Pape L (1961) Total-body irradiation chamber. Radiology 77:788–791

Jurcic JG, Ravandi F, Pagel JM et al (2015) Phase I trial of targeted alpha-particle immunotherapy with actinium-225 (225Ac)-lintuzumab (anti-CD33) and low-dose cytarabine (LDAC) in older patients with untreated acute myeloid leukemia (AML). Blood 126(23):3794

Jurcic JG, Wong JYC, Knox SJ et al (2016) Targeted radionuclide therapy. In: Philadelphia: LL, Gunderson J, Tepper E Clinical radiation oncology, 399–418

Kal HB, van Kempen-Harteveld ML, Heijenbrok MH et al (2006) Biologically effective dose in total-body irradiation and hematopoietic stem cell transplantation. Strahlenther Onkol 182:679

Kim JH, Stein A, Tsai N et al (2014) Extramedullary relapse following total marrow and lymphoid irradiation in patinets undergoing allogenejic hematopoietic cell transplantation. Int J Radiat Oncol Biol Phys 89:75–81

Kode A, Manavalan JS, Mosialou I et al (2014) Leukaemogenesis induced by an activating B-catenin mutation in osteoblasts. Nature 506:240–258

Koenecke C, Hofmann M, Bolte O et al (2008) Radioimmunotherapy with [188Re]-labelled anti-CD66 antibody int he conditioning for allogeneic stem cell transplantation for high-risk acute myeloid leukemia. Int J Hematol 87:414–421

Konopleva MY, Jordan CT (2011) Leukemia stem cells and microenvironment: biology and therapeutic targeting. J Clin Oncol 29:591–599

Labar B, Bogdanic V, Nemet D et al (1992) Total body irradiation with or without lung shielding for allogeneic bone marrow transplantation. Bone Marrow Transplant 9:343–347

Lassailly F, Foster K, Lopez-Onieva L et al (2013) Multimodal imaging reveals structural and functional heterogeneity in different bone marrow compartments: functional implications on hematopoietic stem cells. Blood 122:1730–1740

Lauter A, Strumpf A, Platzbecker U et al (2009) 188Re anti-CD66 radioimmunotherapy combined with reduced-intensity conditioning and in-vivo T cell depletion in elderly patients undergoing allogeneic haematopoietic cell transplantation. Br J Haematol 148:910–917

Magome T, Froelich J, Takahashi Y et al (2016) Evaluation of functional marrow irradiation based on skeletal marrow composition obtained using dual-energy CT. Int J Radiat Oncol Biol Phys 96:679–687

Marks DI, Forman SJ, Blume KG et al (2006) A comparison of cyclophosphamide and total body irradiation with etoposide and total body irradiation as conditioning regimens for patients undergoing sibling allografting for acute lymphoblastic leukemia in first or second complete remission. Biol Blood Marrow Transplant 12:438–453

Matthews DC, Appelbaum FR, Eary JF et al (1999) Phase I Study of 131I-Anti-CD45 antibody plus cyclophosphamide and total body irradiation for advanced acute leukemia and myelodysplastic syndrome. Blood 94:1237–1247

Mawad R, Gooley TA, Rajendran JG et al (2014) Radiolabeled anti-CD45 antibody with reduced-intensity conditioning and allogeneic transplantation for younger patients with advanced acute myeloid leukemia or myelodysplastic syndrome. Biol Blood Marrow Transplant 20:1363–1368

Naveiras O, Nardi V, Wenzel PL et al (2009) Bone-marrow adipocytes as negative regulators of the haematopoietic microenvironment. Nature 460:259–264

Ozsahin M, Pene F, Touboul E et al (1992) Total-body irradiation before bone marrow transplantation. Results of two randomized instantaneous dose rates in 157 patients. Cancer 69:2853–2865

Pagel JM, Appelbaum FR, Eary JF et al (2006) 131I-anti-CD45 antibody plus busulfan and cyclophosphamide before allogeneic hematopoietic cell transplantation for treatment of acute myeloid leukemia in first remission. Blood 107:2184–2191

Pagel JM, Gooley TA, Rajendran J et al (2009) Allogeneic hematopoietic cell transplantation after conditioning with 131I-anti-CD45 antibodyplus fludarabine and low-dose total body irradiation for elderly patients with advanced acute myeloid leukemia or high-risk myelodysplastic syndrome. Blood 114:5444–5453

Scott BL, Pasquini MC, Logan B, Wu J, Devine S et al (2015) Results of a phase III randomized, multi-center study of allogeneic stem cell transplantation after high versus reduced intensity conditioning in patients with myelodysplastic syndrome (MDS) or acute myeloid leukemia (AML): blood and marrow transplant clinical trials network (BMT CTN) 0901. Blood 126 (23):8

Patel P, Aydogan B, Koshy M et al (2014) Combination of linear accelerator-based intensity-modulated total marrow irradiation and myeloablative Fludarabine/Busulfan: a phase I study. Biol Blood Marrow Transplant 20:2034–2041

Petropoulos D, Worth LL, Mullen CA et al (2006) Total body irradiation, fludarabine, melphalan, and allogeneic hematopoietic stem cell transplantation for advanced pediatric hematologic malignancies. Bone Marrow Transplant 37:463–467

Raaijmakers MHGP (2011) Niche contributions to oncogenesis: Emerging concepts and implications for the hematopoietic system. Haematologica 96:1041–1048

Rhoades J, Lawton C, Cohen E et al (1997) Incidence of bone marrow transplant nephropathy (BMT-Np) After twice daily bid hyperfractionated total body irradiation. Am Radium Soc 3:116

Ringden O, Labopin M, Tura S et al (1996) A comparison of busulphan versus total body irradiation combined with cyclophosphamide as conditioning for autograft or allograft bone marrow transplantation in patients with acute leukaemia. Acute Leukaemia Working Party of the European Group for Blood and Marrow Transplantation (EBMT). Br J Haematol 93:637–645

Ringhoffer M, Blumstein N, Neumaier B et al (2005) 188Re or 90Y-labelled anti-CD66 antibody as part of a dose-reduced conditioning regimen for patients with acute leukaemia or myelodysplastic syndrome over the age of 55: results of a phase I–II study. Br J Haematol 130:604–613

Ritchie DS, Morton J, Szer J et al (2003) Graft-versus-host disease, donor chimerism, and organ toxicity in step cell transplantation after conditioning with Fludarabine and Melphalan. Biol Blood Marrow Transplant 9:435–442

Rosenblat TL, McDevitt MRFAU, Mulford D, Mulford DA, Pandit-Taskar FAU et al (2010) Sequential cytarabine and alpha-particle immunotherapy with bismuth-213-lintuzumab (HuM195) for acute myeloid leukemia. Clin Cancer Res 16:5303–5311

Rosenthal J, Wong J, Stein A et al (2011) Phase 1/2 trial of total marrow and lymph node irradiation to augment reduced-intensity transplantation for advanced hematologic malignancies. Blood 117:309–315

Rubini G, Niccoli-Asabella A, Ferrari C et al (2016) Myeloma bone and extra-medullary disease: Role of PET/CT and other whole-body imaging techniques. Crit Rev Oncol Hematol 11:169–183

Salama JK, Chmura SJ, Mehta N et al (2008) An initial report of a radiation dose-escalation trial in patients with one to five sites of metastatic disease. Clin Cancer Res 14:5255–5259

Sampath S, Schultheiss TE, Wong J et al (2005) Dose response and factors related to interstitial pneumonitis after bone marrow transplant. Int J Radiat Oncol Biol Phys 63:876–884

Scarpati D, Frassoni F, Vitale V et al (1989) Total body irradiation in acute myeloid leukemia and chronic myelogenous leukemia: influence of dose and dose-rate on leukemia relapse. Int J Radiat Oncol Biol Phys 17:547–552

Schepers K, Pietras EM, Reynaud D et al (2013) Myeloproliferative neoplasia remodels the endosteal bone marrow niche into a self-reinforcing leukemic niche. Cell Stem Cell 13:285–299

Schultheiss TE, Wong J, Liu A et al (2007) Image-guided total marrow and total lymphatic irradiation using helical tomotherapy. Int J Radiat Oncol Biol Phys 67:1259–1267

Shank B, O'Reilly RJ, Cunningham I et al (1990) Total body irradiation for bone marrow transplantation: the Memorial Sloan-Kettering Cancer Center experience. Radiother Oncol 18 (Suppl 1):68–81

Shueng PW, Lin SC, Chong NS et al (2009) Total marrow irradiation with helical tomotherapy for bone marrow transplantation of multiple myeloma: first experience in Asia. Technol Cancer Res Treat 8:29–38

Somlo G, Spielberger R, Frankel P et al (2011) Total Marrow Irradiation: A new ablative regimen as part of tandem autologous stem cell transplantation for patients with multiple myeloma. Clin Cancer Res 17:174–182

Somlo G, Liu A, Schultheiss TE et al (2015) Total marrow irradiation (TMI) with helical tomotherapy and peripheral blood progenitor cell rescue (PBPC) following high-dose melphalan (Mel) and PBPC as part of tandem autologous transplant (TAT) for patients with multiple myeloma. J Clin Oncol 54:31–67

Speer TW (2013) Radioimmunotherapy and unsealed radionuclide therapy and unsealed radionuclide therapy. Conjugated Therapy 1:525–539

Stein AS, O'Donnell MR, Synold T et al (2011) Phase-2 trial of an intensified conditioning regimen for allogeneic hematopoietic cell transplant for poor-risk leukemia. Bone Marrow Transplant 46:1256–1262

Stein AS, Wong J, Tsia N et al (2012) Phase I trial of escalated doses of targeted marrow/lymphoid radiation delivered by tomotherapy combined with etoposide and cyclophosphamide; an allogeneic HCT preparative regimen for patients with advanced leukemia. In: Conference presented at american society of hematology meeting, Atlanta, GA [Abstract]

Stein AS, Wong JY, Palmer J et al (2015) A Phase I Trial of Total Marrow and Lymphoid Irradiation (TMLI)-Based Transplant Conditioning in Patients (Pts) with Relapsed/Refractory Acute Leukemia. Blood 126(23):735

Tarbell NJ, Amato DA, Down JD et al (1987) Fractionation and dose rate effects in mice: a model for bone marrow transplantation in man. Int J Radiat Oncol Biol Phys 13:1065–1069

Teschendorf W (1927) Uber bestrahlung des ganzen menschlichen Korpers bei Blutkrankheiten. Strahlentherapie 26:720–728

Thomas ED, Lochte HL, Cannon JH et al (1959) Supralethal whole body irradiation and isologous marrow transplantation in man. J Clin Invest 38:1709–1716

Travis EL, Peters LJ, McNeil J et al (1985) Effect of dose-rate on total body irradiation: lethality and pathologic findings. Radiother Oncol 4:341–351

Valls L, Badve C, Avril S et al (2016) FDG-PET imaging in hematological malignancies. Blood Rev 30:317–331

Vanderhoek M, Juckett MB, Perlman SB et al (2011) Early assessment of treatment response in patients with AML using [18F]FLT PET imaging. Leuk Res 35:310–316

Weichselbaum RR, Hellman S (2011) Oligometastases revisted. Nat Rev Clin Oncol 8:378–382

Weiner R, Bortin M, Gale RP et al (1986) Interstitial pneumonitis after bone marrow transplantation. Ann Intern Med 104:168–175

Wong JYC, Liu A, Schultheiss T et al (2006) Targeted total marrow irradiation using three-dimensional image-guided tomographic intensity-modulated radiation therapy: an alternative to standard total body irradiation. Biol Blood Marrow Transplant 12:306–315

Wong JYC, Rosenthal J, Liu A et al (2009) Image guided total marrow irradiation (TMI) using helical tomotherapy in patients with multiple myeloma and acute leukemia undergoing hematopoietic cell transplantation (HCT). Int J Radiat Oncol Biol Phys 73:273–279

Wong JY, Forman S, Somlo G et al (2013) Dose escalation of total marrow irradiation with concurrent chemotherapy in patients with advanced acute leukemia undergoing allogeneic hematopoietic cell transplantation. Int J Radiat Oncol Biol Phys 85:148–156

Zenz T, Glatting G, Schlenk RF et al (2006) Targeted marrow irradiation with radioactively labeled anti-CD66 monoclonal antibody prior to allogeneic stem cell transplantation for patients with leukemia: results of a phase I–II study. Haematologica 91:285–286

Cancer Stem Cells and Tumor Microenvironment in Radiotherapy

Jian Jian Li

Abstract

Ionizing radiation (IR) began to be a powerful medical modality soon after Wilhelm Röntgen's discovery of X-rays in 1895. Today about 60% of cancer patients worldwide receive radiotherapy in their course of cancer control. In the past decades, the technology for precisely delivering tumor IR dose such as stereotactic body radiation therapy (SBRT) has been significantly enhanced, which increases the overall local tumor response and clinical benefit. However, in achieving the goal for long-term cancer control, radiotherapy (RT) has faced several major challenges including the elucidation of the microenvironment causing tumor repopulation and resistance, especially with the most aggressive tumor cells in late phase metastatic lesions. To meet this challenge, a great deal of effort has been devoted to revealing not only the mechanistic insight of tumor heterogeneity, but also the emerging complexity of the irradiated microenvironment. Such new knowledge provides the explanation for the long recognized tumor heterogeneity and tumor cell repopulation, one the major "R"s in tumor radiobiology, which involves cancer stem cells (also termed tumor-imitating cells, cancer stem-like cells, or stem like cancer cells). It is generally accepted that CSCs plays a key role in tumor adaptive radioresistance and are involved in clinical tumor response. The specific cell surface biomarkers as well as the biological topographies of CSCs in many solid tumors have been identified; some of them overlap with those detected in normal stem cells. However, the exact molecular mechanism causing the radioresistant phenotype of CSCs,

J.J. Li (✉)
Department of Radiation Oncology, School of Medicine, NCI-Designated
Comprehensive Cancer Center, University of California Davis,
Sacramento, CA, USA
e-mail: jijli@ucdavis.edu

© Springer International Publishing AG 2017   191
J.Y.C. Wong et al. (eds.), *Advances in Radiation Oncology*,
Cancer Treatment and Research 172, DOI 10.1007/978-3-319-53235-6_9

especially the dynamic nature of CSCs themselves under RT and their communication with the irradiated tumor microenvironment including stromal cells and immune cells, remains to be elucidated. Further elucidation of the complexity of the irradiated local tumor microenvironment in which CSCs reside may generate significant new information to resensitize radioresistant tumor cells and thus to improve therapeutic efficacy. In this chapter, I will describe the general information on normal stem cells, CSCs, CSCs-associated tumor repopulation and energy reprogramming and potential therapeutic targets. The dynamic features of radioresistance-associated factors such as NF-κB and HER2 in some CSCs including breast cancer and GBM will be discussed.

Keywords

Tumor resistance · Radiotherapy · Microenvironment · Cancer stem cells · Tumor repopulation · Metabolic reprogramming · Immunoresponse · Radiosensitization

Abbreviations

ALDH	Aldehyde dehydrogenase
ATRA	All-trans retinoic acid
ATP	Adenosine triphosphate
BCSCs	Breast cancer stem cells
CDK1	Cyclin-dependent kinases 1
CDK2	Cyclin-dependent kinases 2
CHK1	Checkpoint kinase 1
Chk1	Checkpoint kinase 1
CSCs	Cancer stem cells
CXCR4	Chemokine C-X-C motif receptor 4
EMT	Epithelial–mesenchymal transition
ESCs	Embryonic stem cells
FAO	Fatty acid oxidation
FIR	Fractionated ionizing radiation
FR	Fractionated radiation
GBM	Glioblastoma multiforme
GSCs	Glioblastoma multiforme stem cells
HIF-1α	Hypoxia inducible factor alpha
HSCs	Hematopoietic stem cells
ICD	IR-induced immunogenic cell death
iPSCs	Induced pluripotent stem cells
IR	Ionizing radiation
ICD	IR-induced immunogenic cell death
LDH	Lactate dehydrogenase
NF-κB	Nuclear factor kappa B
NSCs	Normal stem cells; neural stem cells

MnSOD   Manganese-containing superoxide dismutase
ROS   Reactive oxygen species
SBRT   Stereotactic body radiation therapy
OXPHOS   Oxidative phosphorylation
RT   Radiation therapy
TNBC   Triple-negative breast cancer

1 Introduction

1.1 General Feature of CSCs

Accumulating evidence demonstrates that the inexorable progression towards the resistant phenotype of cancer cells and the dynamic alterations in tumor microenvironment are associated with the overall adaptive tumor response to radiotherapy. Clinic and lab data suggest that tumors contain cancer stem cells (CSCs, or termed stem-like cancer cells, tumor-initiating cells) which play an integral role in the tumor microenvironment and in radioresistance. The existence of cancer stem cells have long been suspected, which is recently supported by the evidence showing that only a small proportion of tumor cells are able to form colonies or new tumors (Bonnet and Dick 1997; Al-Hajj et al. 2003). Increasing numbers of specific CSCs markers such as CD133, CD44, ALDH, are used to identify CSCs. Breast cancer stem cells expressing such CSC biomarkers (Al-Hajj et al. 2003) have been shown to have increased expression of pro-invasive genes required for metastasis such as IL-1α, IL-6, and IL-8 (Sheridan et al. 2006). Additionally, CSCs appear to exhibit notable radioresistance and chemoresistance. Tumor cells undergoing genotoxic stress conditions (such as with IR and chemotherapy), activate pro-survival pathways and inhibit pro-apoptotic pathways resulting in tumor radioresistance. The molecules involved in these CSC pathways are potential targets to enhance tumor radiosensitivity.

In this chapter, I will discuss some key features associated with radioresistance of CSCs, the dynamics of CSCs repopulation during radiotherapy, and the potential targets that may help to eliminate CSCs by RT. Specific pathways in breast cancer stem cells (BCSCs) and glioblastoma multiforme (GBM) stem cells (GSCs) are discussed. Among pro-survival pathways, the role of NF-κB-HER2 in mediating BCSC radioresistance will be discussed with an emphasis on experimental laboratory data. With the recent interest in cancer immunotherapy, RT mediated alterations in tumor immunoreactions such as ascopal effects and tumor bioenergetics such as mitochondrial energetics will be discussed. An understanding of such pro-survival networks activated in CSCs will not only help to develop effective targets to sensitize tumor cells to radiotherapy, but also generate specific diagnostic approaches for the detection of recurrent or metastatic tumors.

1.2   Normal Stem Cells and CSCs

Mammalian cells with stem like feature (stemness) are grouped into three major types according to different functions: (a) Totipotent stem cells (such as ESCs and iPSCs) refer to stem cells that are highly plastic and can potentially be directed to any cell type; (b) Mesenchymal Stem Cells (MSCs) are the stromal cells present in the bone marrow and most connective tissues, capable of differentiation into mesenchymal tissues such as bone and cartilage; and (c) Lineage-Specific Stem Cells that include Hematopoietic Stem Cell (HSCs), Neural Stem Cells (NSCs) etc. (Hu et al. 2016). Cancer stem cells (CSCs) were first isolated in acute myeloid leukemia patients (Lapidot et al. 1994), followed by many other experiments showing the presence of CSCs in solid tumors including breast, lung, prostate, colon, and brain tumors (Al-Hajj et al. 2003; Ashkenazi et al. 2007; Baumann et al. 2008; Dalerba et al. 2007). Similar features are detected in CSCs that are generally defined as a small subpopulation of cancer cells that show a unique capacity of self-renewal and can also generate the heterogeneous cell lineages comprising the tumor (Clarke et al. 2006). Based on the proliferating rate, CSCs can also be divided into two cell subpopulations: the normal and the slow proliferating cells (quiescent or dormant cells) (Skvortsova et al. 2015). It has been suggested that CSCs originate from NSCs and acquire a malignant phenotype due to gene mutations caused by endogenous and exogenous stimuli (Hittelman et al. 2010). Overlapping with major features of NSCs, CSCs are shown to be resistant to proapoptotic factors, rendering them a forbidding adversary to current anti-cancer modalities (Li and Neaves 2006; Frosina 2009; Lou and Dean 2007). CSCs can also originate from cancer cells and recently stemness features have been detected in non-stem cancer cells after radiation (Vlashi et al. 2016). The major phenotype of CSCs is their enhanced growth potential with the ability to form tumors which can locally invade and metastasize (Clarke 2005; Moncharmont et al. 2012; Chen et al. 2013). Figure 1 shows the typical images of three different mammospheres formed by immortalized normal human breast epithelial MCF-10A cells contrasted with the

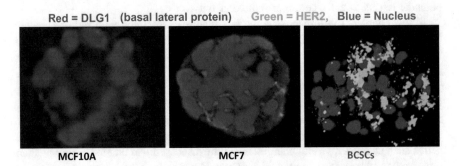

Fig. 1 Representative images showing the different acini structures generated from immortalized normal human breast epithelial MCF10A, breast cancer MCF7 and BCSCs isolated from MCF7 population that survived a course of FR. DLG and HER2 indicate the polarity of cells in the acini

breast cancer MCF7 cells and BCSCs isolated from a surviving MCF7 population after chronic fractionated radiation (FR) (unpublished work of JJ Li's lab).

1.3 Tumor Heterogeneity and CSC-Mediated Tumor Repopulation Under Radiotherapy

Tumor heterogeneity was suspected as early as three hundred years ago when the original microscope was invented (Zellmer and Zhang 2014). As a major tumor response to therapeutic ionizing radiation, repopulation of tumor cells has been defined in experiments and clinic practice (Heppner and Miller 1989). Radiation induced repopulation of tumor cells is recognized as one of the "**R**"s in radiation oncology, which includes **r**epopulation, **r**edistribution, **r**e-oxygenation, and **r**epair. Such repopulation during therapy has been implicated as an important feature in tumor recurrence after radiotherapy (Kim and Tannock 2005). The pioneering work by Dewey's group using long-term observations of irradiated cells via computerized video time-lapse analyses revealed the heterogeneity and different cell fates among irradiated cells (Endlich et al. 2000), demonstrating the heterogeneous IR response in a supposedly homogeneous cell population. Data from our lab also demonstrated that a small fraction of breast cancer MCF7 cells were able survive a course of chronic fractionated radiation (FR) and showed an enhanced profile of genes regulating cell cycle and DNA repair (Li et al. 2001; Guo et al. 2003). This radioresistant breast cancer population was found to be enriched with specific breast cancer stem cells expressing HER2 (Duru et al. 2012). Increased tumorgenicity of CSCs with specific surface markers was first studied in acute myeloid leukemia (Bonnet and Dick 1997).

A CSC is thus defined as a specific tumor cell that has stem-cell like properties including the capacity to self-renew and to generate the heterogeneous lineages of cancer cells that comprise the tumor. A key feature of CSC theory is that only a small subset of tumor cells has the ability to proliferate in an uncontrolled manner which challenges the traditional concept that each tumor cell is able to grow to a new tumor. Al-Hajj et al. demonstrated that BCSCs (CD44$^+$/CD24$^{-/low}$) are more tumorigenic; as few as 100 cells with this phenotype are able to form tumors in mice, while millions of cells without this feature cannot (Al-Hajj et al. 2003). Phillips et al. used the CD44$^+$/CD24$^{-/low}$ BCSCs isolated from breast cancer cells to show that BCSCs can be propagated as mammospheres and enriched after radiation (Phillips et al. 2006). Using xenogeneic tumors treated with chemotherapy, Dylla et al. identified the repopulation of colorectal CSCs with the marker of CD44$^+$ESA$^+$ (Dylla et al. 2008; Dalerba et al. 2007). Firat et al. (Firat et al. 2011) further identified a delayed cell death associated with mitotic catastrophe in irradiated GSCs. These results together with other reports demonstrate that the surviving cancer cells under RT are enriched with CSCs and may contribute to tumor repopulation observed in the clinic. During chemo- and/or radio-therapy, the most resistant CSCs would be selected and continue to sustain the tumor. In clinical studies, the proportion of putative CSCs in a residual tumor has been shown to increase following cytotoxic chemotherapy (Findlay et al. 2014; McClements et al. 2013; Vaz et al. 2014; Duru et al. 2014). These findings shed light on a new conceptual paradigm of how CSCs or tumor-initiating cells contribute to radiation response. Identification of CSC-associated radioresistance needs to be further evaluated in clinical studies.

1.4 GSCs in Brain Tumor Radiotherapy

Glioblastoma multiforme (GBM) is a highly malignant primary brain tumor with a median survival time of approximately 14 months from time of initial diagnosis (Stupp et al. 2009), and radiotherapy has been the major modality for control of this tumor (Brandes et al. 2009; Balasubramaniam et al. 2007; Dhermain 2014). GSCs identified in human GBM showed infinite self-renewal and can differentiate into different cells types such as neurons and glia (Galli et al. 2004; Singh et al. 2004). GSCs also express NSC markers such as CD133, Sox2 and Nestin (Singh et al. 2004). Evidence suggests that GSCs are responsible for the aggressive tumor growth and radiotherapy resistance, although the precise mechanism has yet to be elucidated (Stiles and Rowitch 2008). Not surprisingly, Bao et al. (2006) reported that DNA damage repair capacity was enhanced in isolated GSCs. Using a spontaneous murine glioma model, Chen et al. identified that when temozolomide treatment is discontinued, the first cell population to undergo proliferation and lead to tumor regrowth is the nestin-positive GSCs (Chen et al. 2012). GSCs were also found to be enriched in recurrent gliomas. GSCs isolated from recurrent tumors form more aggressive invasive tumors in athymic mice than GSCs isolated from primary tumors derived from the same patient (Huang et al. 2008), an important result indicating the repopulation of GSCs in recurrent and metastatic tumors. In brief, the radioresistant phenotype of GBM is linked with the following factors seen in GSCs after FR: repopulation, enhancement of DNA repair (Bao et al. 2006), reprogramming of metabolism (Rampazzo et al. 2013), inhibition of apoptosis (Pareja et al. 2014; Zanotto-Filho et al. 2012; Rahaman et al. 2002), and upregulation of pro-survival factors (e.g., Akt and Mcl-1) (Choi et al. 2014; Bruntz et al. 2014). Interference of these pro-surviving signaling pathways is potential approaches to enhance the RT response, especially when recurrent GBM is treated by RT.

1.5 Profiling Radioresistant Biomarkers

IR-responsive gene expression profiles were thoroughly investigated by Amundson and Fornace and their colleagues (Amundson et al. 1999a, b; Amundson and Fornace 2001). Specific proteomics was first investigated by Dritschilo's group in radioresistant and radiosensitive head and neck squamous carcinoma cell lines profiled using two-dimensional polyacrylamide gel electrophoresis followed by computer-assisted quantitative analysis (Ramsamooj et al. 1992). These results provide evidence supporting the fact that differential protein expression is associated with cellular radioresistance or radiosensitivity. To identify the dynamic gene expression profile, i.e., the gene expression pattern of RT-surviving cancer cells, the author's group reported a unique gene expression profile of breast cancer MCF7 cells that survived a clinical regimen of fractionated RT (MCF7+FIR) (Li et al. 2001; Guo et al. 2003; Xia et al. 2004; Fukuda et al. 2004). This preliminary gene profiling of RT-surviving cancer cells demonstrated a cluster of genes involved in DNA repair and cell cycle regulation (Li et al. 2001). Ogawa et al. (2006) further identified a cluster of pro-survival genes in radioresistant pancreatic cancer cell lines that survived FR. Although many gene profiling studies have compared radioresistant and sensitive cancer cells (Fukuda et al. 2004; Ogawa et al. 2006; Kitahara et al. 2002; Guo et al. 2005; Lee et al. 2010), to elucidate the mechanisms causing tumor cell survival after RT, further investigation on dynamic gene and protein expression patterns in surviving cancer cells and recurrent tumors will be highly informative. Using MRM-based targeted proteomics profiling, global kinome signatures of the radioresistant MCF7/C6, a cloned cell line from MCF7 +FIR population has recently been reported. Of 120 kinases studied, kinases involved in cell cycle progression including CHK1, CDK1, CDK2, and the catalytic subunit of DNA-dependent protein kinase are overexpressed and hyperactivated (Guo et al. 2015). To detect the protein expression pattern of CSCs in surviving cancer cells, BCSCs were sorted from MCF7/C6 cells and additionally sorted by HER2 expression. The proteomics of HER2$^+$/CD44$^+$/CD24$^{-/low}$ versus HER2$^-$/CD44$^+$/CD24$^{-/low}$ BCSCs was conducted with two-dimensional differential gel electrophoresis (2-D DIGE) and high-performance liquid chromatography tandem mass spectrometry (HPLC/MS-MS) (Duru et al. 2012). Proteins involved in tumor metastasis, apoptosis, mitochondrial function, and DNA repair were enhanced and the HER2–STAT3 network was identified in the HER2$^+$ BCSCs (Duru et al. 2012). Recently, Yun et al. (2016) reported that a radioresistant H460 (RR-H460) cell line derived from radiosensitive H460 lung cancer cells after chronic FR expressed stem cell markers, CD44, Nanog, Oct4, and Sox2 and enhanced aggressive growth and radioresistance with a short list of new genes detected. Depletion of these genes radiosensitized RR-H460 cells. Additional information by mass spectrometry-based proteomic techniques for profiling radioresistant biomarkers has been recently summarized (Chang et al. 2015) including the proteomics of CSCs (Skvortsov et al. 2014). These studies will continue to provide new information required to accelerate the identification of effective targets for radiosensitization of CSCs.

2 CSCs in the Irradiated Tumor Microenvironment

2.1 Warburg Effect and Its Revisions

Tumor cells require increased adenosine triphosphate (ATP) to support their enhanced anabolism and proliferation (Robertson-Tessi et al. 2015; LeBleu et al. 2014; De Luca et al. 2015; Favre et al. 2010; Sotgia et al. 2012). Two bioenergetics pathways are utilized in mammalian cells to provide cellular fuel demands dependent on oxygen status. Under oxygenated conditions cells can metabolize one molecule of glucose into approximately 34 molecules of ATP via oxidative phosphorylation (OXPHOS) in the mitochondria, producing the major cellular fuel for energy consumption. In contrast under hypoxic conditions, cells metabolize one molecule of glucose into two molecules of lactate and two molecules of ATP. In 1956, Otto Warburg discovered that cancer cells tend to convert glucose into lactate to produce energy rather than utilizing OXPHOS even under aerobic conditions. Warburg's seminal finding has been observed in many tumors that showed mutations in mtDNA and mitochondrial alterations. However, in contrast to Warburg's original hypothesis, many tumor cells showed intact mitochondria function with inducible MnSOD activation and ATP generation (Guo et al. 2003; Gao et al. 2009; Wallace 2012). In fact, fast growing cells showed enhanced mitochondrial metabolism to meet the challenges of macromolecular synthesis. Recently, CDK1 controlled mitochondrial ATP generation which is linked to normal cell cycle progression (Wang et al. 2014), is also involved in mitochondrial bioenergetics required for cellular fuel demands for DNA damage repair and cell survival after radiation (Alexandrou and Li 2014; Lu et al. 2015; Qin et al. 2015), indicating that the mitochondria in cancer cells, especially in the fast-proliferative tumor cells, can be revivid in generating additional cellular fuels for the increased demands of cellular energy consumption, which is to be further investigated.

2.2   IR Induced Cellular Energy Reprogramming

Growing evidence demonstrate that mitochondria are functional in tumor cells and responsible for metastasis and therapy-resistance (Duru et al. 2012, 2014; Lu et al. 2015; Candas et al. 2014; Obre and Rossignol 2015; Chae et al. 2012; Kang et al. 2014). Although mitochondrial dysfunction is linked with radioresistance of some tumor cells (Lynam-Lennon et al. 2014), mitochondrial bioenergetics is shown to be required to boost cellular fuel production for repairing DNA damage and cell survival, and mitochondrial MKP1 is a target for therapy-resistant HER2-positive breast cancer cells (Lu et al. 2015; Candas et al. 2014). A dynamic feature in mitochondrial bioenergetics which has been observed suggests that CDK1 can boost mitochondrial ATP for cell cycle progression and that cancer cells can quickly adjust cellular energy metabolic pathways to enhance their survival under genotoxic stress conditions such as IR (Fig. 2) (Alexandrou and Li 2014; Lu et al. 2015; Qin et al. 2015; Candas and Li 2014). Heat-shock-protein-90 (HSP90) is involved in proper protein folding in mitochondria that is required for cellular bioenergetics in tumor cells (Chae et al. 2012). mTOR, a critical regulator in cell proliferation, is shown to enhance OXPHOS with reduced glycolysis for tumor cells to survive IR. Thus the apparent "quiet" mitochondria in tumor cells can function as a backup to boost cellular fuel supply required for crisis conditions such as IR. Such a pathway for mitochondrial bioenergetics demonstrates the flexibility of energy metabolism pathways in cancer cells (Lu et al. 2015). Additional findings suggest that mitochondria in tumor cells remain functional and play a key role

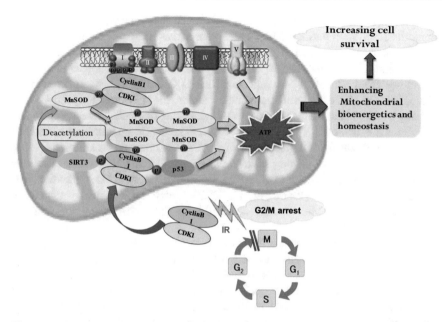

Fig. 2 Proposed mechanism causing mitochondrial bioenergetics for cell survival after radiation

in tumor cell proliferation and metastasis (Zhang et al. 2013; Park et al. 2016). The dynamic programming of energy metabolism in tumor cells especially in CSCs and, iIR-associated cellular energy metabolism as it relates to tumor cell survival undergoing radiotherapy are currently being investigated. These observations are further supported by findings that reprogramming the mitochondrial trafficking can help to fuel tumor cell invasion (LeBleu et al. 2014; Caino et al. 2015), and that mitochondrial respiration is activated in irradiated tumor cells for survival (Lu et al. 2015). Most importantly, mitochondrial energy metabolism has been recently linked with the aggressive pheno-type of triple-negative breast cancer (TNBC) (Park et al. 2016).

2.3 Metabolic Plasticity of NSCS and CSCs

Accumulating data have recently provided a clearer understanding of energy metabolism in normal stem cells (NSCs). When NSCs divide into two daughter cells, older mitochondria are allocated into one cell and younger ones are appor-tioned to another daughter cell so as to maintain stemness in one cell and the other with lineage-specific differentiation (Katajisto et al. 2015; Rossi et al. 2007). The amount of mtDNA and mitochondrial biogenesis are gradually enhanced with the increasing cellular energy demands of the cell during lineage differentiation (Cho et al. 2006; Chung et al. 2010). During this process, the typical spherical and cristae-poor mitochondria of undifferentiated stem cells are transformed into tubular and cristae-rich mitochondria which is required to provide adequate ATP for energy metabolism (Chung et al. 2010). It has been noted that gene production for mito-chondrial respiration and ROS metabolism are activated and genes related to gly-colysis are down-regulated (Chung et al. 2010; Zhang et al. 2013; Urao and Ushio-Fukai 2013; Armstrong et al. 2010; Yanes et al. 2010), indicating a repro-gramming from glycolysis to mitochondrial OXPHOS in NSC differentiation (Panopoulos et al. 2012; Lunt and Vander Heiden 2011; Wanet et al. 2014).

Fatty acid oxidation (FAO) produces one molecule of AcCoA in each cycle and two molecule of AcCoA in the final cycle. The AcCoA-induced oxaloacetate produce the citrate for the generation of NADPH (Carracedo et al. 2013). Thus, FAO participates in maintaining sufficient levels of ATP and NADPH in metabolic stress (Pike et al. 2011; Jeon et al. 2012). Unsaturated fatty acids impair the NSC lineage differentiation (Yanes et al. 2010), and other amino acids and TCA-associated metabolism has been linked with NSC self-renewal and differen-tiation (Lu et al. 2012).

It is far from clear if energy metabolism in CSCs follow the same metabolic adjustments during their self-renewal and/or potential cancer cell differentiation. The question is why cancer cells as well as CSCs can survive the hostile envi-ronment such as low nutrition and pH, and even worse situations such genotoxic IR and/or chemotherapy. CSCs can be induced to differentiate into lingual cell pop-ulation under normal or stress conditions (Vermeulen et al. 2008), and surprisingly, it has been shown that non-cancer stem cells can also be induced back to the stem like feature by radiation with altered cellular bioenergetics (Vlashi and Pajonk 2015). GSCs are found to be less glycolytic and consume less glucose and produce less lactate while maintaining higher ATP levels than their differentiated progeny. However, a higher mitochondrial reserve capacity is detected in GSCs that show radioresistance (Vlashi et al. 2011). Metabolic differences are also identified in BCSCs and differentiated progeny (Vlashi et al. 2014). The metabolic profile which distinguishes the undifferentiated state from the differentiated state of stem cells features a dynamic mitochondrial morphology and a shift from glycolysis to mitochondrial OXPHOS (Westermann 2010; Ferree and Shirihai 2012; Simsek et al. 2010; Suda et al. 2011; Takubo et al. 2013). IR activates mitochondrial OXHPOS (Lu et al. 2015; Candas et al. 2013, 2014), suggesting that mitochondrial bioenergetics can be activated in tumor cells when exposed to genotoxic conditions such as a therapeutic. Thus, mitochondria in tumor cells are functional and can be activated by IR in radioresistant cancer cells and CSCs (Lu et al. 2015; Candas et al. 2014; Candas and Li 2014). A specific population of BCSCs has been identified from surviving breast cancer cells treated by FR (Li et al. 2001; Wang et al. 2005) indicating that BCSCs even from HER2-negative or triple-negative breast cancer (TNBC) cells express not only BCSCs biomarkers (Phillips et al. 2006; Al-Hajj et al. 2004; Reya et al. 2001; Farnie et al. 2007; Cao et al. 2009) but also HER2 (Duru et al. 2012, 2014; Cao et al. 2009). Further analysis revealed that the HER2$^+$ BCSCs are more abundant in the recurrent/metastatic lesions compared to the primary tumors (Duru et al. 2012, 2014) (Fig. 3). All of these results suggest a similar NSC reprogramming of energy metabolism from glycolysis to mitochon-drial respiration when CSCs are undergoing differentiation and/or fast proliferation.

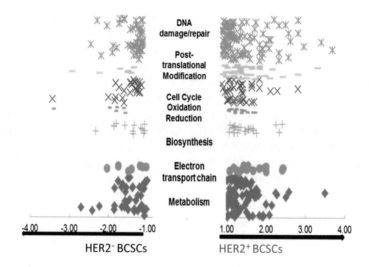

Fig. 3 Proteomics data indiction enhanced proteins in mitochondrial bioenergetics, cell cycle and DNA repair in BCSCs expressing HER2 using HER2negative BCSCs as control

However, the precise dynamics of cellular bioenergetics in CSCs, especially in vivo under anti-cancer therapy conditions, needs to be further investigated.

2.4 Hypoxia as a Biomarker for Radioresistant Cancer Stem Cells

It has long been known that there are hypoxic areas within a solid tumor and that radiation induces re-oxygenation (another R in tumor radiobiology) (Brown and Giaccia 1994). Accumulating data demonstrate a wide range of effects by hypoxia which is associated with chemotherapy and radiation resistance, epithelial–mesenchymal transition (EMT), and tumor metastasis (Erler et al. 2006; Xing et al. 2011; Nantajit et al. 2015). The complexity in tumor metabolism is also linked with the hypoxic and nonhypoxic regions within the tumor as well as the surrounding stroma (Dang 2010). Higher levels of HIF-1α in tumors are associated with a poorer prognosis and up-regulation of markers of EMT due to HIF-1α actions. CSCs are believed to reside in a specific microenvironmental niche in the tumor which is required to maintain the CSC characteristics as well as its potential for self-renewal, metastasis and chemo-radioresistance (Peitzsch et al. 2014). Hypoxia-resistant metabolism has been shown to contribute to the aggressive phenotype in ovarian cancer stem cells (Liao et al. 2014), and GSC (Heddleston et al. 2009). Moreover, hypoxia has been shown to induce non stem cells to acquire GSC characteristics with increased tumorigenesis (Zanotto-Filho et al. 2012). The potential functions of HIF-1α and ROS in cancer and pluripotent stem cells have been summarized (Saito et al. 2015). However, there is limited clinical evidence to date to demonstrate that targeting hypoxic regions during conventional therapy is effective. Gene expression signatures of BCSCs and progenitor cells do not exhibit features of Warburg metabolism (Gordon et al. 2015) and oxygen levels do not determine BCSCs radiation survival (Lagadec et al. 2012). Nevertheless, improved image guided individualized hypoxia targeted therapy directed against appropriate molecular targets may significantly enhance the RT efficacy and eliminate CSCs in the hypoxic areas (Peitzsch et al. 2014; Sheehan et al. 2010). It is felt that if more advanced hypoxia-imaging technologies can be developed to visualize the dynamic events of re-oxygenation and/or de-oxygenation during RT, that this would allow one to monitor hypoxic regions together with CSC-repopulation within the tumor under treatment and thus may enhance the accuracy and ability to target resistant tumor cells in the hypoxic regions.

2.5   Abscopal Effect and IR-Induced Immunoregulation

The abscopal effect, described by Nobler in 1969 (Nobler 1969), refers to the potential inhibition of metastatic lesions at a distance from the tumor site being irradiated. The abscopal effect has recently been further highlighted by a series of studies reported by the Formenti's group demonstrating the benefits of radiotherapy with activation of the immune system by Ipilimumab which inhibits CTLA-4, and also RT combined with granulocyte-macrophage colony-stimulating factor in patients with metastatic solid tumors (Postow et al. 2012; Golden et al. 2013). In the light of the recent growing interest in cancer immunotherapy, there has been increasing interests in the role of the tumor microenvironment on tumor progression and metastasis (Shih et al. 2010; Stefanovic et al. 2014). Although individual immune checkpoint inhibitors have shown clinical benefit, combining these inhibitors with radiation therapy has further enhanced the anti-cancer efficacy. The potential benefits of radiotherapy combined with immunotherapy has been observed (Demaria et al. 2006). In a Phase I clinical trial of 22 patients with metastatic melanoma, radiation combined with inhibition of the programmed cell death protein 1 (PD1) ligand 1 (PDL1)-mediated and CTLA4-mediated immune checkpoints enhanced the tumor responsiveness to immunotherapy. Radiotherapy with double checkpoint blockage of CTLA-4 and PDL-1 enhances T-cell mediated anti-tumor responses outside of the irradiated area (Twyman-Saint Victor et al. 2015). Radiation enhances the diversity of the T-cell receptor (TCR) repertoire of intratumoral T cells (Twyman-Saint Victor et al. 2015). The tumor environment after local irradiation has been suggested to play a key role in tumor immune response after radiation (Golden et al. 2015).

2.6   Tumor Radio-Immunogenicity

The term "tumor radio-immunogenicity" is used here to refer to the observation that specific tumor antigens or epitopes are enhanced or induced after radiotherapy which can then alter the local or systematic tumor immune response. It has been shown that tumors are able to generate an immunosuppressive microenvironment protecting them from host immune surveillance (Schreiber et al. 2011). The selective modulation of Treg in irradiated tumors has been observed which illustrate the immunoregulation occurring in the irradiated tumor microenvironment (Schaue et al. 2008). Radiation induced tumor immune responses are further demonstrated by the fact that irradiated tumors release pro-inflammatory factors such as HSP70 and CXCR6, both of which attract NK cells into the irradiated local tumor environment (Foulds et al. 2013). Derer et al. (2015) recently proposed that increasing the immunogenicity of cancer cells after radiation therapy should be considered as a strategy for systemic cancer immunotherapy and have demonstrated that IR induced tumor phenotypic and tumor microenvironment changes which rendered the cancer cell to be more immunogenic. One of the key immunosuppressive functions of tumor cells has been linked to the expression of CD47, which provides a survival advantage to cancer cells, in particular in CSCs as reported in leukemia, lymphoma, and bladder carcinoma (Chao et al. 2011; Majeti et al. 2009). CD47 is a widely expressed transmembrane protein with multiple functions (Willingham et al. 2012), one of which is to provide a "don't eat me" signal to phagocytic leukocytes. Phagocytosis by macrophages depends on macrophage recognition of pro-phagocytic (eat me) and anti-phagocytic (don't eat me) signals expressed on target cells. CD47 on target cells interacts with the ligand signal regulatory protein α (SIRPα) on macrophages (Willingham et al. 2012; Brown and Frazier 2001) resulting in the phosphorylation of the cytoplasmic tail of SIRPα to initiate a signaling cascade that inhibits phagocytosis (Willingham et al. 2012; Zhao et al. 2011). As expected, anti-CD47 monoclonal antibodies have been shown to enhance macrophage-mediated phagocytosis of cells in an array of cancers including bladder cancer, leukemia, and lymphoma (Willingham et al. 2012; Chan et al. 2009; Majeti et al. 2009). In addition, IR-induced immunogenic cell death (ICD) is believed to make the cells 'visible' to the immune system for phagocytosis and in initiating other antitumor responses (Galluzzi et al. 2012). However, recent data have revealed another side to this. In addition to IR induced abscopal effects, IR also induces CD47 expression to make the tumor cell "invisible" for phagocytosis enabling them to escape immune surveillance and thus may severely compromise the abscopal effect. Data from the author's lab support that NF-κB can co-regulate CD47 and HER2. Co-expression of CD47 and HER2 is a key feature of IR-induced adaptive resistance (Fig. 4). Radiation combined with immunotherapy using anti-CD47 and anti-HER2 showed the most synergy in eliminating clonogenic cancer cells, and local tumor radiation was enhanced by application of anti-CD47 antibody (unpublished data). These results demonstrate the complexity of tumor acquired immunotolerance due to activation of the NF-κB-HER2-CD47 pathway which may be a dominant feature in irradiated CSCs. Thus, a dual inhibition of CD47 and HER2 may enhance the abscopal effect. In addition to the above mentioned HSP70, CXCR6, CD47 and HER2, the specific antigens or epitopes that are enhanced or induced in tumor cells by radiation in CSCs are potential therapeutic targets and thus need to be further explored.

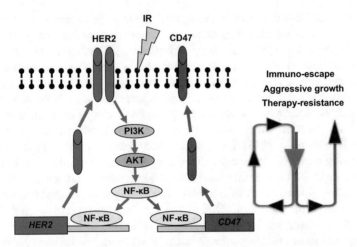

Fig. 4 Proposed co-induction of CD47 and HER2 via NF-κb regulation due to NK-κB binding to both promoters of CD47 and HER2. HER2 is shown to activate NF-κB and radiation accelerates this feed forward loop to further enhance the expression of both. Thus CD47 eqiups the breast cancer cells with HER2-mediated intrinsic pro-survival networks, contributes to the complexity of turn tumor resistance. Radiation combined with immune blocking of CD47 and HER2 may serve as an effective approach to control hard-to treat breast cancer

3 Potential Targets for Radiosensitization of CSCs

3.1 DNA Repair

It has long been proposed that a balance between the degree of DNA damage and activation of pro-survival signaling pathways determines the fate of an irradiated cell. Gene microarray data showed that DNA repair genes are enhanced in the radioresistant fraction of breast cancer cells that survive fractionated radiotherapy (Li et al. 2001). Bao et al. (2006) demonstrate the enhanced DNA repair capacity in GSCs. They also found that the mechanism of radioresistance involves the cell-cycle regulating proteins Chk1/Chk2. Yin et al. showed that ataxia telangectasia mutated (ATM) signaling contributes to radioresistance in CSCs (Frosina 2009). D'Andrea et al. (2011) demonstrated that radioresistance in mesenchymal CSCs is likely due to N-methyltransferase (NNMT) overexpression that is associated with DNA repair mechanisms. Therefore developing small molecules that can specifically bind to CSCs and inhibit the enhanced DNA repair capacity in CSCs will enhance the potential of eliminating CSCs by radiotherapy.

3.2 ROS

Altered ROS metabolism and hypoxia are major features of CSCs. Similarly to NSCs, some CSCs in tumors show lowered ROS levels with enhanced ROS defenses compared to their non-tumorigenic cells (Diehn et al. 2009). Recent studies demonstrate that nuclear factor-erythroid 2-related factor 2 (NRF2), a key regulator of cellular antioxidants and ROS level, is actively involved in maintaining the stemness feature of CSCs (Ryoo et al. 2016). NRF2 regulated ROS level is linked with the growth and resistance of CSCs (Ryoo et al. 2016; Ding et al. 2015). CD44 mediated redox regulation is also suggested in CD44 variant isoforms (Nagano et al. 2013). Blazek et al. showed that Daoy medulloblastoma cells that express CSC features with a low level of ROS can be enhanced under hypoxic condition (Blazek et al. 2007). In agreement with this, Kim et al. (2012) indicated that tumor cells expressing increased CD13 have reduced ROS levels which enhanced the growth of liver CSCs via an EMT-like phenomenon. These results show that ROS levels and redox imbalance are tightly associated with the proliferation status of CSCs which may be altered by IR. Thus the dynamic features of ROS in treated tumor environments need to be further elucidated which may identify approaches to radiosensitization of CSCs.

3.3 MicroRNA

MicroRNA (miRNA; miR) is a small non-coding RNA molecule (containing about 22 nucleotides) involved in gene expression regulation via RNA silencing and post-transcriptional regulation. As epigenetic gene regulators, miRNAs are associated with tumor initiation and progression. An increasing number of reports suggests that miRNAs are promising therapeutic targets of CSCs via epigenetic modification. The function of miRNA in regulation of CSCs is felt to involve a wide array of biological processes involved in CSCs and tumorigenesis (DeSano and Xu 2009; Leal and Lleonart 2013). However, the exact mechanisms underlying miR-regulated CSC biology and therapy-resistance remain to be elucidated. The function of miRNA in NSCs is also linked to CSCs. In addition, miR-504 down-regulates nuclear respiratory factor 1 leading to radioresistance of nasopharyngeal carcinoma (Zhao et al. 2015). It has been shown that the miRNA-153/Nrf-2/GPx1 pathway is involved in the radioresistance and stemness of GSCs (Yang et al. 2015); and knockdown of miR-210 suppresses the hypoxic GSCs and radioresistance (Yang et al. 2014). A nanoparticle conjugated with miR-200c radiosensitized three gastric cancer cell lines and suppressed CD44 and CSCs (Cui et al. 2014).

3.4 IFN-β

Happold et al. reported that GBM cell lines and GSCs (glioma-initiating cells, GICs) express receptors for the immune modulatory cytokine IFN-β. IFN-β treatment remarkably reduced the tumor sphere formation by GSCs (Happold et al. 2014). IFN-β also sensitized GSCs to temozolomide and irradiation. Gene expression profiling showed that IFN-β-associated proapoptotic gene cluster, but not stemness-associated genes were upregulated. Additional analyses revealed the death sensitization mediated by IFN-β is unrelated to chemotherapy or irradiation, indicating that IFN-β is a potential specific GSC target that may be considered in RT of GBM.

3.5   NF-κB and HER2 Crosstalk Pathway

NF-κB activation plays a crucial role in tumor aggressiveness and resistance to anti-cancer therapy (Orlowski and Baldwin 2002; Karin et al. 2002; Bivona et al. 2011; Li et al. 1997). Overexpression of HER2 not only increases cell proliferation and survival (Kurokawa and Arteaga 2001), but also causes NF-κB activation via PI3 K/Akt pathway, which can be inhibited by the tumor suppressor phosphatase PTEN (Pianetti et al. 2001). Radiation induced NF-κB activation can be mediated via nuclear DNA damage through activation of the DNA damage sensor protein ATM (Ataxia Telangiectasia Mutated) (Curry et al. 1999; Locke et al. 2002), and blocking NF-κB inhibits the cell malignant phenotype and radiosensitizes tumor cells (Li and Karin 1998; Brach et al. 1991; Luo et al. 2005; Fan et al. 2007; Ahmed et al. 2006; Braunstein et al. 2008). Rinkenbaugh and Baldwin (2016) recently summarized the NF-κB signaling network in CSCs. Breast cancer cells expressing HER2 were shown to enhance IR-induced NF-κB activation (Guo et al. 2004) and NF-κB in return enhances HER2 gene transcription by activation of ErbB2 promoter (Cao et al. 2009), indicating a positive feedback loop between NF-κB and HER2 (Ahmed et al. 2006; Ahmed and Li 2008). Importantly, HER2-expressing BCSCs (HER2$^+$ BCSCs) are identified in even HER2-negative breast cancer cells that can survive FR (Duru et al. 2012). Recently, persistent activation of NF-κB in BRCA1-deficient mammary progenitors is linked with aggressive phenotype (Sau et al. 2016). In HER2-driven breast cancer mouse models NF-κB pathways contribute to stemness and tumor formation. The canonical NF-κB pathway is required for formation of luminal mammary neoplasia and is activated in the mammary progenitor population (Pratt et al. 2009). Inhibition of NF-κB in a HER2 breast cancer mouse model indicate alterations of gene expression profiles associated with stem cells with NF-κB-dependent changes in the specific stem cell factors Nanog and Sox2 (Liu et al. 2010). Knock-in of a kinase dead IKK led to decreased self-renewal and senescence under mammary stem cell culture conditions (Cao et al. 2007). Thus, it is highly possible that NF-κB and HER2 are mutually activated in CSCs under RT.

3.6   HER2

The HER2 proto-oncogene is located in the long arm of human chromosome 17 and encodes a 185 kD transmembrane glycoprotein in various tissues of epithelial, mesenchymal, and neuronal origin (Soomro et al. 1991; Olayioye 2001). HER2 overexpression is associated with aggressive tumor growth, resistance to treatment, metastasis and a high risk of local relapse and recurrence resulting in poor prognosis (Slamon et al. 1987; Haffty et al. 1996; Holbro et al. 2003). HER2 is valuable both as a prognostic marker and as a predictive factor for therapy response (Haffty et al. 1996; Hicks et al. 2005). The stemness and progenitor cells are increased in normal mammary epithelial cells when HER2 expression is enhanced. The tumorgenicity is also increased with expression of HER2 and ALDH1 (Diehn et al. 2009). These data are significant given that ALDH1 has been suggested as a CSC marker, including in breast cancer (Diehn et al. 2009; Ginestier et al. 2007). Therefore targeting HER2 in breast cancer RT is a promising approach to eliminate HER2-expressing BCSCs, especially for late phase metastatic lesions which are usually multiple tumors and resistant to chemo and radiotherapy.

3.7 MUC13

MUC13 is a transmembrane mucin glycoprotein, is enhanced in many cancers and can activate NF-κB activation. Elevated MUC13 and NF-κB is correlated with colorectal cancer progression and metastases (Sheng et al. 2016). Silencing MUC13 abolished chemotherapy-induced enrichment of CD133+ CD44+ cancer stem cells, slowed xenograft growth in mice, and synergized with 5-fluourouracil to induce tumor regression. Therefore, these data indicate that combining chemotherapy and MUC13 antagonism could improve the treatment of metastatic cancers.

3.8 Wnt/β-Catenin

The Wnt/beta-catenin signaling pathway is associated with the self-renewal of CSC (Reya et al. 2001; Holland et al. 2013). Over-expression of activated β-catenin expands the pool of stem cells (Reya et al. 2003) since it is believed that activation of Wnt leads to the accumulation of β-catenin in cytoplasm and then nuclear translocation to regulate the cluster of genes associated with CSC self-renewal. In a study of myelogenous leukemia, β-catenin was found to accumulate in the nuclei of granulocyte–macrophage progenitors enhancing self-renewal (Jamieson et al. 2004). Thus, dysregulation of Wnt/beta-catenin signaling pathway may be one of approaches worthy of further testing in combination with RT since the self-renewal CSC capacity is enhanced in radioresistant tumors.

3.9 CXCR4

The chemokine C-X-C motif receptor 4 (CXCR4) is found to be a prognostic marker in various types of cancers and is linked with tumor stemness. Interaction of CXCR4 with its ligand, the chemokine C-X-C motif ligand 12 (CXCL12) is believed to function in regulating CSCs and tumor microenvironment. Blocking the CXCR4/CXCL12 axis in CSCs has been evaluated for radiosensitization of CSCs and tumor microenvironment in response to irradiation (Trautmann et al. 2014).

3.10   14-3-3ζ

14-3-3ζ is related to many cancer survival cellular processes. Lee et al. showed that inhibition of 14-3-3ζ reduces the radioresistance of CSCs in HCC (Lee et al. 2014) with reduced capacity of tumor sphere formation and enhanced apoptosis in liver CSCs, indicating that 14-3-3ζ is a candidate CSC target to radiosensitive liver cancer.

3.11   Integrin α6

Integrin α6 which is linked with tumor aggressiveness is found to co-express with GSC markers and enriched in the GSC population (Lathia et al. 2010). Blocking Integrin α6 in GSCs inhibits self-renewal, proliferation, and tumorigenesis of GSCs. These results provide evidence that Integrin α6 can serve not only as an enrichment marker of GSCs but also as a promising radiosensitizer for GSCs.

3.12   YY1

YY1 is a zinc finger transcription factor involved in the regulation of cell growth, development, and differentiation (Seto et al. 1991; Ye et al. 1996). It has also been studied as a potential therapeutic target for anti-cancer therapy (de Nigris et al. 2010; He et al. 2011). YY1 expression is linked with the stemness genes including SOX2, OCT4, BMI1, and NANOG. Proteomics data indicate that co-expression of YY1 and SOX2 as well as SOX2 and OCT4 is regulated by NF-κB pathways (Kaufhold et al. 2016). Therefore, it is possible that dual inhibition of YY1 and NF-κB could be an effective approach to sensitize CSCs to RT.

3.13   Notch

The Notch signaling pathway regulates a wide range of cellular functions in organ development and tissue renewal, and is also highlighted in cancer development due to abnormal Notch functions (Farnie and Clarke 2007). Notch is shown to be able to promote self-renewal and proliferation of mammary stem cells (Dontu et al. 2004) and breast carcinogenesis (Hambardzumyan et al. 2008). Expression of Notch has been associated with radioresistance of GSCs and a potential target for cancer stem cells (Wang et al. 2010; Shen et al. 2015).

3.14   ALDH1A3

Kurth et al. (2013) described that ALDH activity is involved in the radioresistance of CSCs in HNSCC and its isoform ALDH1A3 expression in head and neck squamous cell carcinoma (HNSCC) is suggested to be responsible for tumor relapse after RT. The CSCs in the radioresistant HNSCC cells (SQ20B/SP/CD44$^+$/ ALDH-high) were found to extend G2/M arrest phase after RT. UCN-01, a checkpoint kinase (Chk1) inhibitor, induced the relapse of G2/M arrest and radiosensitization of SQ20B-CSCs. All-trans retinoic acid (ATRA) also resulted in ALDH activity and radiosensitized SQ20B/SP/CD44+/ALDH-high CSCs (Kurth et al. 2013). These results indicate that targeting ALDH together with the inhibition of other cell proliferation factors can radiosensitize CSCs.

4 Conclusion and Perspective

In spite of remarkable advances in the precision of radiation dose delivery, the long-term cancer control by RT remains a challenge. One of the key questions to be addressed in tumor radiobiology is to further elucidate the dynamics of tumor microenvironment causing tumor repopulation and resistance. Although much insight has been gained about cancer stem cells and their resident microenvironment, the complexity of the irradiated tumor microenvironment are just beginning to be understood. The exact molecular mechanisms causing the radioresistant phenotype of CSCs, especially the details of dynamics of cross-talking between CSCs and their stroma cells in the microenvironment, remains to be elucidated. In addition to the well-defined Rs in radiation biology and cancer radiotherapy, such as Repair, Re-oxygenation, Repopulation, accumulating new "Rs" are being defined such as Redox balancing, Reprogramming cellular metabolism, Regulation of immuno-response, etc. With more exciting insights revealed into the biology and radiation response of CSCs, continued efforts are expected to dissect and use the key targets of cancer stem cells and its environment to optimize response to radiotherapy. Further characterization of CSCs interaction with the different components in an irradiated tumor microenvironments will shed new light on the mechanisms underlying tumor adaptive resistance and invent more effective radiosensitizing targets. The most promising topics would be the reprogramming of cellular energy metabolism in cancer stem cells and their resident environment of the "tumor society" which consists of multiple factors involved in radiation response and the fate of irradiated tumor cells. In an era of personalized cancer care, identification of specific tumor biomarkers before, during and after a course of radiotherapy with and without chemotherapy, immunotherapy and other anti-cancer approaches would be important. At this point there are few treatment options that specifically and effectively target CSCs.

Acknowledgements I regret not being able to cite all the important work done in this area due to space restrictions. I'd like to take this opportunity to thank the invaluable input and discussions from all of my colleagues, collaborators and friends who contributed many novel concepts to my research. I thank the graduate students, postdoctoral fellows, and lab personnel who have been involved in the research projects and performed the major of research work in my lab. The author also acknowledges grant support from the National Institutes of Health RO1 CA133402 and CA152313.

References

Ahmed KM, Li JJ (2008) NF-kappa B-mediated adaptive resistance to ionizing radiation. Free Radic Biol Med 44:1–13

Ahmed KM, Dong S, Fan M, Li JJ (2006a) Nuclear factor-kappaB p65 inhibits mitogen-activated protein kinase signaling pathway in radioresistant breast cancer cells. Mol Cancer Res 4:945–955

Ahmed KM, Cao N, Li JJ (2006b) HER-2 and NF-kappaB as the targets for therapy-resistant breast cancer. Anticancer Res 26:4235–4243

Alexandrou AT, Li JJ (2014) Cell cycle regulators guide mitochondrial activity in radiation-induced adaptive response. Antioxid Redox Signal 20:1463–1480

Al-Hajj M, Wicha MS, Benito-Hernandez A, Morrison SJ, Clarke MF (2003a) Prospective identification of tumorigenic breast cancer cells. Proc Natl Acad Sci U S A 100:3983–3988

Al-Hajj M, Wicha MS, Benito-Hernandez A, Morrison SJ, Clarke MF (2003b) Prospective identification of tumorigenic breast cancer cells. Proc Natl Acad Sci U S A 100:3983–3988

Al-Hajj M, Becker MW, Wicha M, Weissman I, Clarke MF (2004) Therapeutic implications of cancer stem cells. Curr Opin Genet Dev 14:43–47

Amundson SA, Fornace AJ Jr (2001) Gene expression profiles for monitoring radiation exposure. Radiat Prot Dosim 97:11–16

Amundson SA, Bittner M, Chen Y, Trent J, Meltzer P, Fornace AJ Jr (1999a) Fluorescent cDNA microarray hybridization reveals complexity and heterogeneity of cellular genotoxic stress responses. Oncogene 18:3666–3672

Amundson SA, Do KT, Fornace AJ Jr (1999b) Induction of stress genes by low doses of gamma rays. Radiat Res 152:225–231

Armstrong L, Tilgner K, Saretzki G, Atkinson SP, Stojkovic M, Moreno R, Przyborski S, Lako M (2010) Human induced pluripotent stem cell lines show stress defense mechanisms and mitochondrial regulation similar to those of human embryonic stem cells. Stem Cells 28:661–673

Ashkenazi R, Jackson TL, Dontu G, Wicha MS (2007) Breast cancer stem cells-research opportunities utilizing mathematical modeling. Stem Cell Rev 3:176–182

Balasubramaniam A, Shannon P, Hodaie M, Laperriere N, Michaels H, Guha A (2007) Glioblastoma multiforme after stereotactic radiotherapy for acoustic neuroma: case report and review of the literature. Neuro Oncol 9:447–453

Bao S, Wu Q, McLendon RE, Hao Y, Shi Q, Hjelmeland AB, Dewhirst MW, Bigner DD, Rich JN (2006) Glioma stem cells promote radioresistance by preferential activation of the DNA damage response. Nature 444:756–760

Baumann M, Krause M, Hill R (2008) Exploring the role of cancer stem cells in radioresistance. Nat Rev Cancer 8:545–554

Bivona TG, Hieronymus H, Parker J, Chang K, Taron M, Rosell R, Moonsamy P, Dahlman K, Miller VA, Costa C, Hannon G, Sawyers CL (2011) FAS and NF-kappaB signalling modulate dependence of lung cancers on mutant EGFR. Nature 471:523–526

Blazek ER, Foutch JL, Maki G (2007) Daoy medulloblastoma cells that express CD133 are radioresistant relative to CD133− cells, and the CD133+ sector is enlarged by hypoxia. Int J Radiat Oncol Biol Phys 67:1–5

Bonnet D, Dick JE (1997) Human acute myeloid leukemia is organized as a hierarchy that originates from a primitive hematopoietic cell. Nat Med 3:730–737

Brach MA, Hass R, Sherman ML, Gunji H, Weichselbaum R, Kufe D (1991) Ionizing radiation induces expression and binding activity of the nuclear factor kappa B. J Clin Invest 88:691–695

Brandes AA, Tosoni A, Franceschi E, Sotti G, Frezza G, Amista P, Morandi L, Spagnolli F, Ermani M (2009) Recurrence pattern after temozolomide concomitant with and adjuvant to radiotherapy in newly diagnosed patients with glioblastoma: correlation with MGMT promoter methylation status. J Clin Oncol 27:1275–1279

Braunstein S, Formenti SC, Schneider RJ (2008) Acquisition of stable inducible up-regulation of nuclear factor-kappaB by tumor necrosis factor exposure confers increased radiation resistance without increased transformation in breast cancer cells. Mol Cancer Res 6:78–88

Brown EJ, Frazier WA (2001) Integrin-associated protein (CD47) and its ligands. Trends Cell Biol 11:130–135

Brown JM, Giaccia AJ (1994) Tumour hypoxia: the picture has changed in the 1990s. Int J Radiat Biol 65:95–102

Bruntz RC, Taylor HE, Lindsley CW, Brown HA (2014) Phospholipase D2 mediates survival signaling through direct regulation of Akt in glioblastoma cells. J Biol Chem 289:600–616

Caino MC, Ghosh JC, Chae YC, Vaira V, Rivadeneira DB, Faversani A, Rampini P, Kossenkov AV, Aird KM, Zhang R, Webster MR, Weeraratna AT, Bosari S, Languino LR, Altieri DC (2015) PI3 K therapy reprograms mitochondrial trafficking to fuel tumor cell invasion. Proc Natl Acad Sci U S A 112:8638–8643

Candas D, Li JJ (2014) MnSOD in oxidative stress response-potential regulation via mitochondrial protein influx. Antioxid Redox Signal 20:1599–1617

Candas D, Fan M, Nantajit D, Vaughan AT, Murley JS, Woloschak GE, Grdina DJ, Li JJ (2013) CyclinB1/Cdk1 phosphorylates mitochondrial antioxidant MnSOD in cell adaptive response to radiation stress. J Mol Cell Biol 5:166–175

Candas D, Lu CL, Fan M, Chuang FY, Sweeney C, Borowsky AD, Li JJ (2014) Mitochondrial MKP1 is a target for therapy-resistant HER2-positive breast cancer cells. Cancer Res 74:7498–7509

Cao Y, Luo JL, Karin M (2007) IkappaB kinase alpha kinase activity is required for self-renewal of ErbB2/Her2-transformed mammary tumor-initiating cells. Proc Natl Acad Sci U S A 104:15852–15857

Cao N, Li S, Wang Z, Ahmed KM, Degnan ME, Fan M, Dynlacht JR, Li JJ (2009) NF-kappaB-mediated HER2 overexpression in radiation-adaptive resistance. Radiat Res 171:9–21

Carracedo A, Cantley LC, Pandolfi PP (2013) Cancer metabolism: fatty acid oxidation in the limelight. Nat Rev Cancer 13:227–232

Chae YC, Caino MC, Lisanti S, Ghosh JC, Dohi T, Danial NN, Villanueva J, Ferrero S, Vaira V, Santambrogio L, Bosari S, Languino LR, Herlyn M, Altieri DC (2012) Control of tumor bioenergetics and survival stress signaling by mitochondrial HSP90s. Cancer Cell 22:331–344

Chan KS, Espinosa I, Chao M, Wong D, Ailles L, Diehn M, Gill H, Presti J Jr, Chang HY, van de Rijn M, Shortliffe L, Weissman IL (2009) Identification, molecular characterization, clinical prognosis, and therapeutic targeting of human bladder tumor-initiating cells. Proc Natl Acad Sci U S A 106:14016–14021

Chang L, Graham P, Hao J, Bucci J, Malouf D, Gillatt D, Li Y (2015) Proteomics discovery of radioresistant cancer biomarkers for radiotherapy. Cancer Lett 369:289–297

Chao MP, Tang C, Pachynski RK, Chin R, Majeti R, Weissman IL (2011) Extranodal dissemination of non-Hodgkin lymphoma requires CD47 and is inhibited by anti-CD47 antibody therapy. Blood 118:4890–4901

Chen J, Li Y, Yu TS, McKay RM, Burns DK, Kernie SG, Parada LF (2012) A restricted cell population propagates glioblastoma growth after chemotherapy. Nature 488:522–526

Chen D, Bhat-Nakshatri P, Goswami C, Badve S, Nakshatri H (2013) ANTXR1, a stem cell-enriched functional biomarker, connects collagen signaling to cancer stem-like cells and metastasis in breast cancer. Cancer Res 73:5821–5833

Cho YM, Kwon S, Pak YK, Seol HW, Choi YM, Park do J, Park KS, Lee HK (2006) Dynamic changes in mitochondrial biogenesis and antioxidant enzymes during the spontaneous differentiation of human embryonic stem cells. Biochem Biophys Res Commun 348:1472–1478

Choi EJ, Cho BJ, Lee DJ, Hwang YH, Chun SH, Kim HH, Kim IA (2014) Enhanced cytotoxic effect of radiation and temozolomide in malignant glioma cells: targeting PI3 K-AKT-mTOR signaling, HSP90 and histone deacetylases. BMC Cancer 14:17

Chung S, Arrell DK, Faustino RS, Terzic A, Dzeja PP (2010) Glycolytic network restructuring integral to the energetics of embryonic stem cell cardiac differentiation. J Mol Cell Cardiol 48:725–734

Clarke MF (2005) A self-renewal assay for cancer stem cells. Cancer Chemother Pharmacol 56 (Suppl 1):64–68

Clarke MF, Dick JE, Dirks PB, Eaves CJ, Jamieson CH, Jones DL, Visvader J, Weissman IL, Wahl GM (2006) Cancer stem cells–perspectives on current status and future directions: AACR workshop on cancer stem cells. Cancer Res 66:9339–9344

Cui FB, Liu Q, Li RT, Shen J, Wu PY, Yu LX, Hu WJ, Wu FL, Jiang CP, Yue GF, Qian XP, Jiang XQ, Liu BR (2014) Enhancement of radiotherapy efficacy by miR-200c-loaded gelatinase-stimuli PEG-Pep-PCL nanoparticles in gastric cancer cells. Int J Nanomedicine 9:2345–2358

Curry HA, Clemens RA, Shah S, Bradbury CM, Botero A, Goswami P, Gius D (1999) Heat shock inhibits radiation-induced activation of NF-kappaB via inhibition of I-kappaB kinase. J Biol Chem 274:23061–23067

D'Andrea FP, Safwat A, Kassem M, Gautier L, Overgaard J, Horsman MR (2011) Cancer stem cell overexpression of nicotinamide N-methyltransferase enhances cellular radiation resistance. Radiother Oncol 99:373–378

Dalerba P, Cho RW, Clarke MF (2007a) Cancer stem cells: models and concepts. Annu Rev Med 58:267–284

Dalerba P, Dylla SJ, Park IK, Liu R, Wang X, Cho RW, Hoey T, Gurney A, Huang EH, Simeone DM, Shelton AA, Parmiani G, Castelli C, Clarke MF (2007b) Phenotypic characterization of human colorectal cancer stem cells. Proc Natl Acad Sci U S A 104:10158–10163

Dang CV (2010) Rethinking the Warburg effect with Myc micromanaging glutamine metabolism. Cancer Res 70:859–862

De Luca A, Fiorillo M, Peiris-Pages M, Ozsvari B, Smith DL, Sanchez-Alvarez R, Martinez-Outschoorn UE, Cappello AR, Pezzi V, Lisanti MP, Sotgia F (2015) Mitochondrial biogenesis is required for the anchorage-independent survival and propagation of stem-like cancer cells. Oncotarget 6:14777–14795

de Nigris F, Crudele V, Giovane A, Casamassimi A, Giordano A, Garban HJ, Cacciatore F, Pentimalli F, Marquez-Garban DC, Petrillo A, Cito L, Sommese L, Fiore A, Petrillo M, Siani A, Barbieri A, Arra C, Rengo F, Hayashi T, Al-Omran M et al (2010) CXCR4/YY1 inhibition impairs VEGF network and angiogenesis during malignancy. Proc Natl Acad Sci U S A 107:14484–14489

Demaria S, Bhardwaj N, McBride WH, Formenti SC (2006) Combining radiotherapy and immunotherapy: a revived partnership. Int J Radiat Oncol Biol Phys 63:655–666

Derer A, Deloch L, Rubner Y, Fietkau R, Frey B, Gaipl US (2015) Radio-immunotherapy-induced immunogenic cancer cells as basis for induction of systemic anti-tumor immune responses—pre-clinical evidence and ongoing clinical applications. Front Immunol 6:505

DeSano JT, Xu L (2009) MicroRNA regulation of cancer stem cells and therapeutic implications. Aaps J 11:682–692

Dhermain F (2014) Radiotherapy of high-grade gliomas: current standards and new concepts, innovations in imaging and radiotherapy, and new therapeutic approaches. Chin J Cancer 33:16–24

Diehn M, Cho RW, Lobo NA, Kalisky T, Dorie MJ, Kulp AN, Qian D, Lam JS, Ailles LE, Wong M, Joshua B, Kaplan MJ, Wapnir I, Dirbas FM, Somlo G, Garberoglio C, Paz B, Shen J, Lau SK, Quake SR et al (2009a) Association of reactive oxygen species levels and radioresistance in cancer stem cells. Nature 458:780–783

Diehn M, Cho RW, Clarke MF (2009b) Therapeutic implications of the cancer stem cell hypothesis. Semin Radiat Oncol 19:78–86

Ding S, Li C, Cheng N, Cui X, Xu X, Zhou G (2015) Redox regulation in cancer stem cells. Oxid Med Cell Longev 2015:750798

Dontu G, Jackson KW, McNicholas E, Kawamura MJ, Abdallah WM, Wicha MS (2004) Role of Notch signaling in cell-fate determination of human mammary stem/progenitor cells. Breast Cancer Res 6:R605–R615

Duru N, Fan M, Candas D, Menaa C, Liu HC, Nantajit D, Wen Y, Xiao K, Eldridge A, Chromy BA, Li S, Spitz DR, Lam KS, Wicha MS, Li JJ (2012) HER2-associated radioresistance of breast cancer stem cells isolated from HER2-negative breast cancer cells. Clin Cancer Res 18:6634–6647

Duru N, Candas D, Jiang G, Li JJ (2014) Breast cancer adaptive resistance: HER2 and cancer stem cell repopulation in a heterogeneous tumor society. J Cancer Res Clin Oncol 140:1–14

Dylla SJ, Beviglia L, Park IK, Chartier C, Raval J, Ngan L, Pickell K, Aguilar J, Lazetic S, Smith-Berdan S, Clarke MF, Hoey T, Lewicki J, Gurney AL (2008) Colorectal cancer stem cells are enriched in xenogeneic tumors following chemotherapy. PLoS ONE 3:e2428

Endlich B, Radford IR, Forrester HB, Dewey WC (2000) Computerized video time-lapse microscopy studies of ionizing radiation-induced rapid-interphase and mitosis-related apoptosis in lymphoid cells. Radiat Res 153:36–48

Erler JT, Bennewith KL, Nicolau M, Dornhofer N, Kong C, Le QT, Chi JT, Jeffrey SS, Giaccia AJ (2006) Lysyl oxidase is essential for hypoxia-induced metastasis. Nature 440:1222–1226

Fan M, Ahmed KM, Coleman MC, Spitz DR, Li JJ (2007) Nuclear factor-kappaB and manganese superoxide dismutase mediate adaptive radioresistance in low-dose irradiated mouse skin epithelial cells. Cancer Res 67:3220–3228

Farnie G, Clarke RB (2007) Mammary stem cells and breast cancer–role of Notch signalling. Stem Cell Rev 3:169–175

Farnie G, Clarke RB, Spence K, Pinnock N, Brennan K, Anderson NG, Bundred NJ (2007) Novel cell culture technique for primary ductal carcinoma in situ: role of Notch and epidermal growth factor receptor signaling pathways. J Natl Cancer Inst 99:616–627

Favre C, Zhdanov A, Leahy M, Papkovsky D, O'Connor R (2010) Mitochondrial pyrimidine nucleotide carrier (PNC1) regulates mitochondrial biogenesis and the invasive phenotype of cancer cells. Oncogene 29:3964–3976

Ferree A, Shirihai O (2012) Mitochondrial dynamics: the intersection of form and function. Adv Exp Med Biol 748:13–40

Findlay VJ, Wang C, Watson DK, Camp ER (2014) Epithelial-to-mesenchymal transition and the cancer stem cell phenotype: insights from cancer biology with therapeutic implications for colorectal cancer. Cancer Gene Ther 21:181–187

Firat E, Gaedicke S, Tsurumi C, Esser N, Weyerbrock A, Niedermann G (2011) Delayed cell death associated with mitotic catastrophe in gamma-irradiated stem-like glioma cells. Radiat Oncol 6:71

Foulds GA, Radons J, Kreuzer M, Multhoff G, Pockley AG (2013) Influence of tumors on protective anti-tumor immunity and the effects of irradiation. Front Oncol 3:14

Frosina G (2009) DNA repair in normal and cancer stem cells, with special reference to the central nervous system. Curr Med Chem 16:854–866

Fukuda K, Sakakura C, Miyagawa K, Kuriu Y, Kin S, Nakase Y, Hagiwara A, Mitsufuji S, Okazaki Y, Hayashizaki Y, Yamagishi H (2004) Differential gene expression profiles of radioresistant oesophageal cancer cell lines established by continuous fractionated irradiation. Br J Cancer 91:1543–1550

Galli R, Binda E, Orfanelli U, Cipelletti B, Gritti A, De Vitis S, Fiocco R, Foroni C, Dimeco F, Vescovi A (2004) Isolation and characterization of tumorigenic, stem-like neural precursors from human glioblastoma. Cancer Res 64:7011–7021

Galluzzi L, Senovilla L, Zitvogel L, Kroemer G (2012) The secret ally: immunostimulation by anticancer drugs. Nat Rev Drug Discov 11:215–233

Gao P, Tchernyshyov I, Chang TC, Lee YS, Kita K, Ochi T, Zeller KI, De Marzo AM, Van Eyk JE, Mendell JT, Dang CV (2009) c-Myc suppression of miR-23a/b enhances mitochondrial glutaminase expression and glutamine metabolism. Nature 458:762–765

Ginestier C, Hur MH, Charafe-Jauffret E, Monville F, Dutcher J, Brown M, Jacquemier J, Viens P, Kleer CG, Liu S, Schott A, Hayes D, Birnbaum D, Wicha MS, Dontu G (2007) ALDH1 is a marker of normal and malignant human mammary stem cells and a predictor of poor clinical outcome. Cell Stem Cell 1:555–567

Golden EB, Demaria S, Schiff PB, Chachoua A, Formenti SC (2013) An abscopal response to radiation and ipilimumab in a patient with metastatic non-small cell lung cancer. Cancer Immunol Res 1:365–372

Golden EB, Chhabra A, Chachoua A, Adams S, Donach M, Fenton-Kerimian M, Friedman K, Ponzo F, Babb JS, Goldberg J, Demaria S, Formenti SC (2015) Local radiotherapy and granulocyte-macrophage colony-stimulating factor to generate abscopal responses in patients with metastatic solid tumours: a proof-of-principle trial. Lancet Oncol 16:795–803

Gordon N, Skinner AM, Pommier RF, Schillace RV, O'Neill S, Peckham JL, Muller P, Condron ME, Donovan C, Naik A, Hansen J, Pommier SJ (2015) Gene expression signatures of breast cancer stem and progenitor cells do not exhibit features of Warburg metabolism. Stem Cell Res Ther 6:157

Guo G, Yan-Sanders Y, Lyn-Cook BD, Wang T, Tamae D, Ogi J, Khaletskiy A, Li Z, Weydert C, Longmate JA, Huang TT, Spitz DR, Oberley LW, Li JJ (2003) Manganese superoxide dismutase-mediated gene expression in radiation-induced adaptive responses. Mol Cell Biol 23:2362–2378

Guo G, Wang T, Gao Q, Tamae D, Wong P, Chen T, Chen WC, Shively JE, Wong JY, Li JJ (2004) Expression of ErbB2 enhances radiation-induced NF-kappaB activation. Oncogene 23:535–545

Guo WF, Lin RX, Huang J, Zhou Z, Yang J, Guo GZ, Wang SQ (2005) Identification of differentially expressed genes contributing to radioresistance in lung cancer cells using microarray analysis. Radiat Res 164:27–35

Guo L, Xiao Y, Fan M, Li JJ, Wang Y (2015) Profiling global kinome signatures of the radioresistant MCF-7/C6 breast cancer cells using MRM-based targeted proteomics. J Proteome Res 14:193–201

Haffty BG, Brown F, Carter D, Flynn S (1996) Evaluation of HER-2 neu oncoprotein expression as a prognostic indicator of local recurrence in conservatively treated breast cancer: a case-control study. Int J Radiat Oncol Biol Phys 35:751–757

Hambardzumyan D, Becher OJ, Holland EC (2008) Cancer stem cells and survival pathways. Cell Cycle 7:1371–1378

Happold C, Roth P, Silginer M, Florea AM, Lamszus K, Frei K, Deenen R, Reifenberger G, Weller M (2014) Interferon-beta induces loss of spherogenicity and overcomes therapy resistance of glioblastoma stem cells. Mol Cancer Ther 13:948–961

He G, Wang Q, Zhou Y, Wu X, Wang L, Duru N, Kong X, Zhang P, Wan B, Sui L, Guo Q, Li JJ, Yu L (2011) YY1 is a novel potential therapeutic target for the treatment of HPV infection-induced cervical cancer by arsenic trioxide. Int J Gynecol Cancer 21:1097–1104

Heddleston JM, Li Z, McLendon RE, Hjelmeland AB, Rich JN (2009) The hypoxic microenvironment maintains glioblastoma stem cells and promotes reprogramming towards a cancer stem cell phenotype. Cell Cycle 8:3274–3284

Heppner GH, Miller BE (1989) Therapeutic implications of tumor heterogeneity. Semin Oncol 16:91–105

Hicks DG, Yoder BJ, Pettay J, Swain E, Tarr S, Hartke M, Skacel M, Crowe JP, Budd GT, Tubbs RR (2005) The incidence of topoisomerase II-alpha genomic alterations in adenocarcinoma of the breast and their relationship to human epidermal growth factor receptor-2 gene amplification: a fluorescence in situ hybridization study. Hum Pathol 36:348–356

Hittelman WN, Liao Y, Wang L, Milas L (2010) Are cancer stem cells radioresistant? Future Oncol 6:1563–1576

Holbro T, Beerli RR, Maurer F, Koziczak M, Barbas CF 3rd, Hynes NE (2003) The ErbB2/ErbB3 heterodimer functions as an oncogenic unit: ErbB2 requires ErbB3 to drive breast tumor cell proliferation. Proc Natl Acad Sci U S A 100:8933–8938

Holland JD, Klaus A, Garratt AN, Birchmeier W (2013) Wnt signaling in stem and cancer stem cells. Curr Opin Cell Biol 25:254–264

Hu C, Fan L, Cen P, Chen E, Jiang Z, Li L (2016) Energy metabolism plays a critical role in stem cell maintenance and differentiation. Int J Mol Sci 17

Huang Q, Zhang QB, Dong J, Wu YY, Shen YT, Zhao YD, Zhu YD, Diao Y, Wang AD, Lan Q (2008) Glioma stem cells are more aggressive in recurrent tumors with malignant progression than in the primary tumor, and both can be maintained long-term in vitro. BMC Cancer 8:304

Jamieson CH, Ailles LE, Dylla SJ, Muijtjens M, Jones C, Zehnder JL, Gotlib J, Li K, Manz MG, Keating A, Sawyers CL, Weissman IL (2004) Granulocyte-macrophage progenitors as candidate leukemic stem cells in blast-crisis CML. N Engl J Med 351:657–667

Jeon SM, Chandel NS, Hay N (2012) AMPK regulates NADPH homeostasis to promote tumour cell survival during energy stress. Nature 485:661–665

Kang R, Tang D, Schapiro NE, Loux T, Livesey KM, Billiar TR, Wang H, Van Houten B, Lotze MT, Zeh HJ (2014) The HMGB1/RAGE inflammatory pathway promotes pancreatic tumor growth by regulating mitochondrial bioenergetics. Oncogene 33:567–577

Karin M, Cao Y, Greten FR, Li ZW (2002) NF-kappaB in cancer: from innocent bystander to major culprit. Nat Rev Cancer 2:301–310

Katajisto P, Dohla J, Chaffer CL, Pentinmikko N, Marjanovic N, Iqbal S, Zoncu R, Chen W, Weinberg RA, Sabatini DM (2015) Stem cells. Asymmetric apportioning of aged mitochondria between daughter cells is required for stemness. Science 348:340–343

Kaufhold S, Garban H, Bonavida B (2016) Yin Yang 1 is associated with cancer stem cell transcription factors (SOX$_2$, OCT$_4$, BMI$_1$) and clinical implication. J Exp Clin Cancer Res 35:84

Kim JJ, Tannock IF (2005) Repopulation of cancer cells during therapy: an important cause of treatment failure. Nat Rev Cancer 5:516–525

Kim HM, Haraguchi N, Ishii H, Ohkuma M, Okano M, Mimori K, Eguchi H, Yamamoto H, Nagano H, Sekimoto M, Doki Y, Mori M (2012) Increased CD13 expression reduces reactive oxygen species, promoting survival of liver cancer stem cells via an epithelial-mesenchymal transition-like phenomenon. Ann Surg Oncol 19(Suppl 3):S539–S548

Kitahara O, Katagiri T, Tsunoda T, Harima Y, Nakamura Y (2002) Classification of sensitivity or resistance of cervical cancers to ionizing radiation according to expression profiles of 62 genes selected by cDNA microarray analysis. Neoplasia 4:295–303

Kurokawa H, Arteaga CL (2001) Inhibition of erbB receptor (HER) tyrosine kinases as a strategy to abrogate antiestrogen resistance in human breast cancer. Clin Cancer Res 7:4436s–4442s; discussion 4411s–4412s

Kurth I, Hein L, Mabert K, Peitzsch C, Koi L, Cojoc M, Kunz-Schughart L, Baumann M, Dubrovska A (2013) Cancer stem cell related markers of radioresistance in head and neck squamous cell carcinoma. Oncotarget 6:34494–34509

Lagadec C, Dekmezian C, Bauche L, Pajonk F (2012) Oxygen levels do not determine radiation survival of breast cancer stem cells. PLoS ONE 7:e34545

Lapidot T, Sirard C, Vormoor J, Murdoch B, Hoang T, Caceres-Cortes J, Minden M, Paterson B, Caligiuri MA, Dick JE (1994) A cell initiating human acute myeloid leukaemia after transplantation into SCID mice. Nature 367:645–648

Lathia JD, Gallagher J, Heddleston JM, Wang J, Eyler CE, Macswords J, Wu Q, Vasanji A, McLendon RE, Hjelmeland AB, Rich JN (2010) Integrin alpha 6 regulates glioblastoma stem cells. Cell Stem Cell 6:421–432

Leal JA, Lleonart ME (2013) MicroRNAs and cancer stem cells: therapeutic approaches and future perspectives. Cancer Lett 338:174–183

LeBleu VS, O'Connell JT, Gonzalez Herrera KN, Wikman H, Pantel K, Haigis MC, de Carvalho FM, Damascena A, Domingos Chinen LT, Rocha RM, Asara JM, Kalluri R (2014) PGC-1alpha mediates mitochondrial biogenesis and oxidative phosphorylation in cancer cells to promote metastasis. Nat Cell Biol 16(992–1003):1001–1015

Lee YS, Oh JH, Yoon S, Kwon MS, Song CW, Kim KH, Cho MJ, Mollah ML, Je YJ, Kim YD, Kim CD, Lee JH (2010) Differential gene expression profiles of radioresistant non-small-cell lung cancer cell lines established by fractionated irradiation: tumor protein p53-inducible protein 3 confers sensitivity to ionizing radiation. Int J Radiat Oncol Biol Phys 77:858–866

Lee YK, Hur W, Lee SW, Hong SW, Kim SW, Choi JE, Yoon SK (2014) Knockdown of 14-3-3zeta enhances radiosensitivity and radio-induced apoptosis in CD133(+) liver cancer stem cells. Exp Mol Med 46:e77

Li N, Karin M (1998) Ionizing radiation and short wavelength UV activate NF-kappaB through two distinct mechanisms. Proc Natl Acad Sci U S A 95:13012–13017

Li L, Neaves WB (2006) Normal stem cells and cancer stem cells: the niche matters. Cancer Res 66:4553–4557

Li JJ, Westergaard C, Ghosh P, Colburn NH (1997) Inhibitors of both nuclear factor-kappaB and activator protein-1 activation block the neoplastic transformation response. Cancer Res 57:3569–3576

Li Z, Xia L, Lee LM, Khaletskiy A, Wang J, Wong JY, Li JJ (2001) Effector genes altered in MCF-7 human breast cancer cells after exposure to fractionated ionizing radiation. Radiat Res 155:543–553

Liao J, Qian F, Tchabo N, Mhawech-Fauceglia P, Beck A, Qian Z, Wang X, Huss WJ, Lele SB, Morrison CD, Odunsi K (2014) Ovarian cancer spheroid cells with stem cell-like properties contribute to tumor generation, metastasis and chemotherapy resistance through hypoxia-resistant metabolism. PLoS ONE 9:e84941

Liu M, Sakamaki T, Casimiro MC, Willmarth NE, Quong AA, Ju X, Ojeifo J, Jiao X, Yeow WS, Katiyar S, Shirley LA, Joyce D, Lisanti MP, Albanese C, Pestell RG (2010) The canonical NF-kappaB pathway governs mammary tumorigenesis in transgenic mice and tumor stem cell expansion. Cancer Res 70:10464–10473

Locke JE, Bradbury CM, Wei SJ, Shah S, Rene LM, Clemens RA, Roti Roti J, Horikoshi N, Gius D (2002) Indomethacin lowers the threshold thermal exposure for hyperthermic radiosensitization and heat-shock inhibition of ionizing radiation-induced activation of NF-kappaB. Int J Radiat Biol 78:493–502

Lou H, Dean M (2007) Targeted therapy for cancer stem cells: the patched pathway and ABC transporters. Oncogene 26:1357–1360

Lu C, Ward PS, Kapoor GS, Rohle D, Turcan S, Abdel-Wahab O, Edwards CR, Khanin R, Figueroa ME, Melnick A, Wellen KE, O'Rourke DM, Berger SL, Chan TA, Levine RL, Mellinghoff IK, Thompson CB (2012) IDH mutation impairs histone demethylation and results in a block to cell differentiation. Nature 483:474–478

Lu CL, Qin L, Liu HC, Candas D, Fan M, Li JJ (2015) Tumor cells switch to mitochondrial oxidative phosphorylation under radiation via mTOR-mediated hexokinase II inhibition—a Warburg-reversing effect. PLoS ONE 10:e0121046

Lunt SY, Vander Heiden MG (2011) Aerobic glycolysis: meeting the metabolic requirements of cell proliferation. Annu Rev Cell Dev Biol 27:441–464

Luo J-L, Kamata H, Karin M (2005) IKK/NF-kappaB signaling: balancing life and death—a new approach to cancer therapy. J Clin Invest 115:2625–2632

Lynam-Lennon N, Connaughton R, Carr E, Mongan AM, O'Farrell NJ, Porter RK, Brennan L, Pidgeon GP, Lysaght J, Reynolds JV, O'Sullivan J (2014) Excess visceral adiposity induces alterations in mitochondrial function and energy metabolism in esophageal adenocarcinoma. BMC Cancer 14:907

Majeti R, Chao MP, Alizadeh AA, Pang WW, Jaiswal S, Gibbs KD Jr, van Rooijen N, Weissman IL (2009a) CD47 is an adverse prognostic factor and therapeutic antibody target on human acute myeloid leukemia stem cells. Cell 138:286–299

Majeti R, Becker MW, Tian Q, Lee TL, Yan X, Liu R, Chiang JH, Hood L, Clarke MF, Weissman IL (2009b) Dysregulated gene expression networks in human acute myelogenous leukemia stem cells. Proc Natl Acad Sci U S A 106:3396–3401

McClements L, Yakkundi A, Papaspyropoulos A, Harrison H, Ablett MP, Jithesh PV, McKeen HD, Bennett R, Donley C, Kissenpfennig A, McIntosh S, McCarthy HO, O'Neill E, Clarke RB, Robson T (2013) Targeting treatment-resistant breast cancer stem cells with FKBPL and its peptide derivative, AD-01, via the CD44 pathway. Clin Cancer Res 19:3881–3893

Moncharmont C, Levy A, Gilormini M, Bertrand G, Chargari C, Alphonse G, Ardail D, Rodriguez-Lafrasse C, Magne N (2012) Targeting a cornerstone of radiation resistance: cancer stem cell. Cancer Lett 322:139–147

Nagano O, Okazaki S, Saya H (2013) Redox regulation in stem-like cancer cells by CD44 variant isoforms. Oncogene 32:5191–5198

Nantajit D, Lin D, Li JJ (2015) The network of epithelial–mesenchymal transition: potential new targets for tumor resistance. J Cancer Res Clin Oncol 141:1697–1713

Nobler MP (1969) The abscopal effect in malignant lymphoma and its relationship to lymphocyte circulation. Radiology 93:410–412

Obre E, Rossignol R (2015) Emerging concepts in bioenergetics and cancer research: metabolic flexibility, coupling, symbiosis, switch, oxidative tumors, metabolic remodeling, signaling and bioenergetic therapy. Int J Biochem Cell Biol 59:167–181

Ogawa K, Utsunomiya T, Mimori K, Tanaka F, Haraguchi N, Inoue H, Murayama S, Mori M (2006) Differential gene expression profiles of radioresistant pancreatic cancer cell lines established by fractionated irradiation. Int J Oncol 28:705–713

Olayioye MA (2001) Update on HER-2 as a target for cancer therapy: intracellular signaling pathways of ErbB2/HER-2 and family members. Breast Cancer Res 3:385–389

Orlowski RZ, Baldwin AS Jr (2002) NF-kappaB as a therapeutic target in cancer. Trends Mol Med 8:385–389

Panopoulos AD, Yanes O, Ruiz S, Kida YS, Diep D, Tautenhahn R, Herrerias A, Batchelder EM, Plongthongkum N, Lutz M, Berggren WT, Zhang K, Evans RM, Siuzdak G, Izpisua Belmonte JC (2012) The metabolome of induced pluripotent stem cells reveals metabolic changes occurring in somatic cell reprogramming. Cell Res 22:168–177

Pareja F, Macleod D, Shu C, Crary JF, Canoll PD, Ross AH, Siegelin MD (2014) PI3 K and Bcl-2 inhibition primes glioblastoma cells to apoptosis through down-regulation of Mcl-1 and phospho-BAD. Mol Cancer Res

Park JH, Vithayathil S, Kumar S, Sung PL, Dobrolecki LE, Putluri V, Bhat VB, Bhowmik SK, Gupta V, Arora K, Wu D, Tsouko E, Zhang Y, Maity S, Donti TR, Graham BH, Frigo DE, Coarfa C, Yotnda P, Putluri N et al (2016) Fatty acid oxidation-driven Src links mitochondrial energy reprogramming and oncogenic properties in triple-negative breast cancer. Cell Rep 14:2154–2165

Peitzsch C, Perrin R, Hill RP, Dubrovska A, Kurth I (2014) Hypoxia as a biomarker for radioresistant cancer stem cells. Int J Radiat Biol 90:636–652

Phillips TM, McBride WH, Pajonk F (2006) The response of CD24(-/low)/CD44+ breast cancer-initiating cells to radiation. J Natl Cancer Inst 98:1777–1785

Pianetti S, Arsura M, Romieu-Mourez R, Coffey RJ, Sonenshein GE (2001) Her-2/neu overexpression induces NF-kappaB via a PI3-kinase/Akt pathway involving calpain-mediated degradation of IkappaB-alpha that can be inhibited by the tumor suppressor PTEN. Oncogene 20:1287–1299

Pike LS, Smift AL, Croteau NJ, Ferrick DA, Wu M (2011) Inhibition of fatty acid oxidation by etomoxir impairs NADPH production and increases reactive oxygen species resulting in ATP depletion and cell death in human glioblastoma cells. Biochim Biophys Acta 1807:726–734

Postow MA, Callahan MK, Barker CA, Yamada Y, Yuan J, Kitano S, Mu Z, Rasalan T, Adamow M, Ritter E, Sedrak C, Jungbluth AA, Chua R, Yang AS, Roman RA, Rosner S, Benson B, Allison JP, Lesokhin AM, Gnjatic S et al (2012) Immunologic correlates of the abscopal effect in a patient with melanoma. N Engl J Med 366:925–931

Pratt MA, Tibbo E, Robertson SJ, Jansson D, Hurst K, Perez-Iratxeta C, Lau R, Niu MY (2009) The canonical NF-kappaB pathway is required for formation of luminal mammary neoplasias and is activated in the mammary progenitor population. Oncogene 28:2710–2722

Qin L, Fan M, Candas D, Jiang G, Papadopoulos S, Tian L, Woloschak G, Grdina DJ, Li JJ (2015) CDK1 enhances mitochondrial bioenergetics for radiation-induced DNA repair. Cell Rep 13:2056–2063

Rahaman SO, Harbor PC, Chernova O, Barnett GH, Vogelbaum MA, Haque SJ (2002) Inhibition of constitutively active Stat3 suppresses proliferation and induces apoptosis in glioblastoma multiforme cells. Oncogene 21:8404–8413

Rampazzo E, Persano L, Pistollato F, Moro E, Frasson C, Porazzi P, Della Puppa A, Bresolin S, Battilana G, Indraccolo S, Te Kronnie G, Argenton F, Tiso N, Basso G (2013) Wnt activation promotes neuronal differentiation of glioblastoma. Cell Death Dis 4:e500

Ramsamooj P, Kasid U, Dritschilo A (1992) Differential expression of proteins in radioresistant and radiosensitive human squamous carcinoma cells. J Natl Cancer Inst 84:622–628

Reya T, Morrison SJ, Clarke MF, Weissman IL (2001) Stem cells, cancer, and cancer stem cells. Nature 414:105–111

Reya T, Duncan AW, Ailles L, Domen J, Scherer DC, Willert K, Hintz L, Nusse R, Weissman IL (2003) A role for Wnt signalling in self-renewal of haematopoietic stem cells. Nature 423:409–414

Rinkenbaugh AL, Baldwin AS (2016) The NF-kappaB pathway and cancer stem cells. Cells 5

Robertson-Tessi M, Gillies RJ, Gatenby RA, Anderson AR (2015) Impact of metabolic heterogeneity on tumor growth, invasion, and treatment outcomes. Cancer Res 75:1567–1579

Rossi DJ, Bryder D, Seita J, Nussenzweig A, Hoeijmakers J, Weissman IL (2007) Deficiencies in DNA damage repair limit the function of haematopoietic stem cells with age. Nature 447:725–729

Ryoo IG, Lee SH, Kwak MK (2016) Redox modulating NRF2: a potential mediator of cancer stem cell resistance. Oxid Med Cell Longev 2016:2428153

Saito S, Lin YC, Tsai MH, Lin CS, Murayama Y, Sato R, Yokoyama KK (2015) Emerging roles of hypoxia-inducible factors and reactive oxygen species in cancer and pluripotent stem cells. Kaohsiung J Med Sci 31:279–286

Sau A, Lau R, Cabrita MA, Nolan E, Crooks PA, Visvader JE, Pratt MA (2016) Persistent activation of NF-kappaB in BRCA1-deficient mammary progenitors drives aberrant proliferation and accumulation of DNA damage. Cell Stem Cell 19:52–65

Schaue D, Comin-Anduix B, Ribas A, Zhang L, Goodglick L, Sayre JW, Debucquoy A, Haustermans K, McBride WH (2008) T-cell responses to survivin in cancer patients undergoing radiation therapy. Clin Cancer Res 14:4883–4890

Schreiber RD, Old LJ, Smyth MJ (2011) Cancer immunoediting: integrating immunity's roles in cancer suppression and promotion. Science 331:1565–1570

Seto E, Shi Y, Shenk T (1991) YY1 is an initiator sequence-binding protein that directs and activates transcription in vitro. Nature 354:241–245

Sheehan JP, Shaffrey ME, Gupta B, Larner J, Rich JN, Park DM (2010) Improving the radiosensitivity of radioresistant and hypoxic glioblastoma. Future Oncol 6:1591–1601

Shen Y, Chen H, Zhang J, Chen Y, Wang M, Ma J, Hong L, Liu N, Fan Q, Lu X, Tian Y, Wang A, Dong J, Lan Q, Huang Q (2015) Increased notch signaling enhances radioresistance of malignant stromal cells induced by glioma stem/progenitor cells. PLoS ONE 10:e0142594

Sheng YH, He Y, Hasnain SZ, Wang R, Tong H, Clarke DT, Lourie R, Oancea I, Wong KY, Lumley JW, Florin TH, Sutton P, Hooper JD, McMillan NA, McGuckin MA (2016) MUC13 protects colorectal cancer cells from death by activating the NF-kappaB pathway and is a potential therapeutic target. Oncogene

Sheridan C, Kishimoto H, Fuchs RK, Mehrotra S, Bhat-Nakshatri P, Turner CH, Goulet R Jr, Badve S, Nakshatri H (2006) CD44+/CD24− breast cancer cells exhibit enhanced invasive properties: an early step necessary for metastasis. Breast Cancer Res 8:R59

Shih YC, Elting LS, Pavluck AL, Stewart A, Halpern MT (2010) Immunotherapy in the initial treatment of newly diagnosed cancer patients: utilization trend and cost projections for non-Hodgkin's lymphoma, metastatic breast cancer, and metastatic colorectal cancer. Cancer Invest 28:46–53

Simsek T, Kocabas F, Zheng J, Deberardinis RJ, Mahmoud AI, Olson EN, Schneider JW, Zhang CC, Sadek HA (2010) The distinct metabolic profile of hematopoietic stem cells reflects their location in a hypoxic niche. Cell Stem Cell 7:380–390

Singh SK, Hawkins C, Clarke ID, Squire JA, Bayani J, Hide T, Henkelman RM, Cusimano MD, Dirks PB (2004) Identification of human brain tumour initiating cells. Nature 432:396–401

Skvortsov S, Debbage P, Skvortsova I (2014) Proteomics of cancer stem cells. Int J Radiat Biol 90:653–658

Skvortsova I, Debbage P, Kumar V, Skvortsov S (2015) Radiation resistance: cancer stem cells (CSCs) and their enigmatic pro-survival signaling. Semin Cancer Biol 35:39–44

Slamon DJ, Clark GM, Wong SG, Levin WJ, Ullrich A, McGuire WL (1987) Human breast cancer: correlation of relapse and survival with amplification of the HER-2/neu oncogene. Science 235:177–182

Soomro S, Shousha S, Taylor P, Shepard HM, Feldmann M (1991) c-erbB-2 expression in different histological types of invasive breast carcinoma. J Clin Pathol 44:211–214

Sotgia F, Whitaker-Menezes D, Martinez-Outschoorn UE, Salem AF, Tsirigos A, Lamb R, Sneddon S, Hulit J, Howell A, Lisanti MP (2012) Mitochondria "fuel" breast cancer metabolism: fifteen markers of mitochondrial biogenesis label epithelial cancer cells, but are excluded from adjacent stromal cells. Cell Cycle 11:4390–4401

Stefanovic S, Schuetz F, Sohn C, Beckhove P, Domschke C (2014) Adoptive immunotherapy of metastatic breast cancer: present and future. Cancer Metastasis Rev 33:309–320

Stiles CD, Rowitch DH (2008) Glioma stem cells: a midterm exam. Neuron 58:832–846

Stupp R, Hegi ME, Mason WP, van den Bent MJ, Taphoorn MJ, Janzer RC, Ludwin SK, Allgeier A, Fisher B, Belanger K, Hau P, Brandes AA, Gijtenbeek J, Marosi C, Vecht CJ, Mokhtari K, Wesseling P, Villa S, Eisenhauer E, Gorlia T et al (2009) Effects of radiotherapy with concomitant and adjuvant temozolomide versus radiotherapy alone on survival in glioblastoma in a randomised phase III study: 5-year analysis of the EORTC-NCIC trial. Lancet Oncol 10:459–466

Suda T, Takubo K, Semenza GL (2011) Metabolic regulation of hematopoietic stem cells in the hypoxic niche. Cell Stem Cell 9:298–310

Takubo K, Nagamatsu G, Kobayashi CI, Nakamura-Ishizu A, Kobayashi H, Ikeda E, Goda N, Rahimi Y, Johnson RS, Soga T, Hirao A, Suematsu M, Suda T (2013) Regulation of glycolysis by Pdk functions as a metabolic checkpoint for cell cycle quiescence in hematopoietic stem cells. Cell Stem Cell 12:49–61

Trautmann F, Cojoc M, Kurth I, Melin N, Bouchez LC, Dubrovska A, Peitzsch C (2014) CXCR4 as biomarker for radioresistant cancer stem cells. Int J Radiat Biol 90:687–699

Twyman-Saint Victor C, Rech AJ, Maity A, Rengan R, Pauken KE, Stelekati E, Benci JL, Xu B, Dada H, Odorizzi PM, Herati RS, Mansfield KD, Patsch D, Amaravadi RK, Schuchter LM, Ishwaran H, Mick R, Pryma DA, Xu X, Feldman MD et al (2015) Radiation and dual checkpoint blockade activate non-redundant immune mechanisms in cancer. Nature 520:373–377

Urao N, Ushio-Fukai M (2013) Redox regulation of stem/progenitor cells and bone marrow niche. Free Radic Biol Med 54:26–39

Vaz AP, Ponnusamy MP, Seshacharyulu P, Batra SK (2014) A concise review on the current understanding of pancreatic cancer stem cells. J Cancer Stem Cell Res 2

Vermeulen L, Todaro M, de Sousa Mello F, Sprick MR, Kemper K, Perez Alea M, Richel DJ, Stassi G, Medema JP (2008) Single-cell cloning of colon cancer stem cells reveals a multi-lineage differentiation capacity. Proc Natl Acad Sci U S A 105:13427–13432

Vlashi E, Pajonk F (2015) Cancer stem cells, cancer cell plasticity and radiation therapy. Semin Cancer Biol 31:28–35

Vlashi E, Lagadec C, Vergnes L, Matsutani T, Masui K, Poulou M, Popescu R, Della Donna L, Evers P, Dekmezian C, Reue K, Christofk H, Mischel PS, Pajonk F (2011) Metabolic state of glioma stem cells and nontumorigenic cells. Proc Natl Acad Sci U S A 108:16062–16067

Vlashi E, Lagadec C, Vergnes L, Reue K, Frohnen P, Chan M, Alhiyari Y, Dratver MB, Pajonk F (2014) Metabolic differences in breast cancer stem cells and differentiated progeny. Breast Cancer Res Treat 146:525–534

Vlashi E, Chen AM, Boyrie S, Yu G, Nguyen A, Brower PA, Hess CB, Pajonk F (2016) Radiation-induced dedifferentiation of head and neck cancer cells into cancer stem cells depends on human papillomavirus status. Int J Radiat Oncol Biol Phys 94:1198–1206

Wallace DC (2012) Mitochondria and cancer. Nat Rev Cancer 12:685–698

Wanet A, Remacle N, Najar M, Sokal E, Arnould T, Najimi M, Renard P (2014) Mitochondrial remodeling in hepatic differentiation and dedifferentiation. Int J Biochem Cell Biol 54:174–185

Wang T, Tamae D, LeBon T, Shively JE, Yen Y, Li JJ (2005) The role of peroxiredoxin II in radiation-resistant MCF-7 breast cancer cells. Cancer Res 65:10338–10346

Wang J, Wakeman TP, Lathia JD, Hjelmeland AB, Wang XF, White RR, Rich JN, Sullenger BA (2010) Notch promotes radioresistance of glioma stem cells. Stem Cells 28:17–28

Wang Z, Fan M, Candas D, Zhang TQ, Qin L, Eldridge A, Wachsmann-Hogiu S, Ahmed KM, Chromy BA, Nantajit D, Duru N, He F, Chen M, Finkel T, Weinstein LS, Li JJ (2014) Cyclin B1/Cdk1 coordinates mitochondrial respiration for cell-cycle G2/M progression. Dev Cell 29:217–232

Westermann B (2010) Mitochondrial fusion and fission in cell life and death. Nat Rev Mol Cell Biol 11:872–884

Willingham SB, Volkmer JP, Gentles AJ, Sahoo D, Dalerba P, Mitra SS, Wang J, Contreras-Trujillo H, Martin R, Cohen JD, Lovelace P, Scheeren FA, Chao MP, Weiskopf K, Tang C, Volkmer AK, Naik TJ, Storm TA, Mosley AR, Edris B et al (2012) The CD47-signal regulatory protein alpha (SIRPa) interaction is a therapeutic target for human solid tumors. Proc Natl Acad Sci U S A 109:6662–6667

Xia L, Paik A, Li JJ (2004) p53 activation in chronic radiation-treated breast cancer cells: regulation of MDM2/p14ARF. Cancer Res 64:221–228

Xing F, Okuda H, Watabe M, Kobayashi A, Pai SK, Liu W, Pandey PR, Fukuda K, Hirota S, Sugai T, Wakabayshi G, Koeda K, Kashiwaba M, Suzuki K, Chiba T, Endo M, Mo YY, Watabe K (2011) Hypoxia-induced Jagged2 promotes breast cancer metastasis and self-renewal of cancer stem-like cells. Oncogene 30:4075–4086

Yanes O, Clark J, Wong DM, Patti GJ, Sanchez-Ruiz A, Benton HP, Trauger SA, Desponts C, Ding S, Siuzdak G (2010) Metabolic oxidation regulates embryonic stem cell differentiation. Nat Chem Biol 6:411–417

Yang W, Wei J, Guo T, Shen Y, Liu F (2014) Knockdown of miR-210 decreases hypoxic glioma stem cells stemness and radioresistance. Exp Cell Res 326:22–35

Yang W, Shen Y, Wei J, Liu F (2015) MicroRNA-153/Nrf-2/GPx1 pathway regulates radiosensitivity and stemness of glioma stem cells via reactive oxygen species. Oncotarget 6:22006–22027

Ye J, Cippetelli M, Dorman L, Ortaldo JR, Young HA (1996) The nuclear factor YY1 suppresses the human gamma interferon promoter through two mechanisms: inhibition of AP1 binding and activation of a silencer element. Mol Cell Biol 16:4744–4753

Yun HS, Baek JH, Yim JH, Um HD, Park JK, Song JY, Park IC, Kim JS, Lee SJ, Lee CW, Hwang SG (2016) Radiotherapy diagnostic biomarkers in radioresistant human H460 lung cancer stem-like cells. Cancer Biol Ther 17:208–218

Zanotto-Filho A, Braganhol E, Battastini AM, Moreira JC (2012) Proteasome inhibitor MG132 induces selective apoptosis in glioblastoma cells through inhibition of PI3 K/Akt and NFkappaB pathways, mitochondrial dysfunction, and activation of p38-JNK1/2 signaling. Invest New Drugs 30:2252–2262

Zellmer VR, Zhang S (2014) Evolving concepts of tumor heterogeneity. Cell Biosci 4:69

Zhang Q, Raje V, Yakovlev VA, Yacoub A, Szczepanek K, Meier J, Derecka M, Chen Q, Hu Y, Sisler J, Hamed H, Lesnefsky EJ, Valerie K, Dent P, Larner AC (2013a) Mitochondrial localized Stat3 promotes breast cancer growth via phosphorylation of serine 727. J Biol Chem 288:31280–31288

Zhang Y, Marsboom G, Toth PT, Rehman J (2013b) Mitochondrial respiration regulates adipogenic differentiation of human mesenchymal stem cells. PLoS ONE 8:e77077

Zhao XW, van Beek EM, Schornagel K, Van der Maaden H, Van Houdt M, Otten MA, Finetti P, Van Egmond M, Matozaki T, Kraal G, Birnbaum D, van Elsas A, Kuijpers TW, Bertucci F, van den Berg TK (2011) CD47-signal regulatory protein-alpha (SIRPalpha) interactions form a barrier for antibody-mediated tumor cell destruction. Proc Natl Acad Sci U S A 108:18342–18347

Zhao L, Tang M, Hu Z, Yan B, Pi W, Li Z, Zhang J, Zhang L, Jiang W, Li G, Qiu Y, Hu F, Liu F, Lu J, Chen X, Xiao L, Xu Z, Tao Y, Yang L, Bode AM et al (2015) miR-504 mediated down-regulation of nuclear respiratory factor 1 leads to radio-resistance in nasopharyngeal carcinoma. Oncotarget 6:15995–16018

Biomarkers and Radiotherapy

Savita V. Dandapani

Abstract

For a biomarker to be clinically useful there must be adequate preclinical data and have prevalence in the disease of interest. Early research focused on molecules implicated in the cell cycle, DNA repair pathways, and apoptosis as radiation is known to affect such pathways. More recent data has focused on big data, i.e.—omics (genomics, proteomics, etc.) to find a molecular signature that predicts response to radiation as well as identify those who may have increased risk of radiation induced toxicities. While many potential biomarkers in assessing radiation response have been researched this chapter is a start to providing information on biomarkers used in clinical practice.

Keywords

Biomarker · EGFR · HPV · MGMT · PSA · ATM · TGF1-beta · Genomics · Proteomics

1 Introduction

A current goal in medicine is to individualize treatment to eradicate disease while reducing toxicity and improving quality of life. Currently radiation doses are generalized with consensus statements for dose tolerance of normal tissues and local control of tumor based on histology and organ/location. Current radiation dose guidelines are based on laboratory studies of the general radiosensitivity/radioresistance of a

S.V. Dandapani (✉)
Department of Radiation Oncology, City of Hope, Duarte, CA 91010, USA
e-mail: sdandapani@coh.org

© Springer International Publishing AG 2017
J.Y.C. Wong et al. (eds.), *Advances in Radiation Oncology*,
Cancer Treatment and Research 172, DOI 10.1007/978-3-319-53235-6_10

particular tumor and modeling the tumor control probability (TCP) based on growth characteristics of a tumor. Recently molecular biomarkers allow for personalized treatment approaches and potentially adaptive radiotherapy and or radiation dose escalation/de-intensification. This chapter gives a review of known common biomarkers used in clinical practice today and is sectioned by organ site. The chapter also presents data on the more recent large scale analysis of a patient's molecular profile, i.e.–omics profiling of tumors (genomics SNPs, proteomics, etc.) to predict radiation effects. The goal of biomarker research is to one-day tailor treatment based on an individual's genetic and molecular profile. This book chapter aims to highlight various biomarkers in each cancer type by histology.

2   Head and Neck Cancers

HPV (human papilloma virus)/p16: predictive biomarker. HPV is the most well-known and reproducible predictive marker in head and neck cancer to date (Wierzbicka et al. 2015). It is the most widely discussed marker researched in radiation oncology today. This section focuses on head and neck biomarkers with an emphasis on HPV. Radiation dose de-escalation trials are ongoing in patients with HPV/p16+ head and neck cancer based on the breadth of research on this virus (Wierzbicka et al. 2015).

Traditionally all squamous cell cancers of the head and neck were treated the same with dose guidelines based on tumor size and surgical lymph node drainage patterns. Historically risk factors for head and neck cancer included excessive smoking and alcohol history. More recently there has been an increase in non-smokers with head and neck cancer. The common thread in this subtype of patients has been the prevalence of HPV/p16 in the tumor cells (Chau et al. 2014). HPV is a DNA virus; there are many subtypes. The one subtype of HPV consistently found to correlate with head and neck cancer is HPV/p16. HPV positivity is confirmed by both presence of HPV DNA using PCR and protein overexpression of p16 on immunohistochemical stains (Lee et al. 2015).

In patients with cancer of the oropharynx patients that have HPV p16 positivity tend to present with more locally advanced disease (Ang et al. 2010). In spite of this HPV p16 expression imparts a better response to radiation both standard fractionation and altered fractionation (Lassen et al. 2011, 2014). Lau et al. (2011) demonstrated that p16+ head and neck squamous cell cancer patients had improved overall survival, disease-free survival, and less locoregional recurrence when compared to p16-patients (Lau et al. 2011). Hong et al. (2010) demonstrated that HPV-patients had 13-fold increased risk of locoregional failure and 4-fold increased risk of death as compared to HPV+ patients (Hong et al. 2010). Lassen et al. (2014) showed that the HPV/p16 expression only positively correlates with response in oropharynx patients; p16 expression did not affect outcome of non-oropharynx patients (larynx, hypopharynx) (Lassen et al. 2014). HPV/p16 seems to be more predictive of response to radiation over surgery; Quon et al. (2013) analyzed p16 expression in resectable oropharyngeal carcinoma and found no difference in surgical outcomes of p16+ and p16-patients treated with surgery first (Quon et al. 2013). Future trials underway in head and neck cancer use radiation dose de-escalation in HPV p16 positive oropharynx patients due to this correlation as a predictive biomarker (Ang and Sturgis 2012).

As HPV positivity is established as a predictive biomarker of response to radiation, there are now studies trying to delineate biomarkers that predict for failure in the HPV+ subset (Lee et al. 2015). Inflammatory cells have been evaluated as a marker for predicting treatment failure in HPV+ tonsil cancer and Lee et al. (2015) demonstrated that both overall survival and disease specific survival was affected by high CD68+ and low CD8/CD4 T lymphocyte ratio (Lee et al. 2015). Neither T stage nor N stage were related to outcomes in this HPV+ tonsil cohort (Lee et al. 2015). Extent of inflammation and response to radiation is a common theme and this paper attempts to start the further subtype characterization of HPV+ patients. Other studies have tried to identify a panel of biomarkers that will predict treatment failure, Thibodeau et al. (2015) found that upregulation of LCE3D (late cornified envelope 3D) and KRTDAP (keratinocyte differentiation-associated protein) and down regulation of KRT19 (keratin 19) was observed in posttreatment failures of HPV+ patients (Thibodeau et al. 2015). These biomarkers haven't been extensively studied in radiation and so future studies will be needed to validate these results.

EGFR is another biomarker analyzed in head and neck patients. There have been mixed reports in its ability to predict locoregional control from radiation therapy (Lassen et al. 2013). While the signal for prediction is not as strong as HPV p16 expression, upregulation of EGFR has been shown to correlate with tumor growth and benefits from accelerated radiotherapy (Eriksen et al. 2004). In the DAHANCA 6 and 7 studies, low EGFR expression correlates with high HPV/p16 expression which seems reasonable given that HPV/p16 expression patients respond better to treatment (Lassen et al. 2013). However the signal for EGFR predicting head and neck cancer was not as strong as HPV/p16 expression and so is not routinely recommended for monitoring at this time (Lassen et al. 2013). Recently EGFR was reassessed in HPV+ and HPV-head and neck patients and again demonstrated that EGFR expression did not affect outcomes in HPV+ patients. In HPV-patients, EGFR expression correlated with worse locoregional failure but only in univariate analysis with T and N stage playing more prominent role (Vainshtein et al. 2014).

Similar to EGFR, p53 mutational status has also been analyzed in head and neck cancer patients. Alone p53 mutational status did not affect local control or overall survival but there was a suggestion that p53 mutant head and neck cancer patients may benefit from shortened treatment time similar to EGFR overexpressing patients (Eriksen et al. 2005). Future studies are underway examining EGFR expression, p53 mutational status, HPV/p16 expression, and smoking status to see if there are further subsets of head and neck cancer patients.

Hypoxia molecules have also been studied as predictive biomarkers of radiation resistance mostly because it is known that lack of oxygen makes tumor cells less sensitive to radiation (Overgaard et al. 2005). Osteopontin is one such biomarker associated with tumor hypoxia. In studies by the DAHANCA group, Overgaard et al. 2005demonstrated head and neck cancer patients with high levels of osteopontin (>167 ug/L) had poorer responses to radiation with higher levels of locoregional failure (Overgaard et al. 2005). In a parallel study at Stanford Petrik et al. (2006) demonstrated that high levels of osteopontin (>450 ng/ml) correlated with higher rates of locoregional failure (3 yr FFR was 72% for patients with osteopontin <450 ng/ml versus 48% for patients with >450 ng/ml (Petrik et al. 2006). Other markers of hypoxia being investigated as markers of radiation resistance include hypoxia inducible factor HIF-2 alpha (HIF-2) and carbonic anhydrase CA9; CA9 is actually one indicator of HIF-1alpha (HIF-1) function. HIF-1 and HIF-2 are thought to be two separate response pathways (Koukourakis et al. 2006). Using data from the CHART trial (continuous hyperfractionated accelerated radiotherapy), Koukourakis et al. (2006) demonstrated that head and neck cancer patients with high levels of HIF-2 and CA9 had worse locoregional control (Koukourakis et al. 2006). These studies haven't led to routine measurement of hypoxic markers or use of hypoxia modifiable treatments such as nimorazole but overcoming hypoxia is still an active area of research in radiation resistance. Future patient samples may well be tested for these hypoxic markers.

From all these various markers only HPV is used routinely in radiation oncology clinical practice in head and neck cancers. Research studies are still underway with these other biomarkers and it is yet to be determined which will be of clinical use in the future.

3 Gynecologic Cancers

Gynecologic and head and neck cancers share many similar biomarkers and thus this next section will highlight some studies of biomarkers in the gynecology literature.

Similar to head and neck cancer, HPV has been implicated in cervical cancer as well and is used as a biomarker. The high-risk HPV 16 and HPV 18 are the most common HPV strains implicated in cervical cancer (Song et al. 2011; Qin et al. 2014). Currently the standard treatment of cervical cancer is concurrent chemotherapy and radiation therapy (Qin et al. 2014). There has been suggestion that for a subset that is radioresistant treatment intensification is needed but finding that subset has remained elusive thus far. Some reports suggest that there is difference response to chemoradiation among the HPV strains (Ferdousi et al. 2010). In one small study of 113 cervical cancer patients, response to radiation was better in HPV-58 and HPV-31 versus HPV 16 and HPV-33 (Ferdousi et al. 2010). There have been reports that persistent HPV after definitive radiation for cervical cancer may predict worse local control of disease (Song et al. 2011). Song et al. (2011) showed that persistent HPV DNA 24 months after radiation predicted risk of local recurrence and HPV persistence at just 3 months alone was the earliest predictor of local recurrence (Song et al. 2011). Testing for HPV is routinely done in clinical practice and this data suggests that all patients treated for cervical cancer with radiation should have HPV testing after radiation is complete as well. Patients with persistent HPV may need treatment intensification either in form of altered radiation treatment regimens, or adjuvant chemotherapy. This data still needs to be validated in multi-institutional trials before becoming routine use in clinical practice.

EGFR has also been explored as a biomarker in cervical cancer in the same manner as it has been studied in head and neck cancer (Qin et al. 2014). Overexpression of EGFR has been shown to lead to more failures after definitive radiation suggesting it is a predictive biomarker of radiation resistance (Pérez-Regadera et al. 2011). Perez-Regadera et al. (2011) examined 112 cervical cancer biopsies and found that patients with high overexpression of EGFR on biopsy had more pelvic relapses and decreased disease free survival with hazard ratio of 2.31 (Pérez-Regadera et al. 2011). Cerciello et al. (2007) demonstrated that changing EGFR levels during radiotherapy administration did not have any correlation with response though they did not mention quantification of initial expression of EGFR (Cerciello et al. 2007). Thus, EGFR may be a biomarker only of inherent radiation resistance and from these studies it suggests that initial EGFR expression of tumor may be more significant in predicting radiation resistance. EGFR testing in cervical cancer is not routinely done currently but may be considered in future trials arguing for more intensive treatment of radioresistant tumors.

Other biomarkers being tested include the bcl2 apoptotic family members such as BAX, prostaglandin pathway molecules such as COX, and hypoxic markers such as HIF1alpha (Qin et al. 2014). Currently only HPV is routinely screened prior to radiation therapy in cervical cancer but these other biomarkers may become significant as we try to individualize treatment or argue for treatment intensification in radiation resistant cervical cancer subtypes.

4   CNS

Glioblastomas are the most aggressive brain tumor. Historically treatment was surgery and whole brain radiation. With the advent of chemotherapy and better imaging with MRI brain, radiation in glioblastoma is directed at the tumor. A landmark trial demonstrated the benefit of temozolomide with limited field radiation in improving overall survival (Stupp et al. 2009).

Current evidence has demonstrated that not all glioblastomas are the same and survival varies widely. New reports suggest specific molecular subtypes have better survival. In the landmark Stupp trial, subset analysis of this trial demonstrated that patients with MGMT methylation have double the survival at 5 years (Stupp et al. 2009). The MGMT (O6-methylguanine-DNA-methyltransferase) gene encodes a DNA repair protein. Methylation of the MGMT promoter silences the gene and prevents DNA repair namely of damage caused by alkylating agents. Thus, this gene is important for regulating the DNA integrity of the cell. MGMT methylation has been shown to sensitize glioblastoma cells to temozolomide, an alkylating agent and is thus a predictive biomarker of the chemotherapy response. Rivera et al. (2010) asked the question if MGMT methylation also sensitizes cells to radiation as radiation also works primarily through DNA damage (Rivera et al. 2010). 225 patients were analyzed in their study of glioblastoma patients who received radiation alone after maximal safe surgical resection (i.e. no chemotherapy such as temozolomide) (Rivera et al. 2010). They demonstrated that patients with MGMT methylated had better response to radiation and that unmethylated tumors were twice as likely to progress during radiation treatment. On multivariate analysis, methylation was independent of age, KPS, and extent of surgical resection (Rivera et al. 2010).

MGMT is now used routinely in clinical practice as both a predictive and prognostic biomarker for chemotherapy. New strategies in glioblastoma treatment involve using MGMT methylation to alter upfront therapy, i.e. adding other targeted agents such as everolimus, etc. that work through pathways different than temozolomide to sensitize glioblastoma cells to radiation. The goal is more tailored treatment for glioblastoma subtypes in an effort to more efficiently eradicate tumor cells. Recently a Phase III randomized control study (GLARIUS trial) was published showing that altering chemotherapy in MGMT methylated patients could improve progression free survival (Herrlinger et al. 2016). In this study, non-MGMT methylated (i.e. predicted temozolomide and radiation resistant) patients with newly diagnosed glioblastoma were randomized to standard of care temozolomide + radiation versus bevacizumab+irinotecan+radiation (Herrlinger et al. 2016). However, the study failed to show improved overall survival as the original Stupp trial so temozolomide and radiation is still the standard for glioblastoma patients (Stupp et al. 2009; Herrlinger et al. 2016). Future studies may target radiation dose escalation or altered radiation fractionation schedules such as hypofractionation or stereotactic body radiation doses.

Recent studies by Ahmed et al. (2015) have looked into generating a radiosensitivity index (RSI) for different cancer subtypes including glioblastoma (Ahmed et al. 2015). The RSI described previously by the same group uses gene expression patterns, tissue histology, and ras and p53 status when cells are treated with radiation (Ahmed et al. 2015; Eschrich et al. 2009). The RSI index directly correlates with tumor radioresistance (high RSI = radioresistance) (Ahmed et al. 2015; Eschrich et al. 2009). Ahmed et al. (2015) used the TCGA (the cancer genome atlas) which has large population data based on histology and centralized at the NIH to see if RSI could predict radiation response (Ahmed et al. 2015). RSI was a predictor of overall survival for the glioblastoma cohort (Ahmed et al. 2015). For radiosensitivity predictions RSI correlated with response in patients with high MGMT expression (Ahmed et al. 2015). MGMT is already known to predict radiation response so it will be interesting to see if the further information from RSI can help delineate earlier which patients will need treatment intensification.

There are now known to be three subclasses of glioma: proneural, proliferative, and mesenchymal. By using these subtypes, known biomarkers such as MGMT and new genomic profiles such as RSI we can begin to tailor treatment for glioblastoma.

5 GU

Prostate cancer is the second leading cause of cancer deaths. Although prognostic factors such as clinical T stage, Gleason score and pretreatment PSA aid in prognosis of prostate cancer there are still many outliers. Early risk prostate cancer can fail localized therapy such as radiation earlier than planned and high risk prostate cancer can remain seemingly indolent for years. Other prognostic and predictors of radiation response in prostate radiation therapy are needed.

PSA is the single most used test in prostate cancer. It is used to screen men though its use as a screening tool has come into question given its high sensitivity and over-diagnosis of slow growing prostate cancers. Elevated PSA (generally >4) prompts urological consult and prostate biopsy. PSA response after definitive treatment (i.e. either surgery or radiation) is the most sensitive test and predicts progression free survival long before patient develops any recurrent tumor or metastases.

Kabarriti et al. (2014) and colleagues wanted to test if PSA can be used during radiation treatment to predict response. Such a marker would give patients confidence in radiation alone as salvage treatment and less worry about earlier need for additional salvage treatment such as hormonal treatment (i.e. lupron) or chemotherapy (i.e. docetaxel). Kabarriti et al. (2014) demonstrated that PSA response during radiation is a predictive biomarker of outcome of salvage prostatectomy patients (Kabarriti et al. 2014). 5 year biochemical control rate for PSA responders was 81% compared to 37% for non-responders (Kabarriti et al. 2014). This suggests that PSA should be used during radiation treatment to give an earlier predictor of patient outcome. If PSA is not responding adequately during radiation dose escalation could be considered or earlier use of additional chemotherapy may be warranted.

Another more recent biomarker is the genome prostate cancer classifier (GC) (Den et al. 2014). The GC score developed by Den et al. (2014) utilizes-omics data, specifically gene expression patterns with microarrays (Den et al. 2014). This GC score helps to predict which men would benefit from earlier adjuvant radiation versus delayed salvage radiation when frequently PSA is higher and radiation may be of less benefit (Den et al. 2014). The A high GC score predicted increased biochemical failure and metastases thus suggesting these men need more aggressive systemic therapy (i.e. long term hormones) (Den et al. 2014).

In lines with the GC score, research has focused on pretreatment molecular characteristics of the prostate cancer to determine if radiation as localized treatment should even be attempted or if patient should go to surgery. P53 accumulation and high expression in prostate cancer cells seems to predict radiation treatment failure in many prostate studies reported by independent research groups (Ritter et al. 2002; Scherr et al. 1999). Abnormal p53 expression was then analyzed in a multi-institutional RTOG trial, RTOG 8610 (Grignon et al. 1997). In this trial, all patients received radiation as the local treatment for prostate cancer and the phase III randomization was for ± addition of androgen deprivation (i.e. zoladex and flutamide) (Grignon et al. 1997). Abnormal p53 expression led to decreased time to development of distant metastases and increased incidence of distant metastases though these results must be taken with caution as they only demonstrated that p53 expression only affected response in patients who received both androgen deprivation and radiation and this was in an era without prostate radiation dose escalation which is standard today (Grignon et al. 1997).

Although in general prostate cancer is thought to be slow growing and with low proliferation index, there is a rare subtype of prostate cancer with a high proliferation index as measured by Ki-67 (Pollack et al. 2004). Pollack et al. (2004) analyzed Ki-67 expression in prostate cancer biopsies of men enrolled in a multi-institutional phase III randomized trial RTOG 92-02 (Pollack et al. 2004). In this trial, prostate cancer patients with locally advanced prostate cancer (intermediate and high risk) where randomized to long-term or short-term androgen deprivation concurrent with radiation therapy (Pollack et al. 2004). Pollack et al. (2004) demonstrated that high Ki-67 (cutpoint 7.1%) in prostate predicts poor response to treatment and these patients had higher biochemical failure, distant metastases and cause-specific death (Pollack et al. 2004). Future studies would need to aim at better initial treatment for this aggressive subtype of prostate cancer maybe with upfront plan for trimodality treatment versus trying one localized treatment and watching/waiting.

Most of these studies are looking at biomarkers that can predict response to radiation. There have been recent efforts in prostate cancer to also see if biomarkers can predict radiation toxicities. Genome-wide association studies have been used to identify SNPs (single nucleotide polymorphisms) associated with a common radiation toxicity from prostate cancer, erectile dysfunction (ED) (Kerns et al. 2010). This large scare-omics project genotyped 909,000 SNPs of African-American men treated with external beam radiation for prostate cancer (Kerns et al. 2010). The cohort filled out the Sexual Health Inventory for Men (SHIM) questionnaire. SHIM score of ≤ 7 was used to identify men with ED and to see which SNPs correlated. Kerns et al. (2010) identified SNP rs2268363 which is in the follicle-stimulating hormone receptor (FSHR) gene as correlating with ED (Kerns et al. 2010).

Overall PSA is still the main biomarker for prostate radiation. GC score and SNP profiling which uses large scale genomic data to predict individual patient responses to treatment may become more mainstream in the future for prostate cancer versus trying to identify one or two biomarkers.

In terms of other GU cancers there is emerging data on biomarkers predicting response to radiation. Koukourakis et al. (2016) examined tissue from 66 bladder cancer patients treated with hypofractionated accelerated radiation (Koukourakis et al. 2016). They observed that high expression of two biomarkers they analyzed, HIF1alpha and LDH5 correlated with poor response to radiation (Koukourakis et al. 2016). LDH5 (lactate dehydrogenase 5) is part of the anaerobic glycolysis pathway and does not require oxygen to function. The other, HIF1alpha, is part of the hypoxia signaling pathway discussed above suggesting still a common thread to predicting response to radiation. Future studies are needed to validate these findings in a larger cohort of bladder cancer patients.

6 Breast

It is now known that there are many subtypes of breast cancer (luminal A, luminal B, basal type, Her2Neu subtype) (Langlands et al. 2013). Each subtype of breast cancer has different overall survival, risk of metastases, response to chemotherapy and radiation. Recent data discussed below suggests that the specific subtype of breast cancer can predict radiation response (Langlands et al. 2013).

Although it is known that radiation tends to work better in cells that are undergoing rapid cell division it has also been suggested that radiation is more effective for luminal A and estrogen depending breast cancers in reducing risk of relapse (Wang et al. 2011; Kyndi et al. 2008). One theory is that estrogen hastens the cell cycle in the G1 to S transition and that could make cells with more error-prone DNA. Radiation thus would more effectively kill these cells with impaired DNA. For basal subtype (triple negative) breast cancers, many of which possess DNA damage repair deficiencies by virtue of BRCA mutations, there is still high risk of local recurrence even with radiation. There is speculation that there may be aberrant upregulation of alternate DNA damage repair pathways intrinsic to these BRCA mutant breast cancers that are able to overcome radiation induced DNA damage (Langlands et al. 2013).

Triple negative breast cancer is not as responsive to treatment as hormone positive breast cancer. Biomarkers unique to this breast cancer subtype may impart more information as to the mechanism of radioresistance (Speers et al. 2016). From studies of triple negative breast cancer cell lines a new potential radioresistance marker MELK (maternal embryonic leucine zipper kinase) has shown promise (Speers et al. 2016). MELK is overexpressed in triple negative breast cancer cell lines and when inhibited cells become more radiation sensitive (Speers et al. 2016). These laboratory bench studies could be translated into clinical trials assessing MELK as a biomarker. Langlands et al. (2014) also discussed work documenting that high expression of a proteasome subtype (PSMD9) was associated with increased local recurrence in patients that received adjuvant radiation versus patients that did not receive radiation suggesting some association with radiation treatment (Langlands et al. 2014). Another study demonstrated that high levels of peroxiredoxin-I was associated with high local recurrence after radiation (Woolston et al. 2011). Peroxiredoxin-I is in the pathway that regulates oxidative stress and thus may be another pathway that protects cells from radiation damage (Woolston et al. 2011). These would all need to be validated before use in routine clinical practice.

Known radioresponsive gene pathways have also been investigated in breast cancer. A recent paper highlights this by investigating 22 genetic variants in 18 radioresponsive genes and their association with breast cancer radiation reactions, specifically skin damage severity ($\geq$ grade 2 toxicity by RTOG criteria) (Mumbrekar et al. 2016). The authors found that a SNP in CD44 rs8193 with significantly associated with radiation induced skin reactions (Mumbrekar et al. 2016). CD44 positivity has been implicated before as a potential marker of breast cancer stem cells; there could possibly be a link with CD44 and ability of breast cancer cells to regenerate skin though more work is needed to justify this conclusion (Shao et al. 2016). Further work in specific radioresponsive genes is ongoing.

There has been large scale—omics studies in breast cancer patients to predict toxicities. Ho et al. (2007) initially ran an analysis of DNA sequence alterations in ATM (ataxia-telangiectasia) in breast cancer patients with grade 2 breast fibrosis toxicities from radiation (Ho et al. 2007). ATM is important in regulating the cell cycle and has been implicated in radiosensitivity for many years (Ho et al. 2007). They discovered that a SNP variant of ATM (5557 G $\rightarrow$ A polymorphism) was associated with increased risk of breast fibrosis ($\geq$ grade 2 late radiation response). This SNP results in a non-conservative amino acid substitution from an aspartic acid to an asparagine in exon 37 in the ATM protein (Andreassen et al. 2016). While the study was small with 131 patients, it suggests that genome wide assays may help pinpoint predictive radiation markers in breast cancer (Ho et al. 2007). There have been many small studies exploring this SNP but no definitive data. A more recent study again looked at ATM SNPs and toxicity in a large cohort of 5456 breast and prostate cancer patients; 2759 patients received radiation for breast cancer and 2697 patients received radiation for prostate cancer (Andreassen et al. 2016). The same SNP discussed by Ho et al. (2007) ATM SNP rs1801516 was associated with radiation toxicity; in this study the association was stronger with acute toxicities (odds ratio 1.5) versus late (odds ratio 1.2) (Andreassen et al. 2016). This study was conducted by the International Radiogenomics Consortium (RgC) and more studies are expected on other cancers from this large multi-institutional collaboration (Andreassen et al. 2016). The authors conclude that such large scale studies are needed to detect weak signals in heterogeneous cohorts. These studies will help pinpoint relevant SNPs that could then be tested in the clinical setting.

7   Thoracic

The standard of care for locally advanced lung cancer is radiation or combination of chemotherapy and radiation. It is already known that small cell lung cancer and squamous cell non-small cell lung cancer respond more to chemoradiation versus non-small cell lung cancer with adenocarcinoma histology. Beyond this it is now known through analysis of the TCGA that lung cancer tends to carry more genetic mutations than was previously appreciated with just histology delineation and that mutations in lung cancer are unstable and can change over course of treatment or after 1st line treatment complete (Kan et al. 2010; Pikor et al. 2013). Predicting treatment response with this now appreciated wide array of non small cell lung cancer subtypes will be helpful to individualize treatment strategies.

Due to this plethora of mutations many studies to predict treatment response now use—omics data to find unique molecular signatures. One such study by Walker et al. (2015) used proteomics and assessed locally advanced non small cell lung cancer patients that had survived <14 months versus >18 months (Walker et al. 2015). Of 650 proteins analyzed they found that two proteins, CRP (C-reactive protein) and LRG1 (leucine-rich alpha-2-glycoprotein), were highly significant for extended survival when tested for high expression just one week post completion of standard radiation treatment. Less is known about LRG1 but there have been studies suggesting role in angiogenesis and can modulate TGF-beta, a known marker of inflammation (Walker et al. 2015). CRP is an acute phase reactant along the same pathway as IL-6 and correlates with previous studies implicating IL-6 in predicting survival to radiation (Walker et al. 2015). The hypothesis is that over-expression of acute phase reactants is detrimental to radiation response probably through excess toxicity via inflammation. This is an interesting study because it is trying to find early predictive markers to help guide patient treatment decisions. Generally, our first assessment of lung cancer patient's response to radiation is 3 months after completion of treatment but this early biomarker may help in deciding if treatment intensification is warranted (Bradley et al. 2015). Or as these markers may be involved in acute phase inflammation if early treatment to prevent inflammation such as pneumonitis should be initiated earlier rather than waiting to see if patient develops clinical symptoms.

Another pathway recently implicated in response to radiation is immune system activation especially with the advent of immunomodulator treatments concurrent with radiation for the treatment of advanced non small cell lung cancer. In a small study by Deng et al. (2016), the authors reported that high GM-CSF (granulocyte-macrophage colony stimulating factor) levels during radiation correlated with better overall survival and progression free survival (Deng et al. 2016). They also described a new test called the "integrated factor" that takes into account the degree of upregulation of GM-CSF as well as pre radiation levels of another immune pathway molecule IFN-gamma (interferon-gamma) and found this also correlated with prediction of better overall survival and progression free survival (Deng et al. 2016).

The main concerns of radiation to the lung are toxicities to lung itself or other structures of the mediastinum (esophagus, great vessels, heart). Acute pneumonitis and subsequent lung fibrosis are two main concerns of lung damage. Early studies assessed specific biomarkers known to be associated with inflammation. Zhao et al. analyzed the predictive role of TGF-beta1 a known inflammation maker with stage I-III lung cancer patients (Zhao et al. 2008). High levels of plasma TGF-beta1 4 weeks during radiation treatment was significantly predictive of $\geq$ grade 2 pneumonitis or fibrosis (Zhao et al. 2008). Kim et al. (2009) also observed that TGF-beta1 was significantly higher 4 weeks after radiation in patients who developed symptomatic radiation pneumonitis (Kim et al. 2009). Another more recent study looking at esophageal patients treated with radiation who would also have significant dose to lung also showed that plasma TGF-beta1 levels were elevated in patients who developed radiation pneumonitis (Li et al. 2015). Although these three studies suggested TGF1-beta as a biomarker, another small study could not find a correlation between either TGF1-beta or IL-6 and radiation pneumonitis (Rübe et al. 2008). In this negative study by Rube, the authors said that baseline

TGF1-beta and IL-6 levels were already elevated and there was no significant increase after radiation was complete (Rübe et al. 2008). As mentioned the molecular signature of lung cancer is now known to be highly variable and this can confound the data from these small studies. All these studies had small samples sizes and thus before we could use TGF-beta1 in the clinic, expression of this marker would need to be assessed in large scale lung cancer RTOG studies such as the recently completed RTOG 0617 (Bradley et al. 2015).

The other main toxicity in lung cancer is esophagitis (Bradley et al. 2015). The same biomarker TGF1-beta1 was assessed in lung cancer patients. This time Guerra et al. (2012) assessed SNPs in TGF-beta1 in 97 NSCLC patients (Guerra et al. 2012). They found that the SNP rs1800469: C-509T was significantly associated with higher risk of $\geq$ grade 3 radiation induced esophageal toxicity (Guerra et al. 2012).

Novel biomarker studies in lung cancer involve assessing micro RNAs (miRNA) (Dinh et al. 2016). miRNAs are small-non coding RNAs that are now known to function in silencing of RNA and regulation of gene expression. A small study of five patients with stage IIIA NSCLC at 5 different dose points during radiation was analyzed. miR29a-3p and miR-150-5p were shown to decrease as the radiation dose increased during course of treatment (Dinh et al. 2016). miR-150 has been shown to decrease in plasma in animals exposed to radiation (Dinh et al. 2016). miR-29a has already been associated with fibrosis in heart, lung and kidneys and so the authors hypothesize that extreme outliers of levels of these specific miRNAs may help predict toxicity to radiation (Dinh et al. 2016). Radiation dose could then be adapted based on the individual. This theory will be exciting to test in future studies of miRNAs because it will allow radiation oncologists to sculpt dose to tumor with confidence.

8   Intrinsic Radiosensitivity of Tissue/Organs

To predict response to radiation and to prevent toxicities we can look for predictive biomarkers in multiple ways either with a targeted approach of molecules implicated in affecting radiation or with a large scale, large data "-omics" type approach. The early studies focused on intrinsic cellular radiosensitivity (Williams et al. 2007). These studies formed the basis of calling some histologies radiation sensitive and some histologies radiation resistant. These studies looked at known oncogenes and tumor suppressor genes such as ATM and p53 and categorized cancer cell lines based on these genetic characteristics (Williams et al. 2007). ATM (ataxia telangiectasia mutated) was already implication in radiation sensitivity as individuals with AT (ataxia telangiectasia) are highly sensitive to radiation damage (Tribius et al. 2001). For radiation sensitive cancers there was less push for dose escalation whereas for radiation resistant there was more push for dose escalation and newer radiation techniques such as stereotactic body radiation (SBRT).

Another focus more recently has been on aging and the fact that intrinsic cellular radiosensitivity may actually change over time due to environmental exposures and oxidative damage (Mishra et al. 2012). Pathways studied include IL-6, CRP, TGF-beta1, advanced glycation end products (AGE), markers of inflammation. Telomere length is also being studied as we know that shorter telomere lengths over time lead to chromosomal instability and thus in theory more susceptibility to radiation damage (Mishra et al. 2012). Some of these pathways have been researched to assess a patient's "biological age" versus "chronological age" to aid in treatment management decisions. Historically biological age was a variable used to assess if radiation is warranted in certain cancers such as breast cancer. Chronological age may be more accurate in determining who best benefits from radiation.

9 Assessing Biomarkers in Clinic

Testing for biomarkers includes methods employed in the pathology laboratory including but not limited to: immunohistochemistry, mass spectroscopy, mutational analysis and gene expression analysis. The RTOG has a central storage for biospecimens and is a useful tool for testing biomarkers researched in basic science laboratories. Future assessments frequently use patient's serum which is also being banked in ongoing RTOG/NRG studies and validation of biomarkers with these large multi-institutional patient sample banks is necessary before a biomarker can be considered for routine clinical testing. As shown in sections in this chapter patient serum is being used to detect genomic and or molecular signatures of response to radiation through large scale—omics studies (genomics, proteomics).

10 Conclusion

While this chapter is by no means exhaustive of all biomarkers, this goal of the chapter is to highlight some common biomarkers and or genre of biomarkers researched to date to help guide current radiation practices. The goal of predictive radiation biomarkers is to help with individualizing radiation therapy. It will be exciting to see in coming years how big data, -omics, will help advance the field of radiation biomarkers.

References

Ahmed KA et al (2015) The radiosensitivity index predicts for overall survival in glioblastoma. Oncotarget 6(33):34414–34422

Andreassen CN et al (2016) Individual patient data meta-analysis shows a significant association between the ATM rs1801516 SNP and toxicity after radiotherapy in 5456 breast and prostate cancer patients. Radiother Oncol

Ang KK, Sturgis EM (2012) Human papillomavirus as a marker of the natural history and response to therapy of head and neck squamous cell carcinoma. Semin Radiat Oncol 22 (2):128–142

Ang KK et al (2010) Human papillomavirus and survival of patients with oropharyngeal cancer. N Engl J Med 363(1):24–35

Bradley JD et al (2015) Standard-dose versus high-dose conformal radiotherapy with concurrent and consolidation carboplatin plus paclitaxel with or without cetuximab for patients with stage IIIA or IIIB non-small-cell lung cancer (RTOG 0617): a randomised, two-by-two factorial phase 3 study. Lancet Oncol 16(2):187–199

Cerciello F et al (2007) Is EGFR a moving target during radiotherapy of carcinoma of the uterine cervix? Gynecol Oncol 106(2):394–399

Chau NG, Rabinowits G, Haddad RI (2014) Human papillomavirus-associated oropharynx cancer (HPV-OPC): treatment options. Curr Treat Options Oncol 15(4):595–610

Den RB et al (2014) Genomic prostate cancer classifier predicts biochemical failure and metastases in patients after postoperative radiation therapy. Int J Radiat Oncol Biol Phys 89(5):1038–1046

Deng G et al (2016) Elevated serum granulocyte-macrophage colony-stimulating factor levels during radiotherapy predict favorable outcomes in lung and esophageal cancer. Oncotarget

Dinh TK et al (2016) Circulating miR-29a and miR-150 correlate with delivered dose during thoracic radiation therapy for non-small cell lung cancer. Radiat Oncol 11:61

Eriksen JG et al (2004) The prognostic value of epidermal growth factor receptor is related to tumor differentiation and the overall treatment time of radiotherapy in squamous cell carcinomas of the head and neck. Int J Radiat Oncol Biol Phys 58(2):561–566

Eriksen JG et al (2005) The possible role of TP53 mutation status in the treatment of squamous cell carcinomas of the head and neck (HNSCC) with radiotherapy with different overall treatment times. Radiother Oncol 76(2):135–142

Eschrich SA et al (2009) A gene expression model of intrinsic tumor radiosensitivity: prediction of response and prognosis after chemoradiation. Int J Radiat Oncol Biol Phys 75(2):489–496

Ferdousi J et al (2010) Impact of human papillomavirus genotype on response to treatment and survival in patients receiving radiotherapy for squamous cell carcinoma of the cervix. Exp Ther Med 1(3):525–530

Grignon DJ et al (1997) p53 status and prognosis of locally advanced prostatic adenocarcinoma: a study based on RTOG 8610. J Natl Cancer Inst 89(2):158–165

Guerra JL et al (2012) Association between single nucleotide polymorphisms of the transforming growth factor β1 gene and the risk of severe radiation esophagitis in patients with lung cancer. Radiother Oncol 105(3):299–304

Herrlinger U et al (2016) Bevacizumab plus irinotecan versus temozolomide in newly diagnosed O6-methylguanine-DNA methyltransferase nonmethylated glioblastoma: the randomized GLARIUS trial. J Clin Oncol

Ho AY et al (2007) Possession of ATM sequence variants as predictor for late normal tissue responses in breast cancer patients treated with radiotherapy. Int J Radiat Oncol Biol Phys 69 (3):677–684

Hong A et al (2010) Relationships between epidermal growth factor receptor expression and human papillomavirus status as markers of prognosis in oropharyngeal cancer. Eur J Cancer 46 (11):2088–2096

Kabarriti R et al (2014) Prostate-specific antigen decline during salvage radiation therapy following prostatectomy is associated with reduced biochemical failure. Pract Radiat Oncol 4 (6):409–414

Kan Z et al (2010) Diverse somatic mutation patterns and pathway alterations in human cancers. Nature 466(7308):869–873

Kerns SL et al (2010) Genome-wide association study to identify single nucleotide polymorphisms (SNPs) associated with the development of erectile dysfunction in African-American men after radiotherapy for prostate cancer. Int J Radiat Oncol Biol Phys 78(5):1292–1300

Kim JY et al (2009) The TGF-beta1 dynamics during radiation therapy and its correlation to symptomatic radiation pneumonitis in lung cancer patients. Radiat Oncol 4:59

Koukourakis MI et al (2006) Endogenous markers of two separate hypoxia response pathways (hypoxia inducible factor 2 alpha and carbonic anhydrase 9) are associated with radiotherapy failure in head and neck cancer patients recruited in the CHART randomized trial. J Clin Oncol 24(5):727–735

Koukourakis MI et al (2016) Hypoxia-inducible proteins HIF1α and lactate dehydrogenase LDH5, key markers of anaerobic metabolism, relate with stem cell markers and poor post-radiotherapy outcome in bladder cancer. Int J Radiat Biol 92(7):353–363

Kyndi M et al (2008) Estrogen receptor, progesterone receptor, HER-2, and response to postmastectomy radiotherapy in high-risk breast cancer: the Danish breast cancer cooperative group. J Clin Oncol 26(9):1419–1426

Langlands FE et al (2013) Breast cancer subtypes: response to radiotherapy and potential radiosensitisation. Br J Radiol 86(1023):20120601

Langlands FE et al (2014) PSMD9 expression predicts radiotherapy response in breast cancer. Mol Cancer 13:73

Lassen P et al (2011) The influence of HPV-associated p16-expression on accelerated fractionated radiotherapy in head and neck cancer: evaluation of the randomised DAHANCA 6&7 trial. Radiother Oncol 100(1):49–55

Lassen P, Overgaard J, Eriksen JG (2013) Expression of EGFR and HPV-associated p16 in oropharyngeal carcinoma: correlation and influence on prognosis after radiotherapy in the randomized DAHANCA 5 and 7 trials. Radiother Oncol 108(3):489–494

Lassen P et al (2014) Impact of HPV-associated p16-expression on radiotherapy outcome in advanced oropharynx and non-oropharynx cancer. Radiother Oncol 113(3):310–316

Lau HY et al (2011) Prognostic significance of p16 in locally advanced squamous cell carcinoma of the head and neck treated with concurrent cisplatin and radiotherapy. Head Neck 33(2):251–256

Lee YS et al (2015) Composition of inflammatory cells regulating the response to concurrent chemoradiation therapy for HPV (+) tonsil cancer. Oral Oncol 51(12):1113–1119

Li J et al (2015) Transforming growth factor-beta-1 is a serum biomarker of radiation-induced pneumonitis in esophageal cancer patients treated with thoracic radiotherapy: preliminary results of a prospective study. Onco Targets Ther 8:1129–1136

Mishra MV, Showalter TN, Dicker AP (2012) Biomarkers of aging and radiation therapy tailored to the elderly: future of the field. Semin Radiat Oncol 22(4):334–338

Mumbrekar KD et al (2016) Genetic variants in CD44 and MAT1A confer susceptibility to acute skin reaction in breast cancer patients undergoing radiation therapy. Int J Radiat Oncol Biol Phys

Overgaard J et al (2005) Plasma osteopontin, hypoxia, and response to the hypoxia sensitiser nimorazole in radiotherapy of head and neck cancer: results from the DAHANCA 5 randomised double-blind placebo-controlled trial. Lancet Oncol 6(10):757–764

Pérez-Regadera J et al (2011) Impact of epidermal growth factor receptor expression on disease-free survival and rate of pelvic relapse in patients with advanced cancer of the cervix treated with chemoradiotherapy. Am J Clin Oncol 34(4):395–400

Petrik D et al (2006) Plasma osteopontin is an independent prognostic marker for head and neck cancers. J Clin Oncol 24(33):5291–5297

Pikor LA et al (2013) Genetic alterations defining NSCLC subtypes and their therapeutic implications. Lung Cancer 82(2):179–189

Pollack A et al (2004) Ki-67 staining is a strong predictor of distant metastasis and mortality for men with prostate cancer treated with radiotherapy plus androgen deprivation: radiation therapy oncology group trial 92-02. J Clin Oncol 22(11):2133–2140

Qin C et al (2014) Factors associated with radiosensitivity of cervical cancer. Anticancer Res 34 (9):4649–4656

Quon H et al (2013) Transoral robotic surgery and adjuvant therapy for oropharyngeal carcinomas and the influence of p16 INK4a on treatment outcomes. Laryngoscope 123(3):635–640

Ritter MA et al (2002) The role of p53 in radiation therapy outcomes for favorable-to-intermediate-risk prostate cancer. Int J Radiat Oncol Biol Phys 53(3):574–580

Rivera AL et al (2010) MGMT promoter methylation is predictive of response to radiotherapy and prognostic in the absence of adjuvant alkylating chemotherapy for glioblastoma. Neuro Oncol 12(2):116–121

Rübe CE et al (2008) Cytokine plasma levels: reliable predictors for radiation pneumonitis? PLoS ONE 3(8):e2898

Scherr DS et al (1999) BCL-2 and p 53 expression in clinically localized prostate cancer predicts response to external beam radiotherapy. J Urol 162(1):12–16; discussion 16–7

Shao J et al (2016) Breast cancer stem cells expressing different stem cell markers exhibit distinct biological characteristics. Mol Med Rep

Song YJ et al (2011) Persistent human papillomavirus DNA is associated with local recurrence after radiotherapy of uterine cervical cancer. Int J Cancer 129(4):896–902

Speers C et al (2016) Maternal embryonic leucine zipper kinase (MELK) as a novel mediator and biomarker of radioresistance in human breast cancer. Clin Cancer Res

Stupp R et al (2009) Effects of radiotherapy with concomitant and adjuvant temozolomide versus radiotherapy alone on survival in glioblastoma in a randomised phase III study: 5-year analysis of the EORTC-NCIC trial. Lancet Oncol 10(5):459–466

Thibodeau BJ et al (2015) Gene expression characterization of HPV positive head and neck cancer to predict response to chemoradiation. Head Neck Pathol 9(3):345–353

Tribius S, Pidel A, Casper D (2001) ATM protein expression correlates with radioresistance in primary glioblastoma cells in culture. Int J Radiat Oncol Biol Phys 50(2):511–523

Vainshtein JM et al (2014) Refining risk stratification for locoregional failure after chemoradio-therapy in human papillomavirus-associated oropharyngeal cancer. Oral Oncol 50(5):513–519

Walker MJ et al (2015) Discovery and validation of predictive biomarkers of survival for non-small cell lung cancer patients undergoing radical radiotherapy: two proteins with predictive value. EBioMedicine 2(8):841–850

Wang Y et al (2011) A retrospective study of breast cancer subtypes: the risk of relapse and the relations with treatments. Breast Cancer Res Treat 130(2):489–498

Wierzbicka M et al (2015) The rationale for HPV-related oropharyngeal cancer de-escalation treatment strategies. Contemp Oncol (Pozn) 19(4):313–322

Williams JR et al (2007) Human tumor cells segregate into radiosensitivity groups that associate with ATM and TP53 status. Acta Oncol 46(5):628–638

Woolston CM et al (2011) Expression of thioredoxin system and related peroxiredoxin proteins is associated with clinical outcome in radiotherapy treated early stage breast cancer. Radiother Oncol 100(2):308–313

Zhao L et al (2008) The predictive role of plasma TGF-beta1 during radiation therapy for radiation-induced lung toxicity deserves further study in patients with non-small cell lung cancer. Lung Cancer 59(2):232–239

The Mammalian DNA Damage Response as a Target for Therapeutic Gain in Radiation Oncology

Eric H. Radany

Abstract

Mutant cells that are defective for certain components of the mammalian DNA damage response (DDR) have been shown to display hypersensitivity to killing by ionizing radiations; these findings have prompted the idea that drugs that emulate these DDR deficiencies might serve as clinically useful radiosensitizers for improving results in cancer therapy. In this chapter, the ways in which several agents now established as radiosensitizers do in fact function by inhibiting parts of the DDR are first presented. The various subsystems of the DDR are next reviewed, and several potential molecular targets for discovery or design of chemical modifiers that could lead novel radiosensitizing drugs are discussed.

Keywords

DNA Damage Response (DDR) · DNA Repair · Double Strand Break (DSB) · Homologous Recombination Repair (HR) · Non-homologous End Joining Repair (NHEJ) · Radiation therapy (XRT) · Radiosensitizer · Therapeutic Ratio (TR)

1 The Challenge of Continuing to Improve the Therapeutic Ratio for Radiation Therapy in Human Oncology

Radiation therapy (XRT) continues to be a key modality in modern cancer medicine for both curative and palliative management of a variety of malignant diseases. It has been suggested that the role radiation therapy plays in obtaining local-regional

E.H. Radany (✉)
Department of Radiation Oncology, City of Hope National Medical Center,
1500 E. Duarte Rd., Duarte, CA 91010, USA
e-mail: eradany@coh.org

© Springer International Publishing AG 2017
J.Y.C. Wong et al. (eds.), *Advances in Radiation Oncology*,
Cancer Treatment and Research 172, DOI 10.1007/978-3-319-53235-6_11

control of tumors might in fact become increasingly important in the coming years as innovative systemic therapies, such as molecularly targeted agents and immune checkpoint modulators, improve our ability to eradicate microscopic metastatic disease for some patients (Citrin and Mitchell 2014). The recent 1–2 decades have witnessed impressive technical advances in the planning and delivery of XRT including multiple imaging modality simulation, 4-dimensional treatment planning and delivery, practical multibeam intensity modulated XRT, and daily image guidance for target positioning verification; several of these have supported development of effective new XRT approaches such as stereotactic body radiotherapy. Improving the conformality of XRT dose delivery in both space and time through these approaches is expected to improve the therapeutic ratio (TR) for XRT by minimizing normal tissue toxicity (Citrin and Mitchell 2014).

An improved TR for XRT can also be achieved by selectively enhancing the lethal effects of ionizing radiation (IR) on tumor versus normal tissues (Citrin and Mitchell 2014; Jekimovs et al. 2014; Gavande et al. 2016). Such an outcome might be obtainable by targeting certain features of malignant disease such as intratumoral hypoxia or host antitumor immune responses for example, but much current interest is centered upon manipulating biological IR responses at the level of individual malignant cells (Citrin and Mitchell 2014; Jekimovs et al. 2014; Gavande et al. 2016; Higgins et al. 2015; Raleigh and Haas-Kogan 2013). The term radiosensitizer properly refers to a chemical that increases cell death in response to a given dose of IR while being completely innocuous to cells in the absence of IR treatment (Citrin and Mitchell 2014; Higgins et al. 2015), although the term is often informally applied to agents such a chemotherapeutic drugs that can themselves be toxic to cells at sufficient doses; the latter are instead properly called chemical modifiers of cellular radiation response (Citrin and Mitchell 2014; Higgins et al. 2015). Drugs that usefully enhance tumor responses to IR are already extremely important in the clinic. Recent large gains in our understanding of the molecular genetics of cancer, along with ever-improving approaches to protein structure-based drug design, point to the strong likelihood that new, potent chemical modifiers for use with XRT will contribute to advances in human cancer medicine. This brief chapter will update and expand upon several recent excellent reviews of this topic (Citrin and Mitchell 2014; Jekimovs et al. 2014; Gavande et al. 2016; Higgins et al. 2015; Raleigh and Haas-Kogan 2013; Begg et al. 2011).

2 Radiosensitizing Agents Targeting the DNA Damage Response: Established Radiosensitizing Agents

2.1 Overview

Formation of DNA double strand breaks (DSB) at sufficient levels in human and other mammalian genomes, as by IR or certain chemotherapeutic agents, activates a complex signal transduction cascade—the DNA Damage Response (DDR)—that culminates in a range of cellular outcomes including repair of the DNA damage, cell cycle arrest at specific checkpoints, and programmed cell death; the DDR and these various endpoints have been reviewed extensively (Begg et al. 2011; Goodarzi and Jeggo 2013; Ceccaldi et al. 2016; Jeggo and Lobrich 2015; Waters et al. 2014; Jackson 2009) and will be covered here only briefly. Natural and engineered mammalian cells and animals that have gene mutations causing functional defects for components of the DDR are commonly IR hypersensitive to varying degrees, along with displaying "genomic instability" (see later). Human patients and mutant mouse strains with germline DDR gene defects often display increased susceptibility to various malignancies; some also have immunodeficiency related to a failure to repair the programmed DSB formed during the course of immunoglobulin and T-cell receptor gene maturation (Goodarzi and Jeggo 2013; Jackson 2009; Curtin 2012; Weinberg and Hanahan 2011). The finding that DDR gene mutations can cause mammalian cell IR hypersensitivity has given the impetus in recent years for discovery of chemical compounds that could inhibit the functions of various DDR proteins and emulate the effects of such gene defects (sometimes called "pharmacological phenocopy"); these agents would be expected to be candidate preclinical cellular radio- and chemo-sensitizers that might ultimately lead to useful drugs for human cancer medicine (Citrin and Mitchell 2014; Jekimovs et al. 2014; Gavande et al. 2016; Higgins et al. 2015; Raleigh and Haas-Kogan 2013). The finding that inhibition of different facets of the DDR is in fact the molecular mechanism of action for some radiosensitizers now used clinically, as detailed next, serves to validate this strategy.

2.2 Targeting DNA Damage Sensing/Signaling Pathways

Following induction of DSB in human nuclear DNA, their presence is sensed by the Mre11/Rad50/NBS1 (MRN) protein complex, which is recruited to the break ends by the human single stranded binding protein 1 (hSSB1); MRN then promotes association of the key damage signaling kinase Ataxia Telangiectasia Mutated (ATM) with the DSB (Begg et al. 2011; Goodarzi and Jeggo 2013; Ceccaldi et al. 2016). ATM kinase is thereby activated toward phosphorylation of itself, of the components of the MRN complex, and of the variant histone H2AX (thereby generating γH2AX) (Begg et al. 2011; Goodarzi and Jeggo 2013; Ceccaldi et al. 2016). γH2AX formation then propagates for many thousands of base pairs from the DSB ends into the DNA strands, and initiates assembly of an array of additional DDR proteins to form a molecular macrostructure, the ionizing radiation induced focus (IRIF) (Goodarzi and Jeggo 2013). ATM signaling is amplified by interactions within the IRIF and then transduced to downstream effectors such as the CHK2 kinase-p53 axis to initiate cell cycle arrest or apoptosis (Begg et al. 2011; Goodarzi and Jeggo 2013; Ceccaldi et al. 2016). Cells with deficient MRN function show severely impaired ATM signaling (Begg et al. 2011; Goodarzi and Jeggo 2013; Ceccaldi et al. 2016). The MRN complex (in particular, the Mre11 nuclease) plays an additional key role in the cellular "choice" between utilization of homologous recombination (HR) versus non-homologous end joining (NHEJ) mechanisms for the repair of DSB in the late-S and G2 phases of the cell cycle ((Begg et al. 2011; Goodarzi and Jeggo 2013; Ceccaldi et al. 2016) and see below). The observed IR sensitivity of MRN function-deficient cells thus makes sense.

Heat treatment of sufficient temperature and duration very potently sensitizes malignant human cells to killing by IR, a phenomenon termed hyperthermic radiosensitization (HtRs) (Dewey 2009). Given the magnitude of this effect, clinical application of HtRs has been of interest for decades, but implementation of this has been hindered previously by the engineering challenges connected with heating deep tumors in situ; this obstacle might now be overcome, however, with the development of MR-guided focused ultrasound technology (see Chapter **XX** of this text). The molecular basis of HtRs has been elucidated using a genetic approach termed epistasis analysis; this strategy is predicated on the fact that two separate functional defects ("hits") in the same mechanistic pathway should have no more consequence than either single hit alone does. In contrast, hits to separate pathways that function in parallel in a complementary fashion (for example, the NHEJ and HR mechanisms for DSB repair; see below) typically have a greater impact on cell physiology than either hit alone. Previous work had implicated one or more of the MRN complex protein components in HtRs, possibly via active export of these proteins out of the nucleus in response to heat treatment (Seno and Dynlacht 2004). The effect heating on clonogenic inactivation by IR was next investigated using cells having natural (cells derived from Mre11- or Nbs1-defective patients) or engineered (siRNA knockdown) deficiencies of Mre11, Nbs1, or Rad50 function (Dynlacht et al. 2011). For Nbs1 and Rad50, unheated cells were hypersensitive to killing by IR compared to normal cells, but that sensitivity was increased still further by the heat treatment. In contrast, heating of the Mre11 cells did not alter their already marked sensitivity to IR (Dynlacht et al. 2011). Purified Mre11 protein was also found to be unusually sensitive to heat denaturation in vitro (Dynlacht et al. 2011). The interpretation of these findings is that the Mre11-mutant cells are already maximally deficient for MRN-ATM signaling after DNA damage so that heat denaturation of any residual Mre11 protein has no consequence. In contrast, low levels of Nbs1 or Rad50 activity in the respective mutant cells did support some MRN-ATM signaling after IR, and this was abolished by total heat inactivation of cellular Mre11. In keeping with these findings, recently developed small molecule inhibitors of the Mre11 endo- and exonuclease activities are radiosensitizing agents in vitro (Shibata et al. 2014).

2.3 Targeting DSB Repair Pathways

Repair of DNA DSB in eukaryotic cell relies on two fundamentally distinct mechanisms, nonhomologous end joining (NHEJ) and homologous recombination (HR) repair (sometimes called homology directed repair) (Begg et al. 2011; Goodarzi and Jeggo 2013; Ceccaldi et al. 2016; Waters et al. 2014; Pannunzio et al. 2014; Moynahan and Jasin 2010). NHEJ entails the nucleolytic processing and direct ligation of DSB ends that may approximately restore the original configuration of a stretch of DNA (typically with loss of some of the nucleotides adjacent to the strand breaks). Alternatively, DNA ends from remote parts of the genome might be brought together by NHEJ repair, forming a chromosomal translocation or inversion (Begg et al. 2011; Goodarzi and Jeggo 2013; Ceccaldi et al. 2016). The kinetics of end joining by this mechanism is determined by the chemistry of the DNA termini and by the chromatin configuration of the DNA within which the DSB occurs; chemically complex ends produced by relatively high LET radiations, and the compacted chromatin associated with heterochromatic chromosomal regions lead to slower end rejoining (Begg et al. 2011; Goodarzi and Jeggo 2013; Ceccaldi et al. 2016). Quite recently, it has been possible to distinguish between so-called canonical NHEJ (the mechanism identified first) and one or more "alternative" NHEJ pathways (Begg et al. 2011; Goodarzi and Jeggo 2013; Ceccaldi et al. 2016; Pannunzio et al. 2014); these differ with respect to the specific proteins involved and the precise molecular details of DNA end synapsis during DSB end rejoining (Begg et al. 2011; Goodarzi and Jeggo 2013; Ceccaldi et al. 2016; Pannunzio et al. 2014). How these various NHEJ processes might be differently targeted for achieving radiosensitization remains to be seen.

HR repair of DSB is initiated by quite extensive exonucleolytic degradation of DNA, starting at the break ends and proceeding in the $5' \rightarrow 3'$ direction, thereby forming long single strands having $3'$ hydroxyl termini (Begg et al. 2011; Goodarzi and Jeggo 2013; Ceccaldi et al. 2016; Moynahan and Jasin 2010). Those strands invade nearby intact homologous DNA (this is typically afforded by the adjacent sister chromatid following replication) and prime the synthesis of new DNA corresponding to the regions surrounding the DSB, using the intact complementary strands as templates. The new DNA strands are then extracted from the sister chromatid and reannealed; ligation of the new DNA $3'$ ends to $5'$ ends of the broken chromatid completes repair of the DSB (Begg et al. 2011; Goodarzi and Jeggo 2013; Ceccaldi et al. 2016; Moynahan and Jasin 2010).

HR contrasts with NHEJ in that the latter has no mechanistic requirement for the presence intact homologous DNA nearby (Begg et al. 2011; Goodarzi and Jeggo 2013; Ceccaldi et al. 2016). For this reason, NHEJ is practicable throughout the cell cycle, while HR is confined to the G2 phase and to those genomic regions that have already undergone replication during S phase (Begg et al. 2011; Goodarzi and Jeggo 2013; Ceccaldi et al. 2016). NHEJ appears to be responsible for the majority of DSB repair throughout the cell cycle in mammalian cells, this despite it being much more "error prone" than HR, given the likelihood of small DNA sequence changes in the vicinity of the DSB and the potential to form gross chromosomal aberrations (Begg et al. 2011; Goodarzi and Jeggo 2013; Ceccaldi et al. 2016; Pannunzio et al. 2014). The mechanistic basis for the cellular "decision" between use of NHEJ versus HR for the repair of a given DSB during G2 or S phase is at present poorly understood and is the subject of much research activity, although the MRN complex appears to be intimately involved (Begg et al. 2011; Goodarzi and Jeggo 2013; Ceccaldi et al. 2016; Shibata et al. 2014).

2.3.1 Targeting the NHEJ Pathway

Curative-intent treatment programs combining XRT and a platinum-containing chemotherapeutic drug such as cisplatin (CDDP) are widely used in human oncology, and have led to improved clinical outcomes for different forms of lung cancer, head and neck cancer, and carcinoma of the uterine cervix among other malignancies (Sears et al. 2016). The mechanistic basis for radiosensitization by platinum-containing drugs has been investigated in vitro. An epistasis analysis showed that CDDP treatment did not sensitize the killing of NHEJ-deficient cells by IR, while HR-defective were markedly sensitized (Raaphorst et al. 2005); this result indicates that NHEJ does not function properly in CDDP-treated cells. NHEJ can be assayed in vitro in mammalian cells extracts by following ligation of linear substrate DNA molecules (Sears and Turchi 2012; Diggle et al. 2005). The presence of CDDP damage in the substrate molecules inhibited NHEJ in vitro (Sears and Turchi 2012; Diggle et al. 2005), while extracts prepared from CDDP-treated cells were NHEJ-competent for repair of undamaged substrate DNA molecules (Sears and Turchi 2012); these results support the model that it is CDDP adducts in DNA near DSB are a block to repair by NHEJ. In keeping with this model, so-call host reactivation of transfected substrate DNA molecules by NHEJ is proficient for undamaged substrates transfected into CDDP-treated cells, but deficient for CDDP-damaged substrates transfected into untreated cells (Sears and Turchi 2012).

2.3.2 Targeting the HR Pathway

The HR pathway for DSB repair depends upon synthesis of long stretches of new DNA using an undamaged sister chromatid as the template (Begg et al. 2011; Goodarzi and Jeggo 2013; Ceccaldi et al. 2016; Moynahan and Jasin 2010); it might thus be anticipated that antimetabolite chemotherapy drugs which deprive mammalian cells of DNA synthetic precursors might serve as effective HR repair inhibitors. Gemcitabine is an antimetabolite chemotherapeutic agent that inhibits ribonucleotide reductase and the de novo synthesis of deoxynucleotide DNA precursors. Gemcitabine is also a potent radiosensitizers (Shewach and Lawrence 1995; Van Putten et al. 2001; Wachters et al. 2001). Using epistasis analysis, the mechanism of gemcitabine radiosensitization was investigated in mammalian cells deficient in NHEJ and HR (Van Putten et al. 2001; Wachters et al. 2001). Following treatment with gemcitabine, radiosensitization was observed in the NHEJ-deficient cells, but this was markedly decreased in the HR-deficient cell, demonstrating that this drug blocks the latter pathway (Van Putten et al. 2001; Wachters et al. 2001). Investigation of the mechanism of radiosensitization by various fluoropyrimidine family drugs, another class of clinically useful antimetabolite chemotherapeutic radiosensitizers, has proven to be more complex (Canman et al. 1994). This may be because, while these agents inhibit thymidine (TdR) DNA precursor synthesis, the simultaneously promote incorporation of deoxyuridine (UdR) into nascent DNA in place of TdR (Canman et al. 1994).

2.4 Targeting Prosurvival/Anti-apoptotic Signaling Pathways

Following DNA damage and several other cellular stresses, many normal cells and certain malignant cells undergo a process of programmed cell death termed apoptosis (Balcer-Kubiczek 2012). For cells exposed to IR, DDR signaling through ATM ultimately impinges upon the tumor suppressor protein p53 and activates it as a transcription factor (Begg et al. 2011; Goodarzi and Jeggo 2013; Ceccaldi et al. 2016; Balcer-Kubiczek 2012). Depending upon cellular context, p53 activation promotes either apoptosis or cell cycle arrest in G1 phase by transcriptional regulation of specific genes (Balcer-Kubiczek 2012). In the checks and balances of cellular governance, pro-apoptotic influences are countered by pro-survival signaling; the Akt serine/threonine kinases are key mediators of the latter process (Balcer-Kubiczek 2012; Toulany and Roderman 2015). Loss of proper apoptotic response to cellular stress appears to be an essential component of carcinogenesis for many cell types (Weinberg and Hanahan 2011); enhanced Akt signaling by several different mechanisms has been found to be one means by which malignant cells can achieve this abrogation of apoptosis (Cengel et al. 2007; Mckenna et al. 2003; Cheung and Testa 2013). Akt activation in tumors is associated with chemotherapy and radiotherapy treatment resistance (Cengel et al. 2007; Mckenna et al. 2003; Cheung and Testa 2013; Sekhar et al. 2011; Kao et al. 2007; Misale et al. 2012; Garrido-Laguna et al. 2012), and down regulation of Akt signaling by dominant negative inhibition or drug targeting of its upstream signaling partner PI3 kinase (PI3K) has been shown in some cases to cause radiosensitization (Tanno et al. 2004). These finding are believed to reflect, at least in some cells, mitigation of the killing effects of IR by pro-survival Akt signaling by these inhibitory interventions (Toulany and Roderman 2015; Tanno et al. 2004; Brognard et al. 2001). Importantly, however, more recent results indicate that activated Akt also plays significant, directs role in cellular responses to IR including DNA DSB sensing/signaling and regulation of NHEJ; targeting activated Akt may thus instead (or in addition) radiosensitize some cells by inhibiting DSB repair (Toulany et al. 2008, 2012; Park et al. 2009).

Akt is a downstream effector of several mitogenic (pro-growth) signaling cascades that are frequently found to be corrupted in tumor cells (Toulany and Roderman 2015; Cheung and Testa 2013); prominent among these are activating mutations and amplification of genes encoding cell surface receptor tyrosine kinases (RTKs) such as EGFR (Weinberg and Hanahan 2011; Toulany and Roderman 2015; Cheung and Testa 2013). One target of deregulated EGFR signaling in tumors, via PI3K, is Akt (Toulany and Roderman 2015; Cheung and Testa 2013). Significant correlations have been found for many tumors between EGFR activation and Akt activation (Cheung and Testa 2013; Nijkamp et al. 2011), and between EGFR activation and chemo/radiation resistance (Ang et al. 2002; Nakamura 2007); findings such as these have made EGFR signaling an attractive target for cancer therapy (Seshacharyulu et al. 2012; Dassonville et al. 2007). Cetuximab, a recombinant monoclonal antibody therapeutic that down regulates EGFR signaling has been investigated in combination with XRT patients with colon cancer, non-small cell lung cancer, and head and neck cancers (Seshacharyulu et al. 2012), and is now in routine use for the latter given its efficacy as a radiosensitizer (Bobber et al. 2010). Erlotinib, a small molecule EGFR TK inhibitor also shows radiosensitizing activity for some malignant cells, and has shown this activity in the clinic in a promising way for patients with brain metastases of non-small cell lung cancer (Zheng et al. 2016).

3 DNA Damage Response: Recent Results for Radiosensitizing Agents

3.1 Targeting DNA Damage Sensing/Signaling Pathways

The ataxia telangiectasia-mutated (ATM) protein is defective in that disease and is a pivotal player in the early steps of DSB detection (Jekimovs et al. 2014; Begg et al. 2011; Goodarzi and Jeggo 2013; Ceccaldi et al. 2016; Jeggo and Lobrich 2015). A-T patients inherit two defective germline copies of the ATM gene, and are characteristically both cancer-prone and hypersensitive to IR (Jekimovs et al. 2014; Begg et al. 2011; Goodarzi and Jeggo 2013; Ceccaldi et al. 2016; Jeggo and Lobrich 2015). ATM inactivation by somatic mutation is a common finding in many tumors, and is thought to be a mechanism for the genomic instability that is believed to be required of carcinogenesis (Jekimovs et al. 2014; Jeggo and Lobrich 2015). ATM is a member of the PI3K-like kinase (PIKK) family that also includes ATR (for ATM-mutated and Rad3-related), DNA-PKcs (DNA-dependent protein kinase catalytic subunit, a core component of the canonical NHEJ pathway), and PI3K itself, along with multiple other proteins (Jeggo and Lobrich 2015). The kinase ATP binding pocket has been a common target for discovery of numerous kinase-inhibiting drugs such as erlotinib; this approach has been problematic for the PIKK family proteins due to difficulty in achieving sufficient target specificity to allow clinical use, however (Jekimovs et al. 2014; Gavande et al. 2016; Higgins et al. 2015; Raleigh and Haas-Kogan 2013). Sufficient success in this regard has been obtained to date for the ATR kinase (Jekimovs et al. 2014; Gavande et al. 2016; Higgins et al. 2015; Raleigh and Haas-Kogan 2013; Jeggo and Lobrich 2015; Sanjiv et al. 2016) to allow inhibitory drugs to enter clinical trials, some in combination with XRT.

As is the case for ATM, ATR contributes to maintaining genomic integrity after various genotoxic insults. ATR appears to be activated primarily by single stranded DNA associated with replication forks during periods of replicative stress (Jeggo and Lobrich 2015; Waters et al. 2014; Jackson 2009), such as DNA synthesis using damaged template strands following IR exposure (Jeggo and Lobrich 2015; Waters et al. 2014; Jackson 2009). Like for ATM, ATR activation leads to cell cycle arrest at a specific checkpoint, in this case S/G2 phase. It has been hypothesized that the loss of G1 checkpoint in ATM-deficient tumor cells renders them more dependent upon integrity of the ATR-mediated S/G2 checkpoint after genotoxic insults such as

IR exposure (Sanjiv et al. 2016). The specific ATR kinase inhibitor VX-970 has been shown to sensitize adenocarcinoma cells to IR and to several chemotherapeutic drugs that cause replication stress (Sanjiv et al. 2016). Based on these findings, VX-970 is currently being investigated in combination with whole brain XRT in patients with brain metastases from non-small cell lung cancer (NCI trial designation NCT02589522).

3.2 Targeting DSB Repair Pathways

3.2.1 Targeting the NHEJ Pathway

The Ku70 protein is a core component, along with Ku80 protein and DNA-PKcs, of the DNA-PK complex that mediates the initial steps of canonical NHEJ (Goodarzi and Jeggo 2013; Waters et al. 2014). Ku70 protein was found to interact with the androgen receptor in prostate carcinoma (CaP) cells (Al-Ubaidi et al. 2013), an observation that motivated study of Ku70 levels and endogenous NHEJ activity in biopsies of CaP in patients, both before and after surgical or pharmacological (GnRH treatment) castration (Al-Ubaidi et al. 2013). Ku70 levels were found to be reduced, and spontaneous γH2AX foci (this is a measure of persisting DSB formed during replication, an indication of reduced NHEJ) were increased following castration (Al-Ubaidi et al. 2013). The remarkable result of these findings was the prediction that initial ("neoadjuvant") androgen deprivation, via surgical or pharmacological means, might be a radiosensitizer for subsequent prostate XRT. To test this hypothesis, 48 patients in a small pilot trial were randomly assigned to neoadjuvant androgen deprivation or not prior to receiving XRT as 2 Gy × 5 fractions; biopsies were obtained prior to any intervention or after the 10 Gy XRT (Tarish et al. 2015). Autophosphorylation of DNA-PKcs, a measure of canonical NHEJ activity (Jeggo and Lobrich 2015; Toulany and Roderman 2015), was strongly upregulated following XRT without prior androgen deprivation, but completely abolished with the androgen deprivation (Tarish et al. 2015). An increased number of persisting nuclear γH2AX foci were observed in the trial castration arm, a finding also consistent with failure of DSB repair in the setting of neoadjuvant androgen deprivation (Tarish et al. 2015). Studies with long term follow up and larger patient numbers will be required to determine whether the putative NHEJ inhibition and radiosensitization in this setting leads to superior local control of CaP.

3.2.2 Targeting the HR Pathway

Protein acetylation on lysine residues is a post-translational protein modification that is increasingly appreciated to be a mode of intracellular signaling comparable to protein phosphorylation (Ceccacci and Minucci 2016; West and Johnstone 2014). This modification was first described for chromatin histone proteins, and the enzymes that add and remove these acetyl groups are called histone acetyl transferases (HATs) and histone deacetylases (HDACs), respectively; many non-histone proteins are clearly substrates for HATs and HDACs as well, however (Ceccacci and Minucci 2016; West and Johnstone 2014; Elia et al. 2015). Signaling via protein acetylation/deacetylation has recently been found to play an important role in the mammalian cellular DNA damage response (Elia et al. 2015). A number of HDAC-inhibiting drugs are showing interesting activity as anti-cancer agents, particularly for hematolymphoid malignancies (Ceccacci and Minucci 2016; West and Johnstone 2014). Several HDAC inhibitors have also been shown to act as radiosensitizers (Camphausen et al. 2004; Chinnaiyan et al. 2008; Chen et al. 2012). Although effects on histone modification and chromatin configuration were suggested to be the mechanistic basis for these findings, persisting acetylation of non-histone proteins clearly also plays a role. For example, we and others have shown that HDAC inhibitors reduce DSB repair via the HR pathway (Chen et al. 2012; Adimoolam et al. 2007). In the case of potent and clinically approved drug SAHA, treatment of multiple myeloma cells at low, non-toxic concentrations led to significant radiosensitization, specifically by inhibiting the HR pathway for DSB repair (Chen et al. 2012). This effect is apparently caused by blocking upregulation of the key HR pathway protein Rad51, and inhibiting normal Rad51 association with chromatin, following IR exposure (Chen et al. 2012; Adimoolam et al. 2007). It is not yet known what protein(s) experiences persistent acetylation in the presence of the drug to mediate these events. Concurrent SAHA treatment would thus be a rational approach to enhancing efficacy of XRT for this disease.

The findings noted here support the ideas that small molecule inhibitors of the NHEJ and HR repair pathways may be useful clinically as cytotoxins and radiosensitizers. As regards the former, an inhibitor of DNA-PKcs and the PIKK m-TOR (mammalian target of rapamycin), CC-115 has shown activity as a single agent in chronic lymphocytic leukemia (Thijssen et al. 2016), and is being characterized with respect to dosing and tolerability in a Phase I trial of advanced solid malignancies (NCI trial designation NCT01353625). Use of this agent along with XRT in patients has not yet been reported. Small molecule inhibitors of HR have been reported, and are in the preclinical phase of development (Huang et al. 2011; Budke et al. 2013; Zhu et al. 2013).

3.3 Targeting Pro-apoptotic Signaling

In addition to transcriptional activation of pro-apoptotic nuclear genes (Balcer-Kubiczek 2012), the p53 tumor suppressor protein can also activate apoptosis as a DDR endpoint through processes mediated at the outer mitochondrial membrane (Chipuk et al. 2002; Chen et al. 2011; Sykes et al. 2006). Treatment with the HDAC inhibitor drug Valproic Acid (VPA) was shown to promote radiosensitization via apoptosis after IR exposure—a response not typically displayed–in two CaP cell lines, but not a third one (Chen et al. 2011). The CaP line showing no radiosensitization did not contain any p53 protein, while the other two lines did, perhaps implicating p53 in the radiosensitization mechanism. However, one of the two CaP lines that did display radiosensitization contained only mutant forms of p53 protein having no activity as a transcription factor (Chen et al. 2011); this fact would argue against the model for p53 involvement in the radiosensitization (at least with respect to its best known function as an regulator of nuclear gene expression).

p53 is a substrate for the HAT Tip60, which acetylates a specific p53 lysine residue in response to DNA damage and other pro-apoptotic stresses (Sykes et al. 2006); this modification activates p53 transcription factor activity toward pro-apoptotic gene targets specifically (Sykes et al. 2006). We and others showed that this modification also activates p53 toward its pro-apoptotic interactions at the mitochondrial membrane, and that some mutant forms of p53 that are inactive as transcription factors are proficient for this process (Chen et al. 2011; Mellert et al. 2011). Following IR, p53 in untreated CaP cells is acetylated by Tip60, but it is then promptly deacetylated (by HDAC1 (Mellert et al. 2011)) and an apoptotic response does not ensue. With VPA treatment, p53 acetylation persists and a sufficient quantity of this modified form of the protein accumulates at the mitochondrial membrane to trigger apoptosis (Chen et al. 2011; Mellert et al. 2011). This adds to amount of cell killing produced by a given dose of IR—the definition of radiosensitization. This mechanism appears to be operative in colorectal carcinoma cells as well (Chen et al. 2009).

4 Future Directions and Promise

Statistical analyses and in vitro studies have led to the conclusion that multiple independent mutational genetic changes are required to convert a fully normal human cell into a fully malignant one (Hahn et al. 1999). Loeb was first to recognized that the fidelity of mammalian genomic replication is sufficiently good that this number of mutations could never accumulate in a human cell during a human lifetime and cause a malignant tumor, a conclusion clearly inconsistent with the clinical problem of cancer. Based on this, Loeb proposed the Mutator Phenotype hypothesis (Loeb 2016), which states the premalignant cells must somehow lose mechanisms of replicative fidelity early in the course of neoplastic transformation and thereby become able to acquire the required mutation burden. A number of observations have shown this idea to be correct, notably the findings of recurrent DNA repair pathway defects in a wide range of human tumor types (Jeggo and Lobrich 2015; Waters et al. 2014; Jackson 2009; Curtin 2012; Weinberg and Hanahan 2011). Malignant cells having a mutator phenotype are often said to have developed "genomic instability".

Mutational inactivation of components of the DNA Damage Response is a frequent cause of genomic instability in tumors (Jeggo and Lobrich 2015; Waters et al. 2014; Jackson 2009; Curtin 2012; Weinberg and Hanahan 2011). It has become clear that, in some cases, such mutational events create in malignant cells an absolute dependence upon the integrity of other DDR components for cell survival, a situation termed "synthetic lethality" (Gavande et al. 2016; Sanjiv et al. 2016; Morgan and Lawrecne 2015). The now classic example of this is the dependence of HR pathway-deficient BRCA1/2 tumor cells on integrity of the DNA Base Excision Repair (BER) system (Jackson 2009; Morgan and Lawrecne 2015). The BER system deals with DNA single strand breaks (SSB) that arise in nascent DNA during replication (Jackson 2009; Morgan and Lawrecne 2015) and it is regulated by poly-ADP ribose polymerase (PARP). If nascent strand SSB are left unrepaired, they will be present in some of the template DNA strands during the next round of replication, and cause replication fork collapse. Rescue of collapsed replication forks depends in turn upon function of the HR pathway. If BER is blocked in BRCA1/2 cells by inhibiting PARP with the drug olaparib, cell death results from breakdown of DNA replication (Jackson 2009; Morgan and Lawrecne 2015). Conversely, malignant cells having BER defects resulting from loss of DNA polymerase β (Morgan and Lawrecne 2015) would be expected to experience synthetic lethality with HR pathway inhibition.

As noted before, IR exposure is capable of provoking synthetic lethal interactions: ATR inhibition with VX-970 in malignant cells is tolerated in unstressed cells, but it is lethal in combination with replicative stress provoked by certain chemotherapeutic agents and IR (Sanjiv et al. 2016). It seems likely that other cases of synthetic lethality in tumor cells, in the context of combined IR and DDR inhibitor treatment, will be found, given the enormous range of genotoxic damages that IR causes (Citrin and Mitchell 2014; Jekimovs et al. 2014; Gavande et al. 2016; Higgins et al. 2015; Raleigh and Haas-Kogan 2013; Begg et al. 2011; Goodarzi and Jeggo 2013; Ceccaldi et al. 2016; Jeggo and Lobrich 2015; Waters et al. 2014). This prospect is an exciting one, given the remarkable ability to localize IR dose deposition with modern radiation therapy technology.

References

Adimoolam S, Sirisawad M, Chen J, Thiemann P, Ford JM, Buggy JJ (2007) HDAC inhibitor PCI-24781 decreased RAD51 expression and inhibits homologous recombination. Proc Natl Acad Sci USA 104:19482–19487

Al-Ubaidi FL, Schultz N, Loseva O, Egevad L, Granfors T, Helleday T (2013) Castration therapy results in decreased Ku70 levels in prostate cancer. Clin Cancer Res 19:1547–1556

Ang KK, Berkey BA, Tu X, Zhang HZ, Katz R, Hammond EH et al (2002) Impact of epidermal growth factor receptor expression on survival and pattern of relapse in patients with advanced head and neck carcinoma. Cancer Res 62:7350–7356

Balcer-Kubiczek EK (2012) Apoptosis in radiation therapy: a double-edged sword. Exp Oncol 34:277–285

Begg AC, Stewart FA, Vens C (2011) Strategies to improve radiotherapy with targeted drugs. Nature Rev Cancer 11:239–253

Bobber JA, Harari PM, Giralt J, Cohen RB, Jones CU et al (2010) Radiotherapy plus Cetuximab for locoregionally advanced head and neck cancer: 5-year survival data from a phase 3 randomized trial, and relation between Cetuximab-induced rash and survival. Lancet Oncol 11:21–28

Brognard J, Clark AS, Ni Y, Dennis PA (2001) Akt/protein kinase B is constitutively active in non-small cell lung cancer cells and promotes cellular survival and resistance to chemotherapy and radiation. Cancer Res 61:3986–3997

Budke B, Kalin JH, Pawlowski M, Zelivianskaia AS, Wu M et al (2013) An optimized RAD51 inhibitor that disrupts homologous recombination without requiring Michael acceptor reactivity. J Med Chem 56:254–263

Camphausen K, Burgan W, Cerra M, Oswald KA, Trepel JB et al (2004) Enhanced radiation enhanced-induced killing and prolongation of gammaH2AX foci expression by the histone deacetylase inhibitor MS-275. Cancer Res 64:316–321

Canman CE, Radany EH, Parsels LA, Davis MA, Lawrence TS, Maybaum J (1994) Cancer Res 54:2296–2298

Ceccacci E, Minucci S (2016) Inhibition of histone deacetylases in cancer therapy: lessons from leukaemia. Br J Cancer 114:605–611

Ceccaldi R, Rondinelli B, D'Andrea AD (2016) Repair pathway choices and consequences at the double-strand break. Trends Cell Biol 26:52–63

Cengel KA, Voong KR, Chandrasekaran S, Maggiorella L, Brunner TB, Stanbridge E et al (2007) Oncogenic K-Ras signals through epidermal growth factor receptor and wild-type H-Ras to promote radiation survival in pancreatic and colorectal carcinoma cells. Neoplasia 9:341–348

Chen X, Wong P, Radany E, Wong JY (2009) HDAC inhibitor, valproic acid, induces p53-dependent radiosensitization of colon cancer cells. Cancer Biother Radiopharm 24:689–699

Chen X, Wong JYC, Wong P, Radany EH (2011) Low-dose valproic acid enhances radiosensitivity of prostate cancer through acetylated p53-dependent modulation of mitochondrial membrane potential and apoptosis. Mol Cancer Res 9:448–461

Chen X, Wong P, Radany EH, Stark JM, Laulier C, Wong JY (2012) Suberoylanilide hydroxamic acid as a radiosensitizer through modulation of RAD51 protein and inhibition of homology-directed repair in multiple myeloma. Mol Cancer Res 10:1052–1064

Cheung M, Testa JR (2013) Diverse mechanisms of AKT pathway activation inhuman malignancy. Curr Cancer Drug Targets 13:234–244

Chinnaiyan P, Cerna D, Burgan WE, Beam K, Williams ES et al (2008) Postradiation sensitization by the histone deacetylase inhibitor valproic acid. Clin Cancer Res 14:5410–5415

Chipuk JE, Kuwana T, Bouchier-Hayes L, Droin NM, Newmeyer DD et al (2002) Direct activation of Bax by p53 mediates mitochondrial membrane permeabilization and apoptosis. Science 303:1010–1014

Citrin DE, Mitchell JB (2014) Altering the response to radiation: sensitizers and protectors. Semin Oncol 41:848–859

Curtin N (2012) J DNA repair dysregulation from cancer driver to therapeutic target. Nat Rev Cancer 12:801–817

Dassonville O, Bozec A, Fischel JL, Milano G (2007) EGFR targeting therapies: monoclonal antibodies versus tyrosine kinase inhibitors. Similarities and differences. Crit Rev Oncol Hematol 62:53–61

Dewey WC (2009) Arrhenius relationships from the molecule and cell to the clinic. Int J Hyperthermia 23:3–20

Diggle CP, Bentley J, Knowles MA, Kiltie AE (2005) Inhibition of double-strand break non-homologous end joining by cisplatin adducts in human cell extracts. Nucleic Acids Res 33:2531–2539

Dynlacht JR, Batuello CN, Lopez JT, Kim KK, Turchi JJ (2011) Identification of Mre11 as a target for heat radiosensitization. Radiat Res 176:323–332

Elia AE, Boardman AP, Wang DC, Huttlin EL, Everley RA et al (2015) Quantitative proteomic atlas of ubiquitination and acetylation in the DNA damage response. Mol Cell 59:867–881

Garrido-Laguna I, Hong DS, Janku F, Nguyen LM, Falchook GS, Fu S et al (2012) KRASness and PIK3CAness in patients with advanced colorectal cancer: outcome after treatment with early-phase trials with targeted pathway inhibitors. PLoS ONE 7:e38033

Gavande NS, Vandervere-Carozza PS, Hinshaw HD, Jalal SI, Sears CR et al (2016) DNA repair targeted therapy: the past or future of cancer treatment? Pharmcol Ther 160:65–83

Goodarzi AA, Jeggo PA (2013) The repair and signaling responses to DNA double-strand breks. AnvGenet 82:1–45

Hahn WC, Counter CM, Lundberg AS, Beijersbergen RL, Brooks MW, Weinberg RA (1999) Creation of human tumor cells with defined genetic elements. Nature 400:464–468

Higgins GS, O'Cathail SM, Muschel RJ, McKenna WG (2015) Drug radiotherapy combinations: review of previous failures and reasons for future optimism. Cancer Treat Rev 41:105–113

Huang F, Motlekar NA, Burgwin CM, Napper AD, Diamond SL, Mazin AV (2011) Identification of specific inhibitors of human RAD51 recombinase using high throughput screening. ACS Chem Biol 6:628–635

Jackson SP (2009) Bartek J The DNA damage response in human biology and disease. Nature 461:1071–1078

Jeggo PA, Lobrich M (2015) How cancer cells hijack DNA double-strand break repair pathways to gain genomic instability. Biochem J 471:1–11

Jekimovs C, Bolderson E, Suraweera A, Adams M, O'Byrne KJ, Richard DJ (2014) Chemotherapeutic compounds targeting the DNA double strand break repair pathways. Front Oncol 4:1–18

Kao GD, Jiang Z, Fernandes AM, Gupta AK, Maity A (2007) Inhibition of phosphatidylinositol-3-OH kinase/Akt signaling impairs DNA repair in glioblastoma cells following ionizing radiation. J Biol Chem 282:21206–21212

Loeb LA (2016) Human cancers express a mutator phenotype: hypothesis, origin, and consequences. Cancer Res 76:2057–2059

Mckenna WG, Muchel RJ, Gupta AK, Hahn SM, Bernhard EJ (2003) The RAS signal transduction pathway and its role in radiation sensitivity. Oncogene 22:5866–5875

Mellert HS, Stanek TJ, Sykes SM, Rauscher FJ, Schultz DC, McMahon SB (2011) Deacetylation of the DNA-binding domain regulates p53-mediated apoptosis. J Biol Chem 286:4264–4270

Misale S, Yaeger R, Hobor S, Scala E, Janakiraman M, Liska D et al (2012) Emergence of KRAS mutations and acquired resistance to anti-EGFR therapy in colorectal cancer. Nature 486:532–536

Morgan MA, Lawrecne TS (2015) Molecular pathways: overcoming radiation resistance by targeting DNA damage response pathways. Clin Cancer Res 21:2898–2904

Moynahan ME, Jasin M (2010) Mitotic homologous recombination maintains genomic stability and suppresses tumorigenesis. Nat Rev Mol Cell Biol 11:196–207

Nakamura JL (2007) The epidermal growth factor receptor in malignant gliomas: pathogenesis and therapeutic implications. Expert Opin Ther Targets 11:463–472

Nijkamp MM, Hoogsteen IJ, Span PN, Takes RP, Lok J, Rijken PF et al (2011) Spatial relationship of phosphorylated epidermal growth factor receptor and activated AKT in head and neck squamous cell carcinoma. Radiother Oncol 101:165–170

Pannunzio NR, Li S, Watanabe G, Lieber MR (2014) NHEJ often uses microhomology: implications for alternative end joining. DNA Repair 17:74–80

Park J, Feng J, Li Y, Hammarsten O, Brazil DP, Hemmings BA (2009) DNA-dependent protein kinase-mediated phosphorylation of protein kinase B requires a specific recognition sequence in the C-terminal hydrophobic motif. J Biol Chem 284:6169–6174

Raaphorst GPGP, Leblanc J-M, Li LF (2005) A comparison of response to cisplatin, radiation and combined treatment for cells deficient in recombination repair pathways. Anticancer Res 25:3–58

Raleigh DR, Haas-Kogan DA (2013) Molecular targets and mechanisms of radiosensitization using DNA damage response pathways. Future Oncol 9:219–233

Sanjiv K, Hagenkort A, Calderon-Montano JM, Koolmeister T, Reaper PM et al (2016) Cancer-specific synthetic lethality between ATR and CHK1 kinase activities. Cell Reports 14:298–309

Sears CR, Turchi JJ (2012) Complex cisplatin-double strand break (DSB) lesions directly impair cellular non-homologous end joining (NHEJ) independent of downstream damage response (DDR) pathways. J Biol Chem 287:24263–24272

Sears CR, Cooney SA, Chin-Sinex H, Mendoca MS, Turchi JJ (2016) DNA damage response (DDR) pathway engagement in cisplatin radiosensitization of non-small cell lung cancer. DNA Repair 40:35–46

Sekhar KR, Reddy YT, Reddy PN, Crooks PA, Venkateswaran A, McDonald WH, et al (2011) The novel chemical entity YTR107 inhibits recruitment of nucleophosmin to sites of DNA damage, suppressing repair of DNA double-strand breaks and enhancing radiosensitization. Clin Cancer Res 17:6490–6499

Seno JD, Dynlacht JR (2004) Intracellular redistribution and phosphorylation of proteins of the Mre11/Rad50/Nbs1 repair complex following irradiation and heat shock. J Cell Physiol 199:157–170

Seshacharyulu P, Ponnusamy MP, Harida D, Jain M, Ganti AK, Batra SK (2012) Targeting the EGFR signaling pathway in cancer therapy. Expert Opin Ther Targets 16:15–31

Shewach DS, Lawrence TS (1995) Radiosensitization of human tumor cells by gemcitabine in vitro. Semin Oncol 22:68–71

Shibata A, Moiani D, Arvai AS, Perry J, Harding SM, Genois M-M, Maity R et al (2014) DNA double-strand break repair pathway choice is directed by distinct MRE11 nuclease activities. Mol Cell 53:7–18

Sykes SM, Mellert HS, Holbert MA, Li K, Marmorstein R et al (2006) Acetylation of the p53 DNA binding domain regulates apoptosis induction. Mol Cell 24:841–851

Tanno S, Yanagawa N, Habiro A, Koizumi K, Nakano Y, Osanai M et al (2004) Serine/threonine kinase AKT is frequently activated in human bile duct cancer and is associated with increased radioresistance. Cancer Res 64:3486–3490

Tarish FL, Schultz N, Tanoglidi A, Hamberg H, Letocha H et al (2015) Castration radiosensitizes prostate cancer tissue by impairing DNA double-strand break repair. Science Trans Med 7:1–6

Thijssen R, Ter Burg J, Garrick B, van Bochove GG, Brown JR et al (2016) Dual TORK/DNA-PK inhibition blocks critical signaling pathways in chronic lymphocytic leukemia. Blood 128:574–583

Toulany M, Roderman HP (2015) Phosphatidylinositol 3-kinase/Akt signaling as a key mediation of tumor cell responsiveness to radiation. Semin Can Biol 35:180–190

Toulany M, Kehlbach R, Florczak U, Sak A, Wang S, Chen J et al (2008) Targeting of AKT1 enhances radiation toxicity of human tumor cells by inhibiting DNA-PKcs-dependent DNA double-strand break repair. Mol Cancer Ther 7:1772–1781

Toulany M, Lee KJ, Fattah KR, Lin YF, Fehrenbacher B, Schaller M et al (2012) Akt1 promotes post-irradiation survival of human tumor cells through initiation, progression and termination of DNA-PKcs-dependent DNA-double strand break repair. Mol Cancer Res 10:945–957

Van Putten JW, Groen HJ, Smid K et al (2001) End-joining deficiency and radiosensitization by gemcitabine. Cancer Ras 61:1585–1591

Wachters FM, Van Putten JW, Maring JG, Zdzienicka MZ, Grown HJ, Kampinga HH (2001) Selective targeting of homologous DNA recombination repair by gemcitabine. Int J Rad Oncol Biol Phys 57:553–562

Waters CA, Strande NT, Wyatt DW, Pryor JM, Ramsden DA (2014) Nonhomologous end joining: a good solution for bad ends. DNA Repair 17:39–51

Weinberg R, Hanahan D (2011) Hallmarks of cancer: the next generation. Cell 144:646–674

West AC, Johnstone RW (2014) New and emerging HDAC inhibitors for cancer treatment. J Clin Invest 124:30–39

Zheng M-h, Sun H-t, Xu J-g, Gang Y, Lei-ming H et al (2016) Combining whole brain radiotherapy with Gefitinib/Erlotinib for brain metastases from non-small-cell lung cancer: a meta analysis. RioMed Res Int 2016:5807346

Zhu J, Zhou L, Wu G, Konig H, Lin S et al (2013) A novel small molecule RAD51 inactivator overcomes imatinib resistance in chronic myeloid leukaemia. EMBO Mol Med 5:353–365

Mathematical Modeling in Radiation Oncology

Translating Mathematical Models into the Clinic

Russell C. Rockne and Paul Frankel

Abstract

The goal of precision medicine is to tailor treatments to the individual patient's disease. In radiation oncology, this means tailoring the dose to the boundaries of the tumor, but also to the unique biology of the patient's disease. In recent years, mathematical modeling has made inroads toward achieving these goals, through the optimization of radiation dose based on radiobiological parameters for individual patients. In this chapter, we review recent literature of mathematical models of tumor growth and response to radiation therapy (RT) and discuss the clinical utility of mathematical models, as well as provide a forward-looking perspective into how mathematical models may enhance patient outcomes through well-designed clinical trials.

Keywords

Mathematical oncology · Radiation oncology · Modeling · Clinical trials · Tumor control probability

Abbreviations

BED   Biologically equivalent dose
CT   Computed tomography

R.C. Rockne (✉)
Division of Mathematical Oncology, Department of Information Sciences,
Beckman Research Institute, City of Hope National Medical Center,
1500 E Duarte Rd., Duarte, CA 91010, USA
e-mail: rrockne@coh.org

P. Frankel
Division of Biostatistics, Department of Information Sciences,
Beckman Research Institute, City of Hope National Medical Center,
1500 E Duarte Rd., Duarte, CA 91010, USA
e-mail: pfrankel@coh.org

© Springer International Publishing AG 2017
J.Y.C. Wong et al. (eds.), *Advances in Radiation Oncology*,
Cancer Treatment and Research 172, DOI 10.1007/978-3-319-53235-6_12

DBCRT   Dynamic biologically conformal radiation therapy
IMRT   Intensity modulated radiation therapy
LQ   Linear-quadratic
MOEA   Multi-objective evolutionary algorithm
MRI   Magnetic resonance imaging
OAR   Organ at risk
PET   Positron emission tomography
RT   Radiation therapy
SF   Surviving fraction
TCP   Tumor control probability

1 Introduction: Rationale for Mathematical Models in Radiation Oncology

Mathematics has played a pivotal role in radiobiology ever since the inception of the field (Hall and Giaccia 2011). Fowler provides an excellent historical account of the trials, tribulations, and challenges of translating laboratory-based radiobiology into the clinic in his 2006 perspective piece published in Physics in Medicine and Biology (Fowler 2006). Over the past 50 years, many experiments have been performed to understand and predict the biological effects of radiation in various dose and fraction schemes. Along with these experiments have come mathematical models of biological response that attempt to provide a mechanistic and predictive component to the observed data.

Despite the enormous variability in experimental conditions and mathematical models, consistent patterns between radiation dose and biological responses have emerged. A critical paradigm in the field is the finding that when the surviving fraction of cells is plotted on a log scale against radiation dose, the trend can be reliably predicted by a quadratic model. This observation led Brenner et al. to demonstrate that several mathematical descriptions (e.g., radiation damage, repair, and response to RT) result in predictions of dose-response relationships similar to this central paradigm (Brenner et al. 1998). Thus, the fundamental linear-quadratic (LQ) dose-response relationship has endured and continues to provide the bench-mark assessment of biological response to radiation. The LQ model states that the surviving fraction (SF) of cells after a dose (D) of radiation is given by

$$SF = \exp(-\alpha D - \beta D^2)$$

where α (1/Gy) and β (1/Gy^2) are parameters that determine the shape of the curve. Indeed, a vast literature exists on the mechanistic and empirical history of this famous equation, and entire books have been written about the mathematics of radiobiology (Hall and Giaccia 2011; Dale and Jones 2007).

To underscore the contemporary relevance of mathematical modeling in the spatial and biological optimization of RT, a point-counterpoint piece published in Medical Physics in 2016 (Kim et al. 2016) contends that, "With newly available tools such as functional imaging and mathematical models to better estimate the patient-specific, radiobiological parameters ... spatiotemporal optimization will enhance current efforts to find more effective treatment schedules to improve patient outcome." The argument against the contention only questions the degree of the potential gains with RT optimization alone; suggests that increased use of RT + chemotherapy or RT + radiosensitizers will achieve larger gains; and laments that progress will take at least five years, partially due to the need for validated mathematical models. Both of these arguments are likely true, and both are actually encouraging for the broader view on the role of mathematical modeling in the optimization of RT-based therapies.

Similarly, several authors have previously discussed the clinical and translational relevance of mathematical models to predict tumor growth and response to RT (Yankeelov et al. 2013; Jackson et al. 2014; Baldock et al. 2013; Gallasch et al. 2013). Mathematical models can inform clinical practice in a number of ways: via patient-specific models of tumor growth and response to RT, by guiding the design of preclinical studies to predict radiation sensitivity, by helping select patients for definitive clinical trials on these mathematically-driven treatment enhancements, and ultimately by optimizing radiation dose and treatment planning. The challenges involved with the inter-disciplinary, iterative cycle between development, testing, and application of mathematical models in collaboration with clinicians and experimental biologists, as well as some recent successful examples, are summarized by Michor and Beal (2015).

2 Illustrative Mathematical Models of Cellular- and Tissue-Scale Responses to Radiation

Here we summarize a few tenets and principles of mathematical modeling in radiation oncology. As the intended audience of this review is the clinical radiation oncologist, we omit gratuitous mathematical detail in favor of a more heuristic view, and point the reader to excellent reviews as well as more technical literature for the mathematical details of the models. A schematic overview of mathematical modeling in RT is provided in Fig. 1.

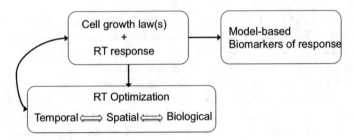

Fig. 1 Mathematical models provide a path to precision medicine in radiation oncology through prediction and optimization of response to RT based on an individual patient's tumor biology. Mathematical models are used to predict cell growth and response to RT, to optimize RT dose, and may also provide biomarkers (metrics) that can be used to identify and predict which patients will respond to a given treatment course

Ultimately, a mathematical model aims to predict response to RT, although the endpoints defining a response may vary from shrinkage in tumor size, to surviving fraction of cells (Powathil et al. 2013; Prokopiou et al. 2015; Rockne et al. 2010), to predictions of overall survival and similar clinical endpoints (Zaw et al. 2014; Baldock et al. 2012). In this section, we survey increasingly complex mathematical models of cellular- and tissue-scale tumor growth and response to RT.

Starting with simple dose-equivalence and dose-response models, the biologically effective dose (BED) and similar concepts date back to the earliest forms of ionizing radiation as a treatment for human maladies. Since then, many mathematical formalisms have been proposed to incorporate additional variables (e.g., cell proliferation, DNA damage, repair, and ultimately the surviving fraction of cells) into a variety of radiation doses and energies. Mathematically, these models tend to take the form of ordinary differential equations that describe the rate of change of the tumor population with and without the effects of radiation, which is described as a negative rate of change. Tumor doubling time (td), which is nominally incorporated in the basic LQ model, is a simplistic interpretation of these concepts. The concept of tumor control, and tumor control probability (TCP), given by

$$TCP = \exp(-N \cdot SF)$$

where N is the number of tumor cells, and SF is the surviving fraction, can be used as a simple measure to evaluate the success of a given treatment protocol. Several different formalisms for evaluating TCP have been proposed, which vary in complexity (Gong et al. 2013).

2.1 Tumor Growth Laws

Tumor cell growth laws often come in variations of a few archetypes: exponential growth, volume-limited logistic growth, or growth rate-limited Gompertzian growth. One or more of these growth models are then paired with mathematical models of response to RT, often based on the LQ model; this subject is thoroughly reviewed with mathematical details by Enderling et al. (2010) and O'Rourke et al. (2009). However, it is debated whether the LQ model is appropriate to describe biological responses to high dose per fraction treatments such as radiosurgery, which can involve doses of up to 20 Gy in a single fraction (Kirkpatrick et al. 2009). As a result, more complex mathematical models have been proposed to account for potentially different biological effects of high dose RT, which include mechanisms of DNA damage and repair kinetics (Siam et al. 2016; Tariq et al. 2015; Watanabe et al. 2016).

2.2 More Complex Multiscale Models

Mathematical models can also include multiple scales in space and time. Models that include cell motility, surrounding tissues, and spatial variations in radiation dose, for example, often take the form of partial differential equations (Stamatakos et al. 2006; Ribba et al. 2006; Powathil et al. 2007) or agent-based models (Scott et al. 2016). These spatial models may include biophysical forces between the tumor and the surrounding tissue, which may influence cell response to radiation-induced damage (Angeli and Stylianopoulos 2016). In addition, environmental factors that influence response to RT can be included in mathematical models. For example, hypoxia, or lack of oxygen, mediates production of DNA-damaging oxygen free radical species in response to radiation. Thus, changes in the spatial and temporal distribution of hypoxia within the tissue can affect cell kill. A number of groups have incorporated hypoxia into both tumor growth and response to RT models (Scott et al. 2016; Malinen et al. 2006; Titz and Jeraj 2008; Jeong et al. 2013; Rockne et al. 2015).

2.3 Pros and Cons of Model Complexity

Although a variety of mathematical models of tumor growth and response to RT exist, a philosophical argument must be considered regarding model complexity and the ability of the model to be parameterized, and to reasonably provide predictive value. In this way, the number of parameters, often a measure of a model's complexity, is weighed relative to the biological assumptions in the model. For instance, models that include environmental factors such as hypoxia tend to be more complex, and involve more equations, more parameters, and more specific assumptions. In contrast, simpler models often involve fewer, but broader, assumptions, and also fewer parameters. Such models can more easily be adapted to individual patient data to make patient-specific models and predictions.

Considering the spectrum of model complexity, along with ease-of-use, and evaluating potential utility in the clinical setting, is a challenge for several reasons. One reason is that complex models are difficult to communicate to non-mathematicians, and are difficult to interpret, even by the mathematicians who craft them. An additional concern is that metrics used for decision-making derived from complex models may be sensitive to small changes in the model's parameters, making the decision-making less robust to variations seen in real data. Finally, more complicated models are not necessarily more effective, as many complicated models make predictions similar to simple models, as shown by Gong et al. (2013).

Simple models, on the other hand, may not include mechanisms or biological detail satisfying to a biologist or clinician, and may miss important features that determine optimal treatment planning, but have the value of being relatively clear to communicate. This highlights just some of the hurdles that support the earlier contention that, even with the ongoing effort in the field, definitive studies on the use of these more complex mathematical models that customize RT to the patient and the patient's disease will most likely not be completed within five years.

3 Personalized Models

Patient-specific mathematical models provide one means of approaching the ultimate goal of precision medicine: to tailor the treatment to the individual patient's disease. Baldock et al. provide a roadmap for translating patient-specific models into precision medicine (Baldock et al. 2013), and describe the application of mathematical models to address a variety of clinical questions, such as prediction of surgical outcomes and response to RT. These applications of patient-specific mathematical modeling are connected to the goals of precision medicine, in that biological characteristics of each patient's disease are incorporated into a tailor-made mathematical model that can provide predictions of response for that individual patient. These predictions can then be used to both better select patients for clinical trials of novel approaches and define cases in which treatment can be rationally modified. In settings with a high cure rate, such as head and neck sarcoma, conventional RT approaches with mathematical models may have a limited value. However, in settings in which the response rate is low or highly variable, personalized mathematical models may provide a means to select patients for a clinical trial, or perhaps modify the treatment plan.

Several methods have been proposed to personalize mathematical models for individual patients. The most common approach is to fit a model to patient data by adjusting parameters in a fixed model. This can be done through a variety of methods, with Bayesian inference (Hawkins-Daarud et al. 2013; Tariq et al. 2016) and model-data fitting procedures (Rockne et al. 2010; Hathout et al. 2015a;

Colombo et al. 2015) being two of the most prevalent methods in recent years. For model-fitting algorithms, the most common forms of input are tumor volume and shape characteristics obtained from magnetic resonance imaging (MRI) (Rockne et al. 2010; Neal et al. 2013; Hathout et al. 2015b), positron emission tomography (PET) (Rockne et al. 2015; Mz et al. 2013), or computed tomography (CT) (Prokopiou et al. 2015; Belfatto et al. 2015). These approaches estimate parameters in the model(s) that correspond to biological characteristics of the tumor, such as cell doubling time, proliferation rate, and rate of migration into the surrounding tissue.

3.1 Proliferation Saturation Index

Prokopiou et al. (2015) have derived a proliferation saturation index (PSI) from a model of tumor cell growth and response to RT with a simple logistic growth law, given by

$$\frac{dV}{dt} = \lambda V(1 - PSI)$$

where PSI is the tumor volume-to-carrying capacity ratio (V/K). Radiation response is determined by the LQ model and is given by

$$V_{postRT} = V - \gamma_D V\left(1 - \frac{V}{K}\right), \quad \gamma_D = 1 - \exp(-\alpha D - \beta D^2).$$

The authors provide a novel perspective on the famous logistic growth equation by using the PSI as a predictive variable for RT response. The patient-specific parameter, PSI, is estimated using regression to fit the logistic growth equation, using data derived from two pre-treatment CT scans. The authors show that PSI correlates with RT response, defined by the post-treatment CT scan, and use their model to simulate different treatment and fractionation schemes that show improved response and tumor control for the individual patient.

3.2 Estimating Radiobiological Parameters

A popular formalism for modeling tumor proliferation, migration, and response to RT takes the form of a partial differential equation to incorporate spatial and temporal variations in the tumor growth, radiation delivery, and radiation response. Although many other models have been proposed, the following model for glioblastoma response to RT provides a means to estimate the LQ radiobiological parameters for individual patients using tumor volume data before and after treatment (Rockne et al. 2009, 2010). The model is given by

$$\frac{\partial c}{\partial t} = \Phi \nabla^2 c + \rho c (1 - c) - R(c, t, D)$$

where the tumor cell density (c(x, t)) is a function of space (x) and time (t), and its rate of change is determined by random Brownian motion in the form of diffusion, with migration rate Φ, and logistic growth with proliferation rate ρ. The parameters of this model can be estimated using serial MRI data prior to treatment (Rockne et al. 2010). The delivery and response to RT is given by the term $R(c, t, D)$, where D is the dose of radiation, and the instantaneous rate of cell kill from radiation is given by $(1 - SF)$, where SF is the surviving fraction determined by the LQ model, as follows:

$$R(c, t, D) = (1 - SF)c(1 - c), \quad SF = \exp(-\alpha(D + (\alpha/\beta)D^2)).$$

Holding the α/β ratio constant, this model may be fitted to tumor volume data to obtain patient-specific estimates of radiation sensitivity, quantified by the LQ parameter α, as we have shown in Rockne et al. (2010). Moreover, a positive correlation is found between the tumor proliferation rate and radiation sensitivity. This correlation provides a prediction of response to RT, since the proliferation rate is calculated with pre-treatment imaging data. This approach enables patient-specific simulations of alternate RT plans that use response to conventional treatment as a reference. Although approaches for estimating patient-specific radiobiological parameters from imaging data have been criticized for being ill-posed (Chvetsov et al. 2015), the technique is formally no different than a parameter estimation algorithm. In this case, the patient-specific radiobiological parameter α may be used to identify patients likely to respond to RT and that may also be validated in observational studies, used in optimization algorithms, and used to select patients for clinical trials, all of which can potentially lead to advances in patient outcome.

4 Treatment Optimization

A logical extension of personalized models of tumor growth and response to RT is optimization of treatment for the patient. Model-based biomarkers may be included along with dose constraints as inputs to algorithms that can maximize response while minimizing dose to normal tissue. Despite the development of patient-specific cell lines and preclinical animal studies, translating in vitro cell survival curves parameterized by the LQ or other mathematical models into optimized RT for individual patients remains problematic. To overcome this, recent literature in radiation treatment optimization has focused on themes of optimizing radiation dose distributions, biological response, and target volume delineation.

4.1 Spatial Dose and Fractionation Optimization

In order to optimize radiation dose, in addition to existing clinical treatment planning which conforms the dose to the target volume, organs at risk (OARs) are identified, and dose to normal tissue is constrained. These spatial optimizations are incremental advances over the routine conformal or intensity-modulated radiation therapy (IMRT) practices currently standard in clinical radiation oncology. Multi-objective evolutionary algorithms (MOEAs) take OARs and normal tissue doses as constraints into the clinical problem of dosimetry, while also maximizing TCP to the target volume (Holdsworth et al. 2010; Kim et al. 2012). These algorithms can also include objectives to be maximized, such as tumor size or cell kill (Corwin et al. 2013). Groups have already demonstrated the feasibility of implementing spatial optimization of dose using multi-objective evolutionary algorithm methods into a clinical workflow (Kim et al. 2015; Smith et al. 2016). The incorporation of patient-specific tumor growth and response models into this paradigm is a reasonable goal.

The temporal optimization of RT through fractionation attempts to minimize normal tissue complications and incorporate cell repair from radiation damage into the mathematical models. Fractionation schemes are often compared with dose equivalence calculations that are typically based upon the LQ model (Holloway and Dale 2013). In addition to BED- and LQ-based calculations of dose equivalence, tumor growth models can be incorporated into optimization algorithms that explicitly model changes in tumor volume. This enables adaptive fractionation schemes that are tailored to the response of the tumor (Unkelbach et al. 2014b) or that include dose to multiple normal tissues (Saberian et al. 2016). Badri et al. (2015) have taken this approach to apply a mathematical optimization for glioblastoma and demonstrate improved tumor control after mathematical model-predicted improved response to an alternative treatment regime in which the treatment fractions were temporally optimized to minimize toxicity to early and late responding normal tissues. The treatment plans suggested by Badri et al. were also constrained by the 8 a.m.–5 p.m. clinical workday, to provide a practical dosing schedule that could be performed in the clinic.

4.2 Tumor Biology Optimization

Perhaps an obvious goal of RT optimization is to maximize tumor cell kill (Zaider and Hanin 2011). In order to tailor optimized RT treatment plans to the biology of the individual patient's tumor, whether that be a genomically adjusted dose as suggested by Alomari et al. (2014), or dynamic biologically conformal radiation therapy (DBCRT) (Kim et al. 2012), one must identify appropriate biological targets. A systems oncology perspective incorporates multiple scales of tumor biology, including proliferation rate, cell signaling, DNA damage repair rate, and organ-level responses as biological targets for optimization (Powathil et al. 2015). Cell phenotypes within the tumor, such as cancer stem cells, and their associated differential responses to RT have also been incorporated into mathematical models and used as biological endpoints for optimization (Leder et al. 2014; Gao et al. 2013).

4.3 Target Volume Delineation

CT imaging is used for dose planning and target volume delineation. However, many cancers are locally invasive, and a portion of the cells beyond the frank lesion are not identified on imaging. This is a particular challenge in glioblastoma, a highly invasive primary brain tumor. In this setting, mathematical models have been used to predict tumor cell invasion not visible with CT or MRI, and have thus improved target delineation (Unkelbach et al. 2014a; Hathout et al. 2016) by including this invisible portion of disease. Mathematical models have also been proposed to adjust target volumes, based on hypoxia predicted within and around the tumor by models and/or inferred from PET imaging (Rockne et al. 2015; Moghaddasi et al. 2016).

4.4 Patient-Specific Optimization

The penultimate optimization is a combination of each of the previously described aspects of RT endpoints—spatial dose distribution, temporal fractionation, normal tissue toxicity, tumor biology, and target volume delineation—on a patient-specific basis. Only a few groups have achieved this penultimate combination of mathematical modeling that incorporates tumor growth rates derived from individual patient's clinical data and adapted to exploit tumor response and treatment. For example, our own work (Rockne) leverages multi-objective optimization, tumor growth and response models, and personalization of model parameters. We use these criteria to suggest, and test, optimal treatment plans for individual patients, and then compare these plans to the standard of care using mathematical model simulations (Corwin et al. 2013). This work demonstrates an improved therapeutic ratio and tumor burden (volume) reduction compared to conventional 2 Gy/day treatment plans. Although these results are purely in silico, they give hope for the continued pursuit of mathematical models to reach the ultimate goal of personalized medicine. In order to translate these studies into patients, the model must be tested in animal systems and in observational clinical trials.

5 Future Directions

Most of the mathematical approaches described in this chapter are focused on the cell and tissue level, with some multi-scale models. An enormous literature in the systems biology field applies mathematical modeling to describe subcellular processes, including cell signaling (McMahon et al. 2013) and DNA repair kinetics (Carlson et al. 2008). Indeed, Craft argues that a more comprehensive, multiscale (subcellular, cell, and tissue level) understanding of radiation response is needed to fully optimize and personalize RT (Kim et al. 2016).

5.1 Combination Therapy and Novel Radiotherapies

The synergy of combining RT with novel therapies, particularly anti-angiogenic therapies, which may impact the tumor microenvironmental variables of hypoxia and blood perfusion, has shown mixed effects in patients. Mathematical models provide a means to interrogate and characterize the hypothetical subset of patients that may benefit from the combination therapy (Hawkins-Daarud et al. 2015). Mathematical models incorporating tumor growth and normal tissue toxicity-related side effects also predict patients that could most benefit from novel RT modalities, such as proton irradiation (Langendijk et al. 2013), particularly for "kill painting" of dose in hypoxic tumors (Tinganelli et al. 2015).

Mathematical models also show promise as tools to investigate the potential roles of phenomena that may be difficult to quantify in a clinical setting, such as the bystander and abscopal effects, in which cells in tissues not directly exposed to ionizing radiation demonstrate behaviours similar to cells that are directly irradiated (Powathil et al. 2016; Poleszczuk et al. 2016). In these cases, mathematical models and simulations can provide novel hypotheses and insights that could be investigated in controlled settings. In this way, models may also provide a bridge between preclinical studies and clinical observations, by providing a mechanistic and general explanation for observations.

5.2 Computational Trials

Mathematical models have also been used to perform "computational trials" which interrogate the impact that varying biological parameters may have in determining outcomes for a given treatment regimen (Raman et al. 2016). In particular, Raman et al. use a mathematical model of glioblastoma growth and response to treatment to quantify motility phenotypes, patterns of progression, and treatment scenarios for various in silico patients that are hypothetically treated. This "phase i" style computational trial—a phrase coined by Jacob G. Scott in the Lancet in 2012 (Scott 2012)—offers a potential application for mathematical models to optimize the efficiency of RT-based clinical trials before they even begin.

5.3 Testing Mathematical Model-Based Biomarkers in Clinical Trials

Although we are not aware of any ongoing prospective clinical studies predicated on mathematical models other than the LQ model (Jones and Dale 2000), these applications are on the horizon. For mathematical models to truly make inroads toward clinical adaptation, a convincing demonstration of the model's utility is needed. Ultimately, there are two ways mathematical models in RT can enhance patient outcomes, the direct and the indirect. The direct means is the simplest to test. A select subset of patients who are eligible for RT in some setting (alone or in combination) are randomized to standard RT planning versus RT planning guided by the addition of a new mathematical model that likely incorporates individual patient and tumor differences obtained from a variety of pre-treatment assessments, and may suggest changes during RT as well. Successful demonstration of utility would be based on outcomes such as response, local disease-free survival, progression-free survival, or overall survival, with the latter being more convincing. If patient benefit is associated with the use of a mathematical model, this would be the clearest and most direct demonstration of the utility of a new mathematical approach. There are, however, other ways in which mathematical models can demonstrate clinical utility. These indirect methods include (1) enhancing our understanding of biology through testing mathematical models that capture our current understanding, and (2) providing a risk stratification of patients. For the latter, there is a large literature on the use of risk scoring and nomograms to help select patients for more aggressive therapy, or to qualify for a clinical trial. These mathematical models can be used in such a scoring system to help characterize patient responsiveness to the standard of care RT-based therapy. This type of biomarker development and use is established by both retrospective and prospective studies, and can lead to innovative prospective studies such as the TAILORx study (clinicaltrials.gov identifier NCT00310180), a **T**rial **A**ssigning **I**ndividua**L**ized **O**ptions for treatment (**Rx**).

6 Summary

Mathematical modeling has played an important role in radiation biology and physics for decades. Similarly, mathematical models have been used to study tumor growth and response to cancer treatments for over a century. Recent advancements in mathematical models have brought these fields together to optimize and improve RT. As summarized in this chapter, models that allow for personalization of tumor growth and response predictions, along with methods to incorporate novel approaches into radiation treatment optimization algorithms, have advanced the role and increased the value of mathematical modeling in clinical radiation oncology. Indeed, as predictive models allow us to to tailor treatments to the individual patient's disease, and provide model-derived biomarkers that may be tested in clinical trials, we move closer to the goal of precision medicine. In radiation oncology, this means not only tailoring the dose to the boundaries of the tumor, but also to the unique biology and stage of the patient's disease. Thus, we believe that mathematical modeling will continue to be a critical element that enables the goal of designing the majority of RT schedules using spatiotemporal optimization "within the next five years ..." (2016) (Kim et al. 2016).

References

Alomari A, Rauch PJ, Orsaria M, Minja FJ, Chiang VL, Vortmeyer AO (2014) Radiologic and histologic consequences of radiosurgery for brain tumors. J Neurooncol [Internet] 117(1): 33–42, March 2014. Available from: http://www.ncbi.nlm.nih.gov/pubmed/24442402

Angeli S, Stylianopoulos T (2016) Biphasic modeling of brain tumor biomechanics and response to radiation treatment. J Biomech [Internet] 49(9):1524–1531. Elsevier. Available from: http:// dx.doi.org/10.1016/j.jbiomech.2016.03.029

Badri H, Pitter K, Holland EC, Michor F, Leder K (2015) Optimization of radiation dosing schedules for proneural glioblastoma. J Math Biol [Internet]. Springer, Berlin, Heidelberg. Available from: http://link.springer.com/10.1007/s00285-015-0908-x

Baldock AL, Anh S, Rockne R, Neal M, Clark-Swanson K, Sterin G et al (2012) Patient-specific invasiveness metric predicts benefit of resection in human gliomas. Neuro Oncol [Internet] 14:131. Available from: https://www.ncbi.nlm.nih.gov/pmc/articles/PMC4211670/

Baldock AL, Rockne RC, Boone AD, Neal ML, Hawkins-Daarud A, Corwin DM et al (2013) From patient-specific mathematical neuro-oncology to precision medicine. Front Oncol [Internet] 3:62, 2013/04/09 ed. Available from: http://www.ncbi.nlm.nih.gov/pubmed/ 23565501

Belfatto A, Riboldi M, Ciardo D, Cecconi A, Lazzari R, Jereczek-Fossa B et al (2015) Adaptive mathematical model of tumor response to radiotherapy based on CBCT data. IEEE J Biomed Heal Informatics [Internet] 2194(c):1–1. Available from: http://ieeexplore.ieee.org/lpdocs/ epic03/wrapper.htm?arnumber=7153523

Brenner DJ, Hlatky LR, Hahnfeldt PJ, Huang Y, Sachs RK (1998) The linear-quadratic model and most other common radiobiological models result in similar predictions of time-dose relationships. Radiat Res [Internet] 150(1):83–91. Available from: http://www.ncbi.nlm.nih. gov/pubmed/9650605

Carlson DJ, Stewart RD, Semenenko VA, Sandison GA (2008) Combined use of Monte Carlo DNA damage simulations and deterministic repair models to examine putative mechanisms of cell killing. Radiat Res [Internet] 169(4):447–459, 2008/03/28 ed. Available from: http://www.ncbi.nlm.nih.gov/pubmed/18363426

Chvetsov AV, Sandison GA, Schwartz JL, Rengan R (2015) Ill-posed problem and regularization in reconstruction of radiobiological parameters from serial tumor imaging data. Phys Med Biol [Internet] 60(21):8491–8503. IOP Publishing

Colombo MC, Giverso C, Faggiano E, Boffano C, Acerbi F, Ciarletta P (2015) Towards the personalized treatment of glioblastoma: integrating patient-specific clinical data in a continuous mechanical model. PLoS One [Internet] 10(7):e0132887. Available from: http://dx.plos.org/10. 1371/journal.pone.0132887

Corwin D, Holdsworth C, Rockne RC, Trister AD, Mrugala MM, Rockhill JK et al (2013) Toward patient-specific, biologically optimized radiation therapy plans for the treatment of glioblastoma. PLoS One [Internet] 8(11):e79115, Jan 2013 [cited 22 Nov 2014]. Available from: http:// www.pubmedcentral.nih.gov/pubmed/3827144

Dale RG, Jones B (2007) British Institute of Radiology. Radiobiological modelling in radiation oncology. British Institute of Radiology, 292 p

Enderling H, Chaplain MA, Hahnfeldt P (2010) Quantitative modeling of tumor dynamics and radiotherapy. Acta Biotheor [Internet] 58(4):341–353. Available from: http://www.ncbi.nlm. nih.gov/pubmed/20658170

Fowler JF (2006) Development of radiobiology for oncology-a personal view. Phys Med Biol [Internet] 51(13):R263–R286, 7 July 2006. Available from: http://www.ncbi.nlm.nih.gov/ pubmed/16790907

Gallasch R, Efremova M, Charoentong P, Hackl H, Trajanoski Z (2013) Mathematical models for translational and clinical oncology. J Clin Bioinf [Internet] 3(1):23. BioMed Central Ltd, 7 Jan 2013. Available from: http://www.jclinbioinformatics.com/content/3/1/23

Gao X, McDonald JT, Hlatky L, Enderling H (2013) Acute and fractionated irradiation differentially modulate glioma stem cell division kinetics. Cancer Res [Internet]. Available from: http://www.ncbi.nlm.nih.gov/pubmed/23269274

Gong J, Dos Santos MM, Finlay C, Hillen T (2013) Are more complicated tumour control probability models better? Math Med Biol 30:1–19

Hall EJ, Giaccia AJ (2011) Radiobiology for the radiologist [Internet], 7th edn. Lippincott Williams & Wilkins, Philadelphia, ix, 546 p. Available from: http://www.loc.gov/catdir/toc/ecip063/2005031128.html

Hathout L, Ellingson B, Cloughesy T, Pope W (2015a) Patient-specific characterization of the invasiveness and proliferation of low-grade gliomas using serial MR imaging and a mathematical model of tumor growth. Oncol Rep [Internet] 2883–2888. Available from: http://www.spandidos-publications.com/10.3892/or.2015.3926

Hathout L, Pope WB, Lai A, Nghiemphu PL, Cloughesy TF, Ellingson BM (2015b) Radial expansion rates and tumor growth kinetics predict malignant transformation in contrast-enhancing low-grade diffuse astrocytoma. CNS Oncol 4:247–256

Hathout L, Patel V, Wen P (2016) A 3-dimensional DTI MRI-based model of GBM growth and response to radiation therapy. Int J Oncol [Internet] 1–7. Available from: http://www.spandidos-publications.com/10.3892/ijo.2016.3595

Hawkins-Daarud A, Prudhomme S, van der Zee KG, Oden JT (2013) Bayesian calibration, validation, and uncertainty quantification of diffuse interface models of tumor growth. J Math Biol 67(6–7):1457–1485

Hawkins-Daarud AJ, Rockne RC, Corwin D, Anderson AR, Kinahan PE, Swanson KR (2015) In silico analysis suggests differential response to bevacizumab and radiation combination therapy in newly diagnosed glioblastoma. J R Soc Interface [Internet] 12(20150388). Available from: http://dx.doi.org/10.1098/rsif.2015.0388

Holdsworth C, Kim M, Liao J, Phillips MH (2010) A hierarchical evolutionary algorithm for multiobjective optimization in IMRT. Med Phys [Internet] 37(9):4986–4997. Available from: http://www.ncbi.nlm.nih.gov/pubmed/20964218

Holloway RP, Dale RG (2013) Theoretical implications of incorporating relative biological effectiveness into radiobiological equivalence relationships. Br J Radiol [Internet] 86 (1022):20120417, 2013/02/07 ed. Available from: http://www.ncbi.nlm.nih.gov/pubmed/23385996

Jackson T, Komarova N, Swanson K (2014) Mathematical oncology: using mathematics to enable cancer discoveries. Am Math Mon 121(November):1–17

Jeong J, Shoghi KI, Deasy JO (2013) Modelling the interplay between hypoxia and proliferation in radiotherapy tumour response. Phys Med Biol [Internet] 58(14):4897–4919, 21 July 2013. Available from: http://www.ncbi.nlm.nih.gov/pubmed/23787766

Jones B, Dale RG (2000) Radiobiological modeling and clinical trials. Int J Radiat Oncol Biol Phys 48(1):259–265

Kim M, Ghate A, Phillips MH (2012) A stochastic control formalism for dynamic biologically conformal radiation therapy. Eur J Oper Res [Internet] 219(3):541–556. Elsevier B.V. Available from: http://dx.doi.org/10.1016/j.ejor.2011.10.039

Kim M, Stewart RD, Phillips MH (2015) A feasibility study: Selection of a personalized radiotherapy fractionation schedule using spatiotemporal optimization. Med Phys [Internet] 42 (11):6671–6678. Available from: http://scitation.aip.org/content/aapm/journal/medphys/42/11/10.1118/1.4934369

Kim M, Craft DL, Orton CG (2016) Within the next five years, most radiotherapy treatment schedules will be designed using spatiotemporal optimization. Med Phys [Internet] 43 (5):2009–2012. Available from: http://scitation.aip.org/content/aapm/journal/medphys/43/5/10.1118/1.4943383

Kirkpatrick JP, Brenner DJ, Orton CG (2009) Point/Counterpoint. The linear-quadratic model is inappropriate to model high dose per fraction effects in radiosurgery. Med Phys [Internet] 36 (8):3381–3384, 2009/09/15 ed. Available from: http://www.ncbi.nlm.nih.gov/pubmed/ 19746770

Langendijk JA, Lambin P, De Ruysscher D, Widder J, Bos M, Verheij M (2013) Selection of patients for radiotherapy with protons aiming at reduction of side effects: the model-based approach. Radiother Oncol [Internet] 107(3):267–273, July 2013. Elsevier Ireland Ltd. Available from: http://www.ncbi.nlm.nih.gov/pubmed/23759662

Leder K, Pitter K, Laplant Q, Hambardzumyan D, Ross BD, Chan TA et al (2014) Mathematical modeling of PDGF-driven glioblastoma reveals optimized radiation dosing schedules. Cell [Internet] 156(3):603–616, 30 Jan 2014. Elsevier. Available from: http://www.ncbi.nlm.nih. gov/pubmed/24485463

Malinen E, Søvik A, Hristov D, Bruland ØS, Olsen DR (2006) Adapting radiotherapy to hypoxic tumours. Phys Med Biol [Internet] 51(19):4903–4921, 7 Oct 2006. Available from: http:// www.ncbi.nlm.nih.gov/pubmed/16985278

McMahon SJ, Butterworth KT, Trainor C, McGarry CK, O'Sullivan JM, Schettino G et al (2013) A kinetic-based model of radiation-induced intercellular signalling. PLoS ONE 8(1):15–18

Michor F, Beal K (2015) Improving cancer treatment via mathematical modeling: surmounting the challenges is worth the effort. Cell [Internet] 163(5):1059–1063. Elsevier Inc. Available from: http://dx.doi.org/10.1016/j.cell.2015.11.002

Moghaddasi L, Bezak E, Harriss-Phillips W (2016) Monte-Carlo model development for evaluation of current clinical target volume definition for heterogeneous and hypoxic glioblastoma. Phys Med Biol [Internet] 61(9):3407–3426. IOP Publishing

Mz H, Petitjean C, Ruan S, Vera P, Dubra B (2013) Predicting lung tumor evolution during radiotherapy from PET images using a patient specific model. IEEE 10th international symposium on biomedical imaging: from nano to macro, San Francisco, CA, pp 1404–1407

Neal ML, Trister AD, Ahn S, Baldock A, Bridge CA, Guyman L et al (2013) Response classification based on a minimal model of glioblastoma growth is prognostic for clinical outcomes and distinguishes progression from pseudoprogression. Cancer Res [Internet] 73 (10):2976–2986, 2013/02/13 ed., 15 May 2013. Available from: http://www.ncbi.nlm.nih.gov/ pubmed/23400596

O'Rourke SFC, McAneney H, Hillen T (2009) Linear quadratic and tumour control probability modelling in external beam radiotherapy. J Math Biol 58(4–5):799–817

Poleszczuk JT, Luddy KA, Prokopiou S, Robertson-Tessi M, Moros EG, Fishman M et al (2016) Abscopal benefits of localized radiotherapy depend on activated T-cell trafficking and distribution between metastatic lesions. Cancer Res 76(5):1009–1018

Powathil G, Kohandel M, Sivaloganathan S, Oza A, Milosevic M (2007) Mathematical modeling of brain tumors: effects of radiotherapy and chemotherapy. Phys Med Biol [Internet] 52 (11):3291–3306. Available from: http://www.ncbi.nlm.nih.gov/pubmed/17505103

Powathil GG, Adamson DJA, Chaplain MAJ (2013) Towards predicting the response of a solid tumour to chemotherapy and radiotherapy treatments: clinical insights from a computational model. PLoS Comput Biol 9(7)

Powathil GG, Swat M, Chaplain MAJ (2015) Systems oncology: towards patient-specific treatment regimes informed by multiscale mathematical modelling. Semin Cancer Biol [Internet] 30C:13–20, Feb 2015. Elsevier Ltd. Available from: http://www.ncbi.nlm.nih.gov/ pubmed/24607841

Powathil GG, Munro AJ, Chaplain MAJ, Swat M (2016) Bystander effects and their implications for clinical radiation therapy: insights from multiscale in silico experiments. J Theor Biol [Internet] 401:1–14. Elsevier. Available from: http://dx.doi.org/10.1016/j.jtbi.2016.04.010

Prokopiou S, Moros EG, Poleszczuk J, Caudell J, Torres-Roca JF, Latifi K et al (2015) A proliferation saturation index to predict radiation response and personalize radiotherapy fractionation. Radiat Oncol [Internet] 10(1):159. Available from: http://www.ro-journal.com/ content/10/1/159

Raman F, Scribner E, Saut O, Wenger C, Colin T, Fathallah-Shaykh HM (2016) Computational trials: unraveling motility phenotypes, progression patterns, and treatment options for glioblastoma multiforme. PLoS One [Internet] 11(1):e0146617. Available from: http://dx. plos.org/10.1371/journal.pone.0146617

Ribba B, Colin T, Schnell S (2006) A multiscale mathematical model of cancer, and its use in analyzing irradiation therapies. Theor Biol Med Mod 3(7)

Rockne R, Alvord EC, Rockhill JK, Swanson KR, Alvord Jr EC, Rockhill JK et al (2009) A mathematical model for brain tumor response to radiation therapy. J Math Biol [Internet] 58(4–5):561–578, April 2009. Available from: http://www.ncbi.nlm.nih.gov/pubmed/18815786

Rockne R, Rockhill JK, Mrugala M, Spence AM, Kalet I, Hendrickson K et al (2010) Predicting efficacy of radiotherapy in individual glioblastoma patients in vivo: a mathematical modeling approach. Phys Med Biol [Internet] 55(12):3271–3285. Available from: http://www.ncbi.nlm. nih.gov/pubmed/20484781

Rockne RC, Trister AD, Jacobs J, Hawkins-daarud AJ, Neal ML, Hendrickson K et al (2015) A patient-specific computational model of hypoxia-modulated radiation resistance in glioblastoma using 18F-FMISO-PET. J R Soc Interface [Internet] 12. Available from: http://classic.rsif. royalsocietypublishing.org/content/12/103/20141174.short

Saberian F, Ghate A, Kim M (2016) Optimal fractionation in radiotherapy with multiple normal tissues. Math Med Biol 33:211–252

Scott J (2012) Phase i trialist. Lancet Oncol [Internet] 13(3):236, March 2012. Elsevier. Available from: http://www.ncbi.nlm.nih.gov/pubmed/22489289

Scott JG, Fletcher AG, Anderson ARA, Maini PK (2016) Spatial metrics of tumour vascular organisation predict radiation efficacy in a computational model. PLoS Comput Biol 12(1):1–24

Siam FM, Grinfeld M, Bahar A, Rahman HA, Ahmad H, Johar F (2016) A mechanistic model of high dose irradiation damage. Math Comput Simul [Internet]. Elsevier B.V. Available from: http://linkinghub.elsevier.com/retrieve/pii/S0378475416000562

Smith WP, Kim M, Holdsworth C, Liao J, Phillips MH (2016) Personalized treatment planning with a model of radiation therapy outcomes for use in multiobjective optimization of IMRT plans for prostate cancer. Radiat Oncol [Internet] 11(1):38. Available from: http://ro-journal. biomedcentral.com/articles/10.1186/s13014-016-0609-7

Stamatakos GS, Antipas VP, Uzunoglu NK, Dale RG (2006) A four-dimensional computer simulation model of the in vivo response to radiotherapy of glioblastoma multiforme: studies on the effect of clonogenic cell density. Brit J Radiol 79:389–400

Tariq I, Humbert-Vidan L, Chen T, South CP, Ezhil V, Kirkby NF et al (2015) Mathematical modelling of tumour volume dynamics in response to stereotactic ablative radiotherapy for non-small cell lung cancer. Phys Med Biol [Internet] 60(9):3695–3713. Available from: http:// iopscience.iop.org/0031-9155/60/9/3695/

Tariq I, Chen T, Kirkby NF, Jena R (2016) Modelling and Bayesian adaptive prediction of individual patients' tumour volume change during radiotherapy. Phys Med Biol [Internet] 61 (5):2145–2161. IOP Publishing. Available from: http://stacks.iop.org/0031-9155/61/i=5/a= 2145?key=crossref.511fc11bdea8efaa5a2bdcb3669ad645

Tinganelli W, Durante M, Hirayama R, Krämer M, Maier A, Kraft-Weyrather W et al (2015) Kill-painting of hypoxic tumours in charged particle therapy. Sci Rep [Internet] 5:17016. Nature Publishing Group. Available from: http://www.nature.com/articles/srep17016

Titz B, Jeraj R (2008) An imaging-based tumour growth and treatment response model: investigating the effect of tumour oxygenation on radiation therapy response. Phys Med Biol [Internet] 53 (17):4471–4488, 7 Sept 2008. Available from: http://www.pubmedcentral.nih.gov/pubmed/ 2819145

Unkelbach J, Menze B, Konukoglu E, Dittmann F, Ayache B, Shih H (2014a) Radiotherapy Planning for Glioblastoma Based on a Tumor Growth Model: improving Target Volume Delineation. Phys Med Biol 59(3):771–789

Unkelbach J, Craft D, Hong T, Papp D, Ramakrishnan J, Salari E et al (2014b) Exploiting tumor shrinkage through temporal optimization of radiotherapy. Phys Med Biol [Internet] 59 (12):3059–79, 21 June 2014. Available from: http://www.ncbi.nlm.nih.gov/pubmed/24839901

Watanabe Y, Dahlman EL, Leder KZ, Hui SK (2016) A mathematical model of tumor growth and its response to single irradiation. Theor Biol Med Model [Internet] 13(1):6. Available from: http://www.tbiomed.com/content/13/1/6

Yankeelov TE, Atuegwu N, Hormuth D, Weis JA, Barnes SL, Miga MI et al (2013) Clinically relevant modeling of tumor growth and treatment response. Sci Transl Med [Internet] 5 (187):187ps9, 2013/05/31 ed. Available from: http://www.ncbi.nlm.nih.gov/pubmed/23720579

Zaider M, Hanin L (2011) Tumor control probability in radiation treatment. Med Phys [Internet] 38(2):574 [cited 14 Jan 2015]. Available from: http://scitation.aip.org/content/aapm/journal/medphys/38/2/10.1118/1.3521406

Zaw TM, Pope WB, Cloughesy TF, Lai A, Nghiemphu PL, Ellingson BM (2014) Short-interval estimation of proliferation rate using serial diffusion MRI predicts progression-free survival in newly diagnosed glioblastoma treated with radiochemotherapy. J Neurooncol [Internet] 116 (3):601–608, Feb 2014. Available from: http://www.ncbi.nlm.nih.gov/pubmed/24395348

Printed in the United States
By Bookmasters